UNLOCK YOUR
MENOPAUSE TYPE

UNLOCK YOUR MENOPAUSE TYPE

Personalized Treatments,
the Last Word on Hormones,
and Remedies that Work

Heather Hirsch, MD, MS, NCMP

with Stacey Colino

ST. MARTIN'S
ESSENTIALS
NEW YORK

First published in the United States by St. Martin's Essentials, an imprint of St. Martin's Publishing Group

UNLOCK YOUR MENOPAUSE TYPE. Copyright © 2023 by Heather Hirsch. All rights reserved. Printed in the United States of America. For information, address St. Martin's Publishing Group, 120 Broadway, New York, NY 10271.

www.stmartins.com

Designed by Steven Seighman

The Library of Congress Cataloging-in-Publication Data is available upon request.

ISBN 978-1-250-85082-9 (hardcover)
ISBN 978-1-250-85083-6 (ebook)

Our books may be purchased in bulk for promotional, educational, or business use. Please contact your local bookseller or the Macmillan Corporate and Premium Sales Department at 1-800-221-7945, extension 5442, or by email at MacmillanSpecialMarkets@macmillan.com.

First Edition: 2023

10 9 8 7 6 5 4 3 2 1

To my daughter DeMille Margaret Hirsch and her generation of women: My hope is that you will experience a greater awareness of women's unique health needs and receive greater quality health care throughout the female reproductive lifespan.

Well-behaved women seldom make history.

—Laurel Thatcher Ulrich, Pulitzer Prize–winning historian specializing in early America and the history of women, and a professor emerita at Harvard University

Contents

Introduction

Whether it's described as puberty in reverse, puberty's evil older sister, or premenstrual syndrome (PMS) on steroids, the menopausal transition is an extremely challenging time for most women. Intense hormonal changes, irregular periods, and mood swings may sound a lot like puberty or even PMS. But this time around, the ovaries are gearing down and heading toward full-time R and R, rather than cranking up their function toward reproduction. And because this transition, called perimenopause, often lasts from four to ten years, it can be hard to tell where you are in the meandering journey toward menopause, which is officially defined as one full year from your last period. Even after their periods are behind them, many women find that menopausal symptoms—including hot flashes, night sweats, vaginal dryness, and/or brain fog—continue for a surprisingly long time. In fact, it's impossible to predict how long they'll last. All of this adds to many women's frustrations with this topsy-turvy physiological phase of life.

Meanwhile, trying to find relief for menopausal symptoms is like navigating the wild, wild West, a terrain that's lawless, un-regulated, and untamed. There's no map, and the landscape is rife with myths and misinformation and self-proclaimed gurus (no, I'm not naming names here; you can probably guess who they are), often with no medical training but claiming to have all the answers and/or the best remedies. Women don't know what to expect or whom to trust for reliable information and advice, nor do they have a realistic sense of what will work and what won't to ease their bothersome symptoms. Too many women suffer due to inconsistent and inaccurate information from both physicians and the media. Honestly, it's a chaotic mess.

In 2010, a small study[1] in the journal *Women's Health Issues* evaluated the needs of midlife women using focus groups and phone interviews with health experts, and found that women in their forties and fifties crave more information about what to expect around menopause and symptom management. *Surprising, huh?* The researchers concluded that a serious knowledge gap exists when it comes to "information about symptoms and how to cope with/reduce them, how to communicate with providers about their experience, [and] what to expect." Sadly, more than a decade later, we haven't made much progress on this front: Recent research[2] reveals that 65 percent of women admit they feel unprepared for the symptoms that menopause may bring.

That comes as no surprise to me. As the clinical program director of the Menopause and Midlife Clinic at the Brigham & Women's Hospital in Boston, I hear this every day. By the time patients come to see me, they're typically at the end of their ropes: They don't feel like their usual selves and they're alarmed because they hardly recognize themselves. They're aggravated because symptoms like hot flashes, sleep disturbances, or brain fog have started dominating their days and nights. And they're often unaware that symptoms like vertigo, pain with urination, hair thinning and hair loss, burning mouth and gums, and heart palpitations may be connected to the hormonal changes their bodies are undergoing. They're frustrated that they haven't been able to find relief and they don't understand why their usual doctors are dismissing their concerns. They're also worried about the future, fearing that the way they're feeling now is their new normal.

I'm here to tell you: It's not—or at least it doesn't have to be. With the right knowledge and interventions, you can reclaim control of your body and mind. You can feel and function well at midlife and beyond. The key is to identify your personal constellation of symptoms, or your "menopause type"—a unique approach that I have cultivated based on the distinct patterns I have seen in my years of clinical experience. Using these types, it's possible to identify and prioritize your symptoms to obtain relief, and to develop an appropriate treatment plan. Many women's experiences will match up with one type; others may experience a combination of types—but either way, the typology approach allows you to pinpoint your unique collection of menopausal symptoms in order to develop a treatment plan that's most likely to work for you.

Just like puberty, menopause is a universal experience for women—at least we hope it is; otherwise, something is wrong with their reproductive systems, or they die prematurely. Given that millions of women enter menopause each year and have since the dawn of time, it's kind of crazy that menopause continues to feel like uncharted territory or a shock to the system for the women who are going through it. I'm deeply committed to changing that. With this book, my goal is to help women cut through the informational noise about menopause and learn how to manage it by identifying their personal menopause type(s) so they can treat their constellation of symptoms more effectively.

After beginning my career as an ob-gyn delivering babies, it didn't take long for me to pivot to internal medicine. I started treating menopausal patients during a two-year fellowship in women's health at the Cleveland Clinic. Women were flying from all over the country to consult with my mentor Holly Thacker, MD, director of the Cleveland Clinic's Center for Specialized Women's Health, about menopause because they were frustrated, confused, and distressed by their symptoms and they weren't getting the care or relief they needed. Many of these women were downright miserable, and some felt as though they were losing their minds. That's when I discovered—to my great surprise!—that much of what I'd learned about menopause in medical school and in my residency was incorrect.

Within the field of medicine, we have cardiac experts, kidney specialists, sleep doctors, and other experts—*why isn't there a menopause specialist?* Women typically talk to their internists or ob-gyns who should be well versed in the physical, mental (cognitive), and psychological changes that accompany this life transition. But in reality many are not because menopausal matters aren't sufficiently addressed in medical school or residency programs. In fact, when researchers[3] recently surveyed medical residents at programs in internal medicine, family medicine, and gynecology, most revealed that they had had only one or two hours of education about menopause in their program, and 20 percent reported that they'd had no menopause education whatsoever. The biggest shocker: Only 7 percent of these doctors in training said they felt adequately prepared to treat menopausal women!

Armed with the information in this book, you will be in a better position to work more effectively with any doctor to address your menopausal and midlife health concerns; you'll have the baseline knowledge about what's happening in your body and the vocabulary to describe it, as well as the options for treating those symptoms, all of which you can bring up with your doctor.

During my fellowship, the more women I treated, the more I realized there are distinct phenotypes to menopause. Based on my clinical experience, I started to see big patterns that couldn't be found in textbooks. The depth and breadth of patient experiences, backgrounds, and histories was truly eye-opening, and I became convinced that treatment for menopausal symptoms needed to be individualized. There isn't one effective way to treat women going through menopause and it's a mistake to pretend there is.

Fast-forward to today: In my work as the clinical program director of the Menopause and Midlife Clinic at the Brigham & Women's Hospital in Boston, I work closely with my midlife patients, going over their most private and emotional symptoms and patterns in close detail, which helps them feel seen and heard. That's very empowering and confidence-building for them, so when we do devise a treatment plan, they're likely to feel invested in it and stick with it, and we can tweak it over time until they feel really good. This approach works wonders, better than anything they've tried before, and it enables them to take control of this topsy-turvy experience. I love helping women through this challenging time. By and large, my patients are smart, curious, and inquisitive, and they often have a strong connection between their minds and bodies—that's part of what makes women excited to take control of this journey.

The reality is, there is no one-size-fits-all approach to managing menopause that works for every woman, and that's because different women have different menopausal experiences. Research has found that the frequency and intensity of menopausal symptoms depend partly on a woman's age, the presence of underlying health conditions, her menopausal status, and sociodemographic variables. That said, the most frequently reported severe symptoms include depressed mood and irritability, physical and mental exhaustion, muscle and joint aches, hot flashes, headaches, sexual problems, and sleep disturbances. But individual women experience different clusters of symptoms, and it's impossible to predict who will experience which ones and for how long. In other words, your mother's, sister's, or best friend's menopausal transition may be quite different from yours, which means it's best to approach your experience in a way that works for you.

When women hear about these types, they often have an "aha" moment and ask, "Why doesn't anyone know about this?" I'm on a mission to change that.

That's where *Unlock Your Menopause Type: A Personalized Guide to Managing Your Menopausal Symptoms and Enhancing Your Health* comes in. By taking matters into your own hands with this book, you'll be able to find your own path to feeling better and protecting your long-term health more effectively. Trust me, because I help women do this day after day, week after week in my clinic. In my practice, I take a uniquely personalized approach to helping women navigate and manage the array of physical and emotional symptoms they're experiencing. But let's face it, I can't help every woman face-to-face or via telemedicine—though I wish I could.

By allowing you to take a personalized approach to feeling better and thriving again, this book will help you discover how simple interventions and lifestyle changes can restore your physical and emotional equilibrium, based on your unique experience with the culmination of your reproductive years. And because it will enable you to take action on your own, it will help you feel more empowered and resilient, which will immediately relieve some of the "what the #$@&%*! is happening to me" feelings that often accompany the menopausal experience. My hope is that this essential, comprehensive guidebook will provide you with all the tools you'll need for getting through this time in your life, happily and healthfully.

In part 1, you will discover what's really happening in your body during the menopausal experience, and you'll learn about the role of hormones in your overall health and how their decline not only results in symptoms like hot flashes, but also impacts everything from your bone health to your cardiovascular system. I'll reveal where myths and misconceptions about this time of life come from. You'll learn about the concept of menopause types and take a quiz to identify which type(s) you have now (spoiler alert—it can evolve over time).

In part 2, I'll help you identify your menopause type(s) and address what's driving the changes in how you're feeling and functioning; then, I'll assist you in picking and choosing the evidence-based treatments that make the most sense for your symptoms, your health history, your needs and preferences, and your priorities. In some instances, hormone therapy may be recommended. I'll walk you through the pros and cons of hormone therapy, as well as what we've learned in the past decade about how women can use hormones effectively—whether orally, vaginally, transdermally, topically, or in long-acting or short-acting formulations—depending on their menopause types, their symptoms, and their long-term goals. But if hormone therapy isn't an option for you, rest assured: There are many other medical and lifestyle-based approaches that can relieve your symptoms and improve your sense of well-being. Each menopause type has its own baseline treatment plan, as well as additional recommendations for dietary, lifestyle, and psychological strategies to help you feel at the top of your game again.

In part 3, I will show you how to personalize your menopause survival plan by adding remedies that address your specific or remaining symptoms. You'll find things you can do without any help from your doctor to mitigate typical challenges like hot flashes and night sweats, less well-known ones like breast tenderness and skin rashes, and the ones you may be embarrassed to talk about like pain during sex or loss of libido. I'll also help you formulate a long-term game plan for taking care of your physical, emotional, and mental (cognitive) health into the future, even as things shift with the different seasons of your life.

What we're going to do is create a customized road map through this often tumultuous transition and put you in the driver's seat: Besides helping you make your way onto steady terrain, this approach will arm you with knowledge about smart detours and troubleshooting measures if unexpected potholes or obstacles arise along the way. One way or another, I promise you, you can get to where you want to go—to a new, healthy, feel-good chapter of your life. These days women spend more than a third of their lives in the postmenopausal zone, given the increasing human life expectancy. Why not feel amazing during those years?!

Using my custom-tailored approach, the majority of my patients feel significantly better and reclaim their health and their ability to lead fulfilling lives throughout the menopausal transition. I'm confident that I can help you do the same because I see these transformations every day in my clinic. With this approach, you'll gain a sense of empowerment as you take ownership of the experience and develop confidence that you can start living your best life from this moment forward. Every woman deserves to feel and function at her best during menopause and after, setting the stage for better health into her sixties, seventies, and eighties. *Let's get started!*

Part I

HORMONAL HAVOC

The Wild, Wild West of Health Experiences

When women come to see me for the first time about their midlife symptoms, they often say things like:

"I don't recognize myself anymore."

"I don't feel like myself."

"I feel like someone has taken over my body."

"I'm at the point where I'm just going to wear elastic pants for the rest of my life because I feel so bloated."

"When will this vaginal dryness, irritability, [fill in the blank] end?!"

"When it comes to sex, I feel dead inside. I miss my libido!"

Sometimes they'll ask, "Is this too much information for you?" or "Have you ever heard this before?" Of course, every woman should feel special because truly they are, but these feelings and experiences are common (almost universal!)—and yet women often feel blindsided by them. This is partly because when it comes to accessing accurate information about a woman's symptoms, menopause can feel like an untamed and unpredictable frontier. In our culture, there is almost a cone of silence around what to expect when you're in the menopausal transition; plus, every woman's experience is personal and unique to her and could be vastly different from her friends' or family members' experiences.

When Lucy, age fifty, first came to see me, the intensity of her hot flashes was off the charts and she was having heart palpitations along with them, which made them feel like panic attacks; naturally she was scared by these symptoms as well as highly uncomfortable. By the time I met Laura, forty-seven, she'd spent months waking up at 2 A.M., drenched in sweat and unable to sleep; as a result, she was muddling through her days in such a heavy brain fog that she was barely able to function and afraid she'd have a car accident. After having chemotherapy for breast cancer, my patient Anna, forty-three, a trial attorney, experienced such severe vaginal dryness that her vulva and labia continuously felt like they were on fire. Lucy, Laura, and Anna's symptoms were different from each other's but all related to menopause—and they were all affecting these women's day-to-day lives in seriously distressing ways and making them absolutely miserable! And these three women are far from alone. Did you know that 75 percent of women have symptoms that disrupt their lives and/or their ability to function during perimenopause and postmenopause—and that these symptoms often last for years? That adds up to millions of women, many of whom feel utterly bewildered, distressed, or pissed off by these life-altering changes and struggle to find safe and sufficient relief from them.

This is especially challenging to handle because there's a lot of informational noise about this time in a woman's life. Women are consistently bombarded with messages about what's normal or not during the menopause transition, and what to do or *not* do for their symptoms (there's a lot of menopause shaming going on out there, too, especially online). The problem is, some of this advice lacks scientific evidence to support it or to refute the claims that are made. And frankly there's a lot of sheer nonsense out there, much of which is passed around through various social media platforms and advertisements for specific products. So, it's important, though not easy, to cut through the myths, old wives' tales, half-truths, and snake-oil promises and zero in on what's really going on with your symptoms and what's likely to actually help you.

Compounding the challenge, the health-care system isn't helping in this respect. In most practices, physicians and nurses haven't adequately prepared women for menopause by giving them even basic information about some of the symptoms and changes they may experience or how long they may last. Currently, there's no such thing as a perimenopause evaluation, where a doctor does an assessment of a woman and comes up with a what-to-expect game plan for how she can address menopause-related symptoms, as there is with a pre-surgery evaluation, for example. Many women are still reluctant to talk to their primary care physicians about their menopausal symptoms, whether it's because they feel embarrassed, they feel like they should just toughen up and stick it out, or because their doctors are dismissive when the subject arises. The reasons for this dismissiveness vary, but research has shown that education about menopause and how to manage it is woefully inadequate in medical schools and residency programs. As a result, it's hardly surprising that when many women who are experiencing serious menopausal discomfort seek help from their physicians, they receive answers like, "There's nothing we can do" or "You'll have to wait it out; this will pass eventually" or, unbelievably, "In previous generations, many women didn't live to see menopause, so we just don't have a lot of research about it."

I want you to know that it doesn't have to be this way. I will help you cultivate a sense of control over the physical and mental chaos you may be experiencing—without falling for bogus treatments, tearing your hair out (or having more fall out), spending a fortune, or hopping from one medical practitioner to another. With this book, we'll be putting you in the driver's seat for this experience and guiding you toward a greater sense of well-being. The first step in this journey is to identify your personal menopause type—a unique approach that I have cultivated based on six distinct patterns I have seen in my years of clinical experience. Using these types, it's easier to pinpoint which of your symptoms are priorities for obtaining relief and develop a treatment plan that will start turning this ship around.

By treating and tracking more than a thousand women in my clinical practice, I've identified the following six menopause types:

The **Premature Menopause Type**, which occurs before age forty, tends to bring a surprising and often abrupt wave of symptoms such as hot flashes, night sweats, mood swings, mental fogginess, vaginal dryness, and decreased sex drive.

The **Sudden Menopause Type**, which often results from surgery or chemotherapy (but can occur for other reasons, as you'll see), is often a shock to a woman's system with its arrival and intensity.

The **Full-Throttle Menopause Type**, which is marked by diverse and often fierce symptoms from pretty much every direction, can be absolutely overwhelming and sometimes downright debilitating.

The **Mind-Altering Menopause Type** primarily involves mood and cognitive changes—such as anxiety, depression, dramatic mood swings, brain fog, difficulty with concentration, and memory challenges.

The **Seemingly Never-Ending Menopause Type** is marked by one or two symptoms (such as the occasional hot flash, persistent vaginal dryness, or low libido, or less common ones like dizziness or olfactory changes) that go on and on and . . . on.

The **Silent Menopause Type**, where you're largely symptom-free but need to pay attention to new health challenges and risks that emerge postmenopause because whether or not menopausal symptoms are present, your body is changing from the drop in hormones.

In the chapters that follow, you'll learn much more about each of these different menopause types. Many women's experiences will match up with one particular type; other women may experience a combination of types—a hybrid type, so to speak. Either way, my unique typology approach allows you to pinpoint your personal collection of menopausal symptoms in order to develop a treatment plan that's most likely to help you feel better ASAP. In my clinical experience, when women discover they have a certain menopause type or a hybrid, it makes them feel seen, heard, and understood— and not alone!—and it gives them a name for what they're experiencing; this in turn lends a sense of order to the seemingly unwieldy experience, which comes as a tremendous relief. Perhaps most important, once you know what you're dealing with, you can develop a plan that caters to *your* personal symptoms and is likely to work for *you*. Let's face it: Your mother's, sister's, neighbor's, or best friend's experience with menopause is likely to be quite different from yours, so interventions that helped them may not help you. This really is all about *you*—and that's a very good thing, as you'll see in the chapters to come.

Personalized medicine (a.k.a. precision medicine) is the wave of the future, and my approach to helping women navigate menopause works within this framework. Only in this case, we're not using an individual woman's genetic profile or specific biomarkers to guide decisions for her care (though some day we may be able to do that, which would be amazing!). At this point, we're using her personal cluster of symptoms and their severity, her health history and current health status, and her personal preferences and goals to inform her treatment plan. The menopause type approach is both reactive and proactive because it addresses a woman's current symptoms and also takes into account her future health risks with preventive measures. Best of all, it involves a unique combination of medical interventions and lifestyle modifications.

THE PHYSIOLOGY OF MENOPAUSE

Before we dive into the details about the different menopause types and their recommended treatment regimens, let me give you a brief refresher about what's happening in your body that triggers the changes you're experiencing. As you approach menopause, your ovaries—which make the vast majority of your estrogen—are downshifting and heading toward retirement. When you're in the phase of life where you still have your period, your estrogen levels fluctuate between 50 and 500 pg/mL every single month. At menopause, which is defined as a full year since a woman's last period, those levels are effectively zero, though some women have a little extra estrogen because adipose (fat) tissue makes some estrogen. Yes, you read that correctly: A woman's fat cells produce some estrogen (we used to think of body fat as an inert substance but now we know that's not true). Throughout the menopausal transition, progesterone levels also decrease—in fact, we now think that progesterone may decline at a faster rate than estrogen throughout perimenopause, which may lead to a lot of the mood and anxiety changes that occur then. Levels of testosterone, which is the sex-drive hormone for women as well as men, also decrease. The majority of symptoms of menopause—such as hot flashes, night sweats, mood changes, and vaginal dryness—stem from the loss of estrogen, while a drop in libido can result from the loss of testosterone.

Estrogen receptors are everywhere in a woman's body, though we have the most estrogen receptors in the vagina and the second largest concentration in our brains. So when estrogen is no longer present after menopause, those estrogen receptors continue to look for their old friend estrogen. When they don't find the hormone, the receptors freak out in a way that's like flicking a thermostat off and on, off and on; this is what we currently think triggers hot flashes, as well as some downstream effects such as mood shifts and cognitive changes. In other words, this flicking effect is what can make you feel like your body and mind aren't quite your own. It's true that eventually your body will adjust to these lower hormone levels and these symptoms will quiet down, but this period of flicking off and on can last for several years.

Researchers and menopause experts aren't sure why menopausal symptoms are more severe in some women than others. The current hypothesis is that it has a lot to do with genetic factors, as well as environmental factors that may turn specific genes "on" or "off"—not just influences that come from your mom but also those that could stem from Dad's side of the family or even second- or third-degree relatives. During this time of life, some women are programmed to have receptors that are more persistent in "looking" for that missing estrogen, which results in more severe or longer-lasting symptoms like hot flashes. By contrast, other women have a genetic predisposition for their estrogen receptors to give up the search, and hence they experience fewer symptoms. The fact that genetics seems to play a significant role should take the feeling of *what am I doing wrong?* off your shoulders—because your symptoms probably aren't being caused by anything you are or aren't doing. But that doesn't mean you can't take steps to ease them, as you'll discover in later chapters.

Let's back up a few steps and consider the in-between time—perimenopause and later stages of the menopausal transition. Perimenopause, which is like a long suspension bridge with an uneven surface, carries a woman from her reproductive years into menopause. The symptoms the transition brings often sneak up on women, catching them by surprise. Some women in their forties haven't even heard the word "perimenopause," so when these disruptive symptoms come on suddenly and make women feel like they're having an out-of-body experience, they're like, *WTH?!* And because these women are typically still menstruating, most don't connect the dots between hormonal changes and the physiologic changes (such as irregular periods, hot flashes, night sweats, and vaginal dryness) and emotional changes they're experiencing.

I can't even tell you how many women have come to me saying things like, "When I had my first hot flash, I thought I was spiking a fever and getting sick." (In 2020 and early 2021, so many women went and got tested for COVID-19 and quarantined until they got their results.) I heard this from women in high-powered professional jobs as well as women who worked at retail stores and fast-food joints.

Not long ago, I read an article in which celebrities shared their experiences with the menopausal transition,[1] and I found actress Kim Cattrall's experience particularly interesting. In her role as Samantha Jones on *Sex and the City*,[2] the actress had to pretend she was experiencing hot flashes on screen before she ever had them in real life. Ironically, she thought the acting experience had prepared her for the real thing—but that just wasn't the case. Two years later, her own experience was significantly more dramatic, as she experienced hot flashes that felt "earth shaking . . . like being put in a vat of boiling water."

Believe it or not, symptoms of perimenopause can start as early as ten years before your final menstrual period. Most women experience menopause between the ages of forty and fifty-eight, with the average age being fifty-one, according to the North American Menopause Society (NAMS).[3] During perimenopause, a woman's hormones really are on a roller-coaster ride. In particular, major swings in estrogen levels—from high to low and back again—can irritate your brain. Simply put, the female brain seems to prefer a steady state of hormones, which is why some women experience premenstrual syndrome (PMS) or even premenstrual dysphoric disorder (PMDD) as their reproductive hormones fluctuate each month with their menstrual cycles. While a woman is still menstruating, estrogen and progesterone levels go up and down in a fairly predictable pattern that resembles rolling hills.

During perimenopause, these hormonal fluctuations turn into sharper and more sporadic peaks and troughs. The brain can really struggle with these dramatic swings, which is why many women experience anxiety, irritability, insomnia, and other mood-related changes during this time.

Complicating matters, because the perimenopause transition can last from four to ten years, it can be hard to tell where you are in the meandering journey to menopause. Before we dive into what's really going on behind the scenes, it's important to understand the key players in the menopausal transition. You've probably heard about the hypothalamic-pituitary-adrenal (HPA) axis, which is the body's central stress response system; it's what leads to the release of the stress hormone cortisol when something stressful happens. But you may not be familiar with the hypothalamic-pituitary-ovarian (HPO) axis, a tightly regulated system that secretes hormones involved in female reproduction. (Keep in mind: Both the hypothalamus and the pituitary gland are in the brain stem.)

When the HPO axis works properly, a woman's body has monthly menstrual cycles that include ovulation and priming of the uterine tissue for possible implantation of a fertilized egg; if conception doesn't occur in a given cycle, the lining of the uterus is shed and a woman gets her period. When the HPO axis *doesn't* work properly, ovulation doesn't occur on a regular basis. Here's where the menopausal transition comes into the picture: During perimenopause, the HPO axis starts to malfunction and eventually its activity comes to a screeching halt once a woman experiences menopause. At that point, the brain recognizes that the HPO axis isn't providing the hormones it wants—namely, estrogen—so it often turns to the HPA axis and activates the adrenal glands. But, because the adrenal glands don't have estrogen, instead they may release cortisol, which can unfortunately contribute to or worsen menopause-related symptoms such as acne, irritability, low libido, and a slowing of metabolism.

It's against this backdrop that the "stages of menopause" come into play.[4] Did you even know there are stages of menopause? They've been around for a while and have been refined over time. In 2011, an international panel of experts revised the criteria for the different stages of perimenopause and menopause that had been established ten years earlier in the Stages of Reproductive Aging Workshop (STRAW). In modifying the staging system, the 2011 group, which came to be known as STRAW+10,[5] reviewed advances in understanding the key changes in hypothalamic-pituitary-ovarian function that occur before and after a woman's final menstrual period. This is important because there are actually several phases in the run-up to menstruation's not-so-grand finale (it's more of a petering out, really), with a great deal of individual variation in terms of when the phases hit, how long they last, and how sensitive women are to the hormonal changes that occur.

Here's a look at how the different stages compare:

Late reproductive stage (Stages-3b and-3a): A sort of pre-transition before perimenopause, this is the final stage of the baby-making years, a time when fertility begins to decline and a woman's ability to have a baby drops significantly. She may start to see subtle changes in the volume and frequency of her menstrual bleeding, often experiencing shorter cycles in Stage-3a.

Early menopausal transition (Stage-2): During this phase, the length of a woman's menstrual cycle becomes erratic and begins to vary by seven or more days from one cycle to the next. Her body is making estrogen but less progesterone. During this stage, which can last an unpredictable amount of time, you may experience an increase in irritability due to declining progesterone levels, and PMS-like symptoms and bleeding patterns can vary.

Late menopausal transition (Stage-1): During this stage, you may begin to skip periods, going for sixty or more days without one. In addition to variability in menstrual cycle length, you may experience extreme fluctuations in hormonal levels (including estrogen and progesterone), and you may frequently have cycles in which you don't ovulate. (These are called anovulatory cycles.) Overall, you'll experience a decline in estrogen but simultaneously there can also be dramatic fluctuations in hormonal levels, including estrogen, progesterone, and testosterone. Vasomotor symptoms like hot flashes are common during this stage, which is estimated to last one to three years on average.

Early postmenopause (Stages +1a, +1b, +1c): These stages occur at least one year after a woman's last period—thus, it corresponds to the end of *perimenopause.* During this stage, estrogen and progesterone levels decline to very low levels, while follicle-stimulating hormone (FSH) levels—FSH is what tells the ovaries to release an egg (a.k.a. ovulate) each month during a woman's reproductive years—continue to increase for approximately another two years. Stage +1a marks the end of the twelve-month span since a woman's final period; Stage +1b also lasts a year, at the end of which levels of FSH stabilize. During these stages, vasomotor symptoms like hot flashes and night sweats are most likely to occur or worsen. During Stage +1c, which can last three to six years, hormone levels tend to stabilize even more to ultra-low levels.

Late postmenopause (Stage +2): During this phase, hormonal shifts and changes in reproductive endocrine function are more limited but some of the processes related to reproductive aging become a greater concern. Symptoms of vaginal dryness (including itching and irritation) and urogenital atrophy (a scary term for changes that occur in tissues in the vulva, vagina, bladder, and urethra due to declining estrogen levels) become more prevalent; these changes can lead to pain with intercourse, recurrent urinary tract infections, urinary frequency and urgency, and other anatomical changes, such as pelvic organ prolapse. Changes that occur to the pelvic floor are now collectively called genitourinary syndrome of menopause (or GSM, for short), a mouthful of a term that inclusively describes all the changes that are occurring to the vulva, vagina, perineum, bladder, and urethra.

What's in a Name?

People are often confused by the terms that are used to describe this reproductive transition in a woman's life. This is partly because they're sometimes used interchangeably when they're actually distinct entities or have specific definitions. Here's what they really mean:

1. Perimenopause: the period of time leading up to menopause, a transition that can last four to ten years.
2. Menopause: the celebratory milestone where a woman has gone a full year without getting a menstrual period. It's a retrospective event, given that a woman won't know when her final period occurred until she has gone twelve months without another one. Some women can't rely on their periods as an indicator—if they've had a hysterectomy or endometrial ablation or have a progesterone-releasing IUD in place, for example—so they should use blood tests showing a persistently elevated FSH level of greater than 35 mIU/mL and an estradiol level of lower than 20 pg/mL as a gauge for when they're postmenopausal.
3. Menopause transition: the time span from perimenopause to your last menstrual period,

which can take up to a decade for some women. Think of this as a broad way to describe the beginning of the maelstrom that will continue until your final period.

4. Premature menopause: menopause that occurs before age forty for one reason or another, including genetic disorders (such as Turner syndrome).[6]

5. Early menopause: menopause that occurs between the ages of forty and forty-five. Research has found that women who've never been pregnant or given birth are considerably more likely to have premature or early menopause; the same is true of those who got their first period at a young age (before eleven). Also, women who have autoimmune diseases[7]—such as rheumatoid arthritis, lupus, or certain thyroid disorders—may have an earlier menopause.

6. Premature ovarian insufficiency (POI): a disorder in which a woman's ovaries stop producing eggs before age forty, which also means they no longer produce sufficient estrogen.

7. Diminished ovarian reserve (DOR): This phrase refers to a condition in which the ovaries lose their normal reproductive potential, thus compromising fertility. This can be a result of the normal aging process but it can also occur due to a medical condition or injury. Women who find out they have DOR often make the discovery when they're trying to get pregnant.

8. Surgical menopause: menopause that's caused by the surgical removal of *both* ovaries (if only one was removed, it's not surgical menopause because the other ovary may keep working).

9. Natural menopause: menopause that occurs spontaneously or without any intervention after age forty-six. This is due to the loss of active follicles in the ovarian tissue and the natural decline in estrogen production.

10. Medication-induced menopause: menopause that's caused by a medically induced cessation of ovarian function, often from chemotherapy, which is known to kill rapidly dividing cells in the ovarian tissue or alkylating agents (also used in cancer treatment). Other medications that can cause menopause to come early include methotrexate (which is often used to treat rheumatoid arthritis) and long-term use of methylprednisolone (used to treat lupus, multiple sclerosis,[8] and other inflammatory conditions) or GnRH therapy (used to treat endometriosis or fibroids); also, radiation to the pelvic area can alter the timing of menopause.

11. Postmenopause: the span of time that follows the day of your official one-year anniversary without menstrual periods and continues into the future; in other words, every day after menopause.

I must confess: I tend to cringe inside when women say they are "done with menopause" or they "already had menopause" because those statements don't make sense. Similarly, saying that you've "reached menopause" isn't accurate because there isn't an endpoint or a destination; technically, menopause is a one-day milestone because it marks one year after your final period. The important thing to recognize is that once you are postmenopausal your body will always be different than it was premenopausally, and that's true regardless of the menopause type(s) you have. It's true even if you never experience menopause-related symptoms (meaning, you have the Silent Menopause Type). So fasten your seatbelt because you're in for a long and possibly bumpy ride!

Whatever stage your symptoms seem to fall in, having a road map, even if it's a somewhat sketchy one, can help you identify what's happening now and what to expect going forward, which can help you make more informed decisions about interventions. The reality is: Every woman's road map is a little bit different. And while the STRAW+10 model presents a useful framework for the progression of menopause-related changes, women's experiences in real life can vary considerably. Rather than follow a linear progression in an orderly fashion, research has found that some women skip a particular stage (or several). Others get stuck in a particular stage for a surprisingly long time, while still others swing back and forth between specific stages. And some women have regular periods until they suddenly and mysteriously stop, almost as if a faucet were turned off for good one day. Simply put, the trajectory from the reproductive years to menopause is not necessarily uniform or predictable.

And there's no one-size-fits-all approach to managing menopause that works for every woman, and that's because women have different menopausal experiences, health goals, and personal priorities for symptom relief. Individual women experience different combinations of symptoms, and it's impossible to foresee who will experience which ones. On a near-daily basis, I see lots of women with vastly different menopausal symptom patterns. Here are snapshots of two patients I recently treated who had contrasting experiences and turned out to have two totally different menopause types.

When Nancy, fifty-four, a history professor, came to me complaining of confusion, brain fog, and depression, she was having trouble staying organized at work and sometimes even misplaced her students' papers; simply put, she felt like she was losing it. During our appointment, it became clear that she had the Mind-Altering Menopause Type. To promote alertness, I recommended she reduce her consumption of starchy carbs and increase her protein intake and do aerobic exercise every day, even if it was just a twenty-minute brisk walk; I also started her on Wellbutrin (an antidepressant with stimulant properties). Within two months, her ability to concentrate and be productive was back on track and her mood had improved.

By contrast, Erin, forty-nine, a physician's assistant in orthopedic surgery, was experiencing up to thirty severe hot flashes per day and drenching night sweats, which disturbed her sleep. Her Full-Throttle Menopause Type was so intense that during surgery, hot flashes were causing her goggles to fog, impairing her ability to assist safely. (I know—yikes!) With the help of hormone therapy, a reduction in her intake of caffeine and other stimulants, and relaxation exercises in the evening, her symptoms improved considerably.

As you're probably starting to realize, the onset and length of the menopausal transition also can vary significantly from one woman to another. A woman is born with all the follicles (egg sacs) she's ever going to have and the rate at which they deteriorate during her life plays a role in the timing of her menopause. Because ovarian follicles are rapidly dividing cells, they are easily susceptible to damage from both environmental factors and medical stressors. So, while a woman's body mass index (BMI), ethnicity, and genetic factors can affect the timing of the menopausal transition, lifestyle factors can also influence when she's likely to experience "the change."

In particular, smoking can push a woman into earlier perimenopause or menopause than she was genetically programmed to have. Both current and former smokers are at risk for earlier menopause, and the intensity, duration, cumulative dose, and earlier initiation of smoking all matter on this front. Research[9] has found that current smokers who have smoked for fifteen or more years have a fifteen-fold increased risk of premature menopause and a six-fold increased risk of having menopause arrive one to two years earlier than it does for non-smokers. Ongoing exposure to secondhand smoke is also associated with an earlier arrival of menopause, even among women who are non-smokers.

Meanwhile, exposure to other chemicals—especially endocrine-disrupting chemicals (EDCs)—which can mimic, block, or interfere with hormones in the body, including estrogen—have been linked with an earlier age of menopause.[10] The chemical culprits that fall into this problematic category of EDCs include dioxins (persistent organic pollutants, meaning they stay in the environment), polychlorinated biphenyls (PCBs, which are no longer produced in the US but also remain in the environment), pesticides, phthalates (which are used to soften plastic and personal care products), and perfluorooctanoic acid (PFOA, which is used in nonstick cookware and stain-repellant applications). These chemicals are ubiquitous in the modern world—but that doesn't mean you can't take steps to minimize or mitigate your exposure to them, as you'll see in later chapters.

The reason the issue of timing matters is because women who enter menopause at a later age have lower risks of cardiovascular disease, osteoporosis, and premature death, which is great news for them. On the other hand, women who enter menopause at an earlier age have increased risks for developing heart disease and osteoporosis and dying young—but we can take steps (thanks to hormone therapy, for example) to reduce those risks and help these women lead long, healthy, vibrant lives.

Of course, various genetic factors also may influence when a woman is likely to become menopausal, though there isn't a clear consensus on them. Research has, however, found some differences in symptom severity during the menopausal transitions in women of various ethnic groups. For example, perimenopausal African American women are twice as likely to report hot flashes and severe hot flashes as Caucasian women, while Hispanic women are more likely to report menopausal mood changes, decreased energy, heart palpitations, and breast tenderness than Caucasian women.[11] The reasons for these variations aren't completely understood—and here's why: Not only is menopause under-researched in general, but the majority of research is focused on Caucasian women—and this is not okay. It's so important to understand how menopause affects women of all races and ethnicities and more dedicated research needs to be done in these areas.

Meanwhile, other factors can influence the *intensity* of a woman's symptoms during the menopausal transition. For example, women who take chemopreventive drugs—such as tamoxifen, raloxifene, or aromatase inhibitors—to lower their cancer risk (because they're at high risk) or prevent a recurrence (if they've already had cancer) may have an increased intensity of menopausal symptoms, especially hot flashes. Also, long-term use of steroids—for a connective tissue disorder, an autoimmune disorder, asthma, or another medical condition—may worsen symptoms, especially hot flashes, for some women as they navigate the transition.

The way I see it, women are on a need-to-know basis when it comes to information about the menopausal transition and what to expect. There shouldn't be a gap between what healthcare providers know (or *should* know) about the final chapters in a woman's reproductive life and the information that's accessible to the women who are going through them. But often there is. That's entirely unacceptable because it's your body and you should be armed with the knowledge and the tools you need to take care of it in an optimal fashion. Rather than feeling like you're on a runaway train, my goal is to put you in the driver's seat for this journey. Rather than feeling distressed or debilitated by your symptoms, I want you to feel empowered to take charge of your health as you navigate this stage of indeterminable length and erratic hormone levels. This really matters because how you treat your body during the menopausal transition can affect your health for decades to come—for better or worse.

(Note: Wherever you are in the menopausal transition, keeping a journal and using it to track your daily symptoms, along with their fluctuations, can help you get a forecast of what your menopause type is and/or a leg up on developing greater body awareness to help you through the transition. If you don't already keep one, I encourage you to start one now—see the appendix for a sample.)

Remember: The menopausal experience is a natural part of a woman's reproductive life, just as puberty was. For many women, as human lifespans increase, *over half their lives* will be spent in a postmenopausal state—meaning they have a *lot* of living still to do. They deserve to have their troublesome menopause symptoms alleviated, so that they can not only feel the best they possibly can, but lead their best lives during these years. *You do, too!* And it can be done.

Trust me, because I help women do this day after day, week after week in my clinic, where I take a uniquely personalized approach to helping women navigate and manage the array of physical and emotional symptoms they're experiencing. Now it's your turn. By reading and using this book, you'll be able to forge your own path to feeling better and protecting your long-term health more effectively into the postmenopausal years. I may not be with you in person but I will be with you in spirit and guiding you with my words, every step of the way.

Myths and Misconceptions About Menopause

You know the old adage that you shouldn't believe everything you hear? Well, that definitely applies to the menopausal experience. There's a lot of misinformation about menopause in the media, as well as passed down from one generation to another or from one girlfriend to another. This is part of the informational noise I mentioned previously. The effects can be misleading, if not downright harmful or dangerous, which is why it's important to separate fact from fiction about this natural life transition.

When it comes to the menopausal experience, women are on a need-to-know basis, whether they're in the midst of the transition or anticipating it. It's your body and you have a need and a right to understand what's happening during this final act of your reproductive years. You shouldn't be led astray by the myriad mistruths about menopause that are running rampant in our world. Not only will getting the unvarnished truth help you allay your worries, it can also help you ease into the transition as smoothly as possible with the help of the trustworthy advice you'll find in the chapters that follow.

Here are common myths about menopause that not only deserve to but *need* to be busted—now!

MYTH: BECOMING MENOPAUSAL MEANS YOU'RE OLD

In our culture, menopause has lots of negative connotations but it really shouldn't. For one thing, "old" reflects a state of mind or poor health but it doesn't have anything to do with your actual age or reproductive status. For another, menopause can be a time of life that can bring new opportunities for growth and flexibility. It can bring a chance to reinvent your relationship with your body or refocus on yourself, especially if you have kids that have grown up and are becoming more independent. By this point in your life, you also probably have a strong sense of your values and what you like or don't like, which can be inspiring and liberating.

Plus, women in general are aging in ways that are different from the way their mothers or grandmothers did. There really is some truth to the notion that fifty or sixty is the new forty. It all depends on how you work with the changes that are happening for you physically, emotionally, socially, and spiritually. It's a mind-set shift, really, and this is a transition that should be embraced and celebrated.

MYTH: MENOPAUSE SYMPTOMS LAST FOR ONE YEAR

This is a misconception more than anything else. Menopause is defined as one year with no periods; after that, a woman is considered postmenopausal *but* she can still have symptoms. I hate to be the bearer of bad news but the average length of menopausal symptoms is five to seven years. A woman can have hot flashes and night sweats during perimenopause, even when she's still getting her period, and women with the lingering type of menopause can have symptoms for longer. Sadly, there's just no way to predict how long they'll last because the menopausal transition operates on its own schedule or timetable for every woman. But that doesn't mean there aren't steps you can take to tame your bothersome symptoms—for however long they do go on.

MYTH: YOU NEED TO HAVE A BLOOD TEST TO DIAGNOSE MENOPAUSE

For many women, the diagnosis of menopause comes clearly and naturally—going a full year without a period tells you what you need to know. This is one of many reasons I recommend that women track their symptoms and periods—your clinical history is much more relevant than any test I could order for you. But it may not be that simple for some women, including those who don't get regular periods, those who have an IUD in place, those who had an endometrial ablation (a procedure to remove the endometrial lining of the uterus), or those who had a hysterectomy (removal of the uterus). In these instances, the diagnosis can be aided by a blood test to measure FSH and estradiol levels—having an elevated FSH (above 35 mIU/mL) along with low estradiol (under 20 pg/mL) on two separate occasions, six to twelve weeks apart, will deliver the news.

MYTH: WEIGHT GAIN IS UNAVOIDABLE WITH MENOPAUSE

Menopause doesn't necessarily cause a woman to gain weight but it can increase belly fat (hence, the dreaded "menopot"). In this case, whether or not the number on the scale actually changes, adipose (fat) tissue can shift to the abdomen and breasts thanks to a drop in estrogen levels, which is why your clothes may fit differently.

Meanwhile, the natural aging process can cause your metabolic rate to slow down as you lose muscle mass; it's true for men and women. But you don't have to take any of these changes sitting or lying down—or be destined to gain weight in your forties, fifties, or sixties. To prevent menopausal weight gain, the keys are to trim your calorie intake by about two hundred calories per day, up your protein consumption, and/or increase your physical activity by aiming for at least 150 minutes of moderate-intensity aerobic activity per week, plus strength training twice a week. Building or preserving lean muscle mass will help keep your metabolic rate humming faster.

MYTH: MENOPAUSE RUINS YOUR SEX LIFE

Some women actually feel sexually liberated after menopause, knowing their days of worrying about getting pregnant are in the rearview mirror. While it's true that vaginal dryness can become a challenge during and after the menopausal transition, that doesn't have to be a deal breaker in the bedroom (or anywhere else). Applying a prescription low-dose estrogen cream or using an estrogen ring or suppository in the vagina can counteract the thinning and dryness of vaginal tissues; similarly, using over-the-counter water-based lubricants during sex can help make the experience more comfortable, while a daily moisturizer can help keep the tissues hydrated in general. And here's the great news: When sex isn't painful, the more often you have it, the healthier and moister your vaginal tissues may become.

As for changes in libido, that can be more of a psychological issue at this stage of life, which means you should consider: Has something changed in your mood or in your relationship? Did you have issues with desire before menopause? Taking into consideration the answers to these questions, there are lots of things you can do to get your sexual groove back and improve your sexual mind—even after menopause. (Spoiler alert: Regular exercise helps improve desire and orgasm potential; so can engaging in self-stimulation with a vibrator.)

MYTH: IF YOU GOT YOUR PERIOD AT AN EARLY AGE, YOU'LL DEFINITELY GO THROUGH MENOPAUSE EARLY

Not necessarily. In the past, some research had reported that women who got their first menstrual period early (a.k.a. early menarche) also had earlier menopause, but other, more recent studies found that women who started getting their periods at younger ages had later menopause.

A major study in a 2018 issue of the journal *Human Reproduction*[1] investigated this issue among 336,788 women in Norway and found that (drumroll, please!) . . . women who started getting their periods at age nine or younger actually had a nine-year-longer reproductive lifespan than those who started menstruating at age seventeen or older.

The take-home message: There isn't a consistent correlation between the age at which a woman starts getting her period and when she's likely to go through menopause. The patterns vary widely, depending on the study (and real life), so it's a mistake to guesstimate when you're likely to become menopausal based on when you got your first period. You'll just have to wait and see how this plays out for you.

MYTH: IF YOU'RE FIT AND STRONG, MENOPAUSE WILL BE A BREEZE FOR YOU

There are no guarantees on this. While there's no question that being fit and strong is beneficial for your overall health and functionality, as far as the menopausal experience goes, there isn't a clear association between fitness levels and the severity of symptoms. In fact, research has yielded some conflicting and often counterintuitive results on this subject. For example, a recent study[2] that examined the physical activity patterns and intensity of hot flashes among pre-, peri-, and postmenopausal women found that sedentary behavior predicted nighttime hot flashes. By contrast, a 2009 study[3] found that higher levels of physical activity among midlife women were significantly linked with a greater likelihood of having moderate to severe hot flashes. Meanwhile, a study published in a November 2021 issue of the journal *Menopause*[4] found that menopausal women with greater muscle mass have *more* vasomotor symptoms, including hot flashes, than women with sarcopenia (loss of muscle mass). That said, many women[5] find that regular physical activity improves their ability to cope with hot flashes and night sweats. (As you'll see in the chapters that follow, I strongly recommend exercise for a variety of reasons.)

MYTH: YOUR ATTITUDE TOWARD MENOPAUSE WILL AFFECT YOUR EXPERIENCE

Maybe it will and maybe it won't. To be honest, I have seen this go both ways among women in my clinical practice. Some women have a lousy attitude toward menopause, often based on their mother's or sisters' negative experiences, and have frustration with their own menopausal transition—but others do just fine. In a

2010 review[6] of the medical literature on this subject, researchers found that ten studies showed that women with more negative attitudes toward menopause reported more symptoms, while three studies found no association between these factors. So there isn't a clear consensus on this. Of course, it's also possible that women who have more menopausal symptoms develop a negative attitude toward menopause—in other words, it's a question of which comes first.

In any case, I strongly believe in the power of cultivating an upbeat attitude because it can't hurt and it might help with your symptoms—and at least you'll be in a better headspace in the meantime. Research[7] has found that midlife women who practice mindfulness—being aware and accepting of your thoughts, feelings, and bodily sensations without being emotionally reactive toward them—tend to have fewer or more mild menopausal symptoms, even if they experience more stress in their lives. Which means that even if your attitude doesn't affect your symptom experience directly, it can affect your emotional reaction to it. So why not swing positive with your attitude?

MYTH: A HOT FLASH IS JUST A NUISANCE

If you have the very occasional hot flash it might just be annoying, but if hot flashes are persistent or chronic, they can have a significant effect on the way you feel and function, and on your health and your life. A hot flash, as we are learning, is more than just a temporarily bothersome experience. During a hot flash the blood vessels can dilate (open up) or constrict (narrow down), which briefly raises blood pressure; you are also not getting great blood flow to the brain, which may compromise your thinking abilities, and possibly the functioning of other organs. Over time, this can take a real toll on the body: There is a growing body of evidence suggesting associations between hot flashes and night sweats with cardiovascular disease,[8] metabolic syndrome, type 2 diabetes, and osteoporosis.

Let's back up a few steps and consider what's actually going on with hot flashes: Described as a feeling of intense warmth that may spread like a wave through the torso and head, a hot flash usually lasts from thirty seconds to three or four minutes. This wave is often accompanied by an increase in heart rate and followed by a flushing of the skin, after which the woman will get sweaty, and in some instances, women report "cold flashes" after the resolution of a hot flash. Hot flashes stem from what's called vasomotor instability—it's as if the thermostat in a woman's brain is being cranked up then down, then up then down again. You get the picture—thermal chaos is in play. And if this process is happening for years on end, these hot flashes can have a profound effect on a woman's health. But you don't have to grin and bear them—you can take steps to find relief.

As an example, consider my patient Maria, fifty-eight, who experienced surgical menopause—after having a hysterectomy, including removal of her ovaries—at thirty-eight. After her surgery, she was put on a very low-dose estrogen patch to replace some of the estrogen she should have been getting but her body was no longer producing. For the last twenty years, she had been having five to ten hot flashes per day—and even though they were distressing, the doctors she had seen hadn't done anything to help her with them, because she was already on estrogen. In the meantime, she had gained weight and developed type 2 diabetes, cholesterol abnormalities, high blood pressure, and sleep apnea. When she came to see me, I increased the dose of her estrogen patch, and four months later, she was having only one or two hot flashes per week, which was fine with her. As she began feeling better, she started sleeping better and exercising regularly, walking at least a mile every day. Her most recent blood sugar and blood pressure measures also were much improved.

MYTH: DURING A HOT FLASH, YOUR CORE BODY TEMPERATURE INCREASES

Nope. It's true that during a hot flash the blood that rushes to the vessels closest to the skin may increase the skin's temperature by 5 to 7 degrees, but your core (internal) body temperature won't usually change[9]; it will likely stay around the normal 98.6 degrees. If a woman breaks out in a sweat in response to a hot flash, her skin temperature will quickly come down—that's the body's inherent cooling system in action.

MYTH: IF YOU DON'T HAVE NIGHT SWEATS, YOUR SLEEP ISN'T LIKELY TO BE DISTURBED DURING THE MENOPAUSAL TRANSITION

Among the less recognized symptoms that can crop up during perimenopause and postmenopause are a decline in sleep quality or an increase in disturbed (or fragmented) sleep or insomnia.[10] Sometimes these persist after menopause. These sleep troubles are *not* insignificant. Getting enough good-quality sleep (seven to nine hours per night) on a consistent basis is important for numerous aspects of your health and well-being, as well as your ability to feel and function optimally, and research suggests that women who regularly get seven to nine hours of quality sleep live longer compared to women who don't!

Also, sleep disruptions during the menopausal transition are linked to changes in women's metabolic health (including insulin sensitivity), as well as their eating behaviors and ability to regulate hunger, satiety, and impulse control; these effects can lead to weight gain, including fat accumulation around the midsection (a.k.a. the dreaded menopot). So it's a mistake to suffer silently with sleep woes. Trying to "tough it out" may end up taking a toll on your health and quality of life.

MYTH: MENOPAUSE INCREASES EVERY WOMAN'S RISK OF DEPRESSION

The truth is: Not every woman will experience mood-related symptoms during the menopausal transition, let alone full-blown depression. For some women, menopause is something they look forward to after years of dealing with hormonal ups and downs and menstrual periods, perhaps including unpleasant symptoms (such as cramps and mood swings) that may accompany them.

But some women do experience depression at this time in their lives. Research has found that a prior history of depression is the strongest predictor of experiencing a subsequent episode of depression in any stage of life. And a study published in *JAMA Psychiatry*[11] found that women who enter the menopausal transition earlier than their peers have an increased risk for the onset of depression even if they've never had it before; the presence of vasomotor symptoms (like hot flashes and night sweats) also elevated the risk.

Having said this, it's not uncommon for women to experience mood changes or irritability during the menopausal transition. This is especially true for women who have a history of sensitivity to hormonal fluctuations (think: bad PMS). But it's important to differentiate between depression and moodiness. One is a clinical diagnosis; the other is not.

MYTH: ONCE YOU GO THROUGH MENOPAUSE, YOUR BODY RETURNS TO NORMAL

Even after menopausal symptoms like hot flashes and night sweats go away, your estrogen levels are not going to return to their pre-menopausal levels. Yes, your body may still make a little bit of estrogen, but it won't affect your body the way it used to. Plus, over time, a woman's estrogen receptors start to downregulate and new ones are no longer made; this means that symptoms you may have had that were related to monthly estrogen fluctuations will stop. Meanwhile, your brain and heart function will still change as a result of the loss of estrogen, as will your pelvic floor function. These changes become your new physiological normal.

MYTH: IF YOU'RE PERIMENOPAUSAL, YOU DON'T NEED BIRTH CONTROL BECAUSE YOU CAN'T GET PREGNANT

Even as your estrogen levels are declining and your ovaries are shifting toward retirement, you're still ovulating if you're still getting even occasional periods. Which means that if a healthy sperm has the chance to meet your viable egg, you could make a baby. It's true that your chances of conceiving decline as you get older: In any given month, a woman between the ages of twenty-five and thirty-five has a 25 to 30 percent likelihood of getting pregnant with unprotected sex; by age forty-five, a woman's chances decrease to 5 percent. But 5 percent isn't 0 percent! So until you've gone at least a full twelve months since your last period—the definition of menopause—you can get pregnant. Which means that if you don't want to get pregnant, you need to use birth control until your periods are history.

MYTH: IF YOU DIDN'T HAVE ANY OF THE TELLTALE SYMPTOMS, YOU DIDN'T GO THROUGH MENOPAUSE

Menopause occurs when the ovaries retire and stop producing estrogen—it's that simple. Your period is simply a marker of what your ovaries are doing—if they're not working, you're not ovulating and you won't get your period. About 75 percent of women have symptoms of menopause but others don't. Symptoms are things you can feel or sense—like hot flashes or sleep disturbances. They are manifestations of what's happening in the body, but not everything that happens in the body causes perceptible changes.

Some women don't feel any different as they go through the menopausal transition but there are still changes going on in their bodies, including changes to their bone density and blood vessels that are tied to the loss of estrogen. Some women who don't think they have symptoms of menopause may have such mild ones that they don't really notice them, or they may not be aware of the changes that are going on. But their bodies are still changing inside, which is important to recognize because their health risks change after menopause. That's when certain preventive strategies become crucial to protect women from chronic diseases that become more common during the postmenopausal years, as you will see in chapter 13.

MYTH: OSTEOPOROSIS IS A NATURAL CONSEQUENCE OF MENOPAUSE

It's true that the loss of estrogen that accompanies the menopausal transition increases the rate of bone loss, but maybe not as much as previously believed. In fact, the longest study[12] of bone loss in postmenopausal women thus far found that bone mineral density (BMD) at the most common location for a hip fracture declined by 10 percent in twenty-five years—considerably less than expected based on other studies.

To help you understand the significance of this, here's a brief summary about the biology of bones: It may surprise you to know that bones are very dynamic—throughout your life, they are continuously being built up and broken down, resorbed and remodeled. The cells that form bone are called osteoblasts, and the ones that break down bone are called osteoclasts. During your reproductive years, estrogen inhibits bone breakdown by acting on both osteoclasts and osteoblasts.[13] Estrogen also regulates bone remodeling by modulating the production of cytokines and growth factors from bone marrow and bone cells. After you become menopausal, your bones no longer have these protective benefits of estrogen, which means bone can break down faster than it can be built back up, leading to a more rapid rate of bone loss.

Whether you develop osteoporosis (a progressive condition where bones become structurally weak and susceptible to fracture) or osteopenia (low bone mineral density that's considered a precursor to osteoporosis) depends on your peak bone mass before the menopausal transition. Your risk is also influenced by lifestyle factors such as getting good nutrition (particularly an adequate intake of protein, calcium, and vitamin D) and regular physical activity, and avoiding smoking and excessive alcohol consumption.

Don't get me wrong: Osteoporosis is a very real concern for women after menopause, especially if you had premature or early menopause (before age forty-five), both ovaries removed, or chemotherapy. Overall, 25 percent of women ages sixty-five and older have osteoporosis, compared to 6 percent of men in the same age group, according to the Centers for Disease Control and Prevention.[14] But it's hardly a foregone conclusion that you'll develop osteoporosis after menopause, and there are preventive steps you can take to protect your bone density.

MYTH: GOING THROUGH THE MENOPAUSAL TRANSITION IS DESTINED TO BE A MISERABLE EXPERIENCE

There's no question that symptoms of menopause can be distressing. But it's hardly universal that with menopause comes misery. Some women feel free knowing they no longer have to deal with periods or PMS or worry about getting pregnant. Some women feel a sense of maturity and wisdom once they reach the menopause milestone. And some women who have difficult symptoms during perimenopause obtain relief once they cross the threshold into postmenopause.

Not long ago, Rachel, forty-nine, came to see me during perimenopause. She was worried because her mother and aunt had a terrible time with the menopausal transition so she was starting to dread what lay ahead for her. She came to me because she wanted to be proactive. When I explained all the different ways we could treat the symptoms that she was especially worried about getting—such as hot flashes and intense mood changes—she breathed a huge sigh of relief. Rachel ended up feeling more empowered and optimistic that it didn't have to be a miserable experience. Instead of worrying about that, she began focusing on what she could do to enhance her health and well-being right now—namely, by embracing a healthy diet, regular exercise, stress management techniques, and plenty of sleep.

MYTH: ONCE YOU'RE POSTMENOPAUSAL, YOUR BODY WON'T PRODUCE HORMONES ANYMORE

First of all, it's important to remember that your body produces lots of different hormones, not just sex hormones like estrogen, progesterone, and testosterone. There's also insulin, melatonin, cortisol, adrenaline, growth hormone, thyroid hormones, oxytocin, and many others that your body will continue to produce as long as you live.

Even when it comes to reproductive (sex) hormones, some postmenopausal women continue to make small amounts of estrogen, either from their adipose (fat) tissue or their adrenal glands. Contrary to popular belief, fat is not an inert tissue in the body; it's now considered an endocrine organ because it produces hormones, particularly estrogen. That's why women with a higher body mass index (BMI) tend to have slightly higher levels of estrogen after menopause. In addition, women's adrenal glands will continue to make testosterone after their ovaries have retired; some testosterone can be converted into estrogen in a woman's body. This is kind of a good news/bad news scenario because having that unexpected estrogen may take the edge off menopausal symptoms, but the estrogen release from fat tissue after menopause could increase the risk of certain kinds of cancers.

MYTH: MEN GO THROUGH MENOPAUSE, TOO

Not exactly. Men do experience a slight decline in testosterone levels as they get older. It's about 1 percent per year after age forty[15]— not nearly as dramatic or sudden a drop-off as women experience with estrogen. It's not inevitable, and it's certainly not the same as a complete end to the reproductive lifespan the way female menopause is when the ovaries shut down permanently. Many older men continue to have testosterone levels within the normal range,[16] and men can, and some do, continue to father children into their seventies and eighties (a case in point: the late actor Tony Randall). So, the idea of male menopause is a myth.

That said, symptoms of declining testosterone levels in men can include irritability, weight gain, low sex drive, erectile dysfunction, sleep problems, depression, fatigue, and loss of strength. A blood test can reveal if a man has low testosterone levels and if testosterone therapy is needed.

After reading this chapter, you've probably discovered that many of the things you believed to be true about the menopausal experience aren't. This reality check is a crucial step toward putting your head in the right space with legitimate expectations and a can-do spirit—and setting you up to navigate this final reproductive transition as comfortably as possible. If menopause were a musical, the title might as well be *Anything Goes* because there's no cookie-cutter template or predictable playbook for the experience. Many women's experiences vary widely, which is why there's no one-size-fits-all treatment plan that works for every woman.

By gaining a better sense of what to expect and more accurate information about this pivotal experience, you'll be in a better position to identify interventions that are appropriate for *your* unique constellation of symptoms and your future health risks. This really is one of those times in life where *knowledge is power*. Rest assured: You are already on your way to boosting yours!

3

The Hormone Conundrum

When it comes to treating menopausal symptoms with hormone therapy, in my clinical experience women tend to have fairly strong beliefs on both sides of the equation. Some have a "Sign me up!" attitude, based on the idea or hope that taking hormones will quell their unpleasant symptoms. Others say, "No way!" often because they're holding on to outdated preconceptions and information about the potential risks of using menopausal hormone therapy.

It's a complicated, often polarizing, issue, and there isn't a single answer that applies to all women. When I talk to women about the possibility of using hormone therapy for their menopausal symptoms, I typically ask them what approaches they've tried already (so I have a sense of what *hasn't* helped them), and if they've thought or read about hormone therapy (so I can get a sense of what they already know, what questions they may have, and whether they might have any preconceived ideas about it).

Some of the confusion surrounding hormone therapy stems from the informational whiplash that has occurred in recent decades regarding the risks versus benefits. I don't want to get lost in the weeds on this so consider this brief snapshot: The Women's Health Initiative (WHI)[1]—which was designed to evaluate the benefits and risks of menopausal hormone therapy in terms of its potential to prevent chronic age-related diseases—was launched in 1991. It followed 160,000 postmenopausal women, ages fifty to seventy-nine, in what was supposed to be a fifteen-year study. (Something many people don't realize: The WHI was not designed to look at the use of hormone therapy to calm menopausal symptoms.) Part of the study was stopped early, in 2002, in the women who were taking combination (estrogen and progestin) hormone therapy because they were found to have an increased risk for breast cancer, heart disease, stroke, blood clots, and urinary incontinence; on the upside, the women using combined hormone therapy had a lower risk of bone fractures and colorectal cancer, but the medical consensus at the time was that these benefits did not outweigh the risks.[2] Not surprisingly, these results scared the bejesus out of many women, who vowed to avoid hormone therapy even if their symptoms were driving them mad. Other studies added to the fear and loathing women were experiencing about this.

Suffice it to say that like many things in life, science evolves, and a lot has been learned about the nuances of hormone therapy (HT) in recent years. For example, in 2017, a newer analysis from the WHI[3] examined all-cause and specific-cause mortality among postmenopausal women who were taking conjugated equine estrogens (CEE) plus medroxyprogesterone acetate (MPA) if they had an intact uterus, or conjugated equine estrogens alone if they'd had a hysterectomy. The researchers found that among postmenopausal women, taking combination hormone therapy for an average of 5.6 years or conjugated equine estrogens alone for an average of 7.2 years was *not* associated with an increased risk of premature death or mortality from cardiovascular disease or cancer during a follow-up period of eighteen years. These findings helped ease many women's fears.

Also, a later analysis of the WHI study data focused on the age of the participants and found that it was primarily women who started hormone therapy after age sixty-five who were at risk from the use of HT. It also found that the benefits of using HT generally outweighed the risks for healthy women under age sixty who were within ten years of the onset of menopause.

Many women are more open-minded about using hormone therapy now than a decade or two ago. These days, for most women who have moderate to severe menopausal symptoms such as hot flashes and vaginal dryness, it's safe to use hormone therapy within ten years of menopause and before age sixty, according to the North American Menopause Society.[4] That's right—there's an optimal therapeutic window in terms of HT's safety profile (meaning the possibility of having the most benefits and the fewest risks). That said, some women will continue to have hot flashes and other va-somotor symptoms even after the ten-year window—menopausal symptoms don't have a natural expiration date—and they may want to continue to use HT, and with clinical supervision, that may be possible if the benefits of relieving their symptoms and/or protecting their bone or pelvic floor health outweigh the risks[5] of ongoing use of hormone therapy. Ultimately, every woman and her health-care provider need to discuss the potential benefits and risks of using HT based not only on a woman's age but also on her individual health status and medical history.[6]

Before we get into the nitty-gritty of who's a candidate for hormone therapy and why (or why not), let's back up a few steps and address what exactly hormone therapy entails at this stage of a woman's life. There are three terms that are often used inter-changeably and confused for each other when they are actually distinct entities: Hormone replacement therapy (HRT) is more appropriately used for women with premature menopause (before age forty), early menopause (which occurs between the ages of forty and forty-five), or premature ovarian insufficiency (POI), because it's essentially providing or replacing the hormones that the woman's body should be making at her age; as a result, slightly higher doses are often indicated for these women than those at the average age of menopause, because we are physiologically replacing the hormones a woman at this age should have. By contrast, hormone therapy (HT) or menopausal hormone therapy (MHT) refers to the use of hormones at low doses to treat menopausal symptoms or otherwise help a woman who is experiencing natural menopause. (I prefer the simplicity of the term "hormone therapy," or HT, so that's what I'll use throughout this book.)

To put all this in perspective, birth control pills, or oral contraceptives, are similar to HT in that they contain an estrogen and a progesterone—but birth control pills contain higher doses of these hormones in order to make a woman stop ovulating (and thus prevent pregnancy). Hormone therapy doesn't prevent ovulation if a woman is still menstruating, so it isn't used for pregnancy prevention. Which means that if you're still getting your period, even if it's irregular, you still need to use a method of contraception along with HT.

This alphabet soup of terminology encompasses the use of estrogen and progesterone if a woman has an intact uterus. Progesterone will protect the uterine lining from uncontrolled growth—and perhaps the growth of abnormal cells—that could happen from taking unopposed estrogen. By contrast, women who've had a hysterectomy can use estrogen on its own. The estrogens used in HT are conjugated equine estrogens (such as Premarin), which come from—you guessed it!—horse urine, or plant-based estradiol or pharmaceutical estradiol, both of which are made in a lab. As far as menopausal symptoms go, taking estrogen supplements can help relieve moderate to severe symptoms like hot flashes and night sweats, as well as improve brain fog, joint pain, genitourinary symptoms (like vaginal dryness, burning, painful intercourse, and urinary frequency and urgency), mood changes, and insomnia. While progesterone is used primarily to counteract the effects of unopposed estrogen in women who have a uterus, it can also be used on its own for sleep disturbances because some formulations (like oral micronized natural progesterone) have a calming effect. For menopausal symptoms, my goal with any type of hormone therapy is to achieve an 80 percent improvement in symptoms for my patients.

There are many different routes of administration for hormone therapy.[7,8] Estrogen can be prescribed and taken as oral preparations, transdermal patches, sprays or gels, vaginal rings, creams, or injectables. Progestogens, including progesterone, can be taken orally, in combination with estrogen in a patch, as a vaginal gel or tablet, or as a monthly intramuscular injection. These are all considered "systemic" therapies because the hormones are delivered throughout the body. With another approach to systemic hormone therapy, there's a pill that combines conjugated estrogens and a compound known as a selective estrogen receptor modulator (SERM), which protects the uterus but isn't a progestogen; the advantage is that it's potentially more targeted to the tissues where we want it to work (namely, the brain, vagina, and bones) and it leaves other tissues (like the breasts and uterus) alone.

The route of administration (oral, transdermal, or vaginal) may make a big difference in the efficacy, depending on the individual woman. Meanwhile, the time at which hormone replacement is started may influence which route of administration is the best one to go with. When it comes to dosing, things can be a bit tricky because we don't have any way to tell what dose a woman will thrive on; unlike prescribing non-hormonal medications, the dosing has nothing to do with a woman's weight or the severity of her symptoms. The optimal dose varies from one woman to another based on individual differences in sensitivity, metabolism, and the ability to break down drugs and make use of them.

I warn my patients that finding the right dose often involves some trial and error; it's a bit like playing Goldilocks with hormones, with the goal of finding the approach that's "just right." All women metabolize hormone supplements and medications differently. And while the goal with hormone therapy is to get an 80 percent improvement in symptoms, an 80 percent improvement for one woman can require a completely different dose than an 80 percent improvement for another woman. If a woman's symptoms are limited to the genitourinary tract—namely, the vagina and bladder—estrogen therapy can be administered right into the vagina with creams or gels, which means that very little goes into the bloodstream.

WHAT THE B-WORD REALLY MEANS

You've probably heard the term "bioidentical" in the context of hormone therapy, and you may be confused about what it means. *You're not alone!* The North American Menopause Society (NAMS) uses the term to refer to "compounds that have the same chemical and molecular structure as hormones that are produced in the body." But not everyone subscribes to that meaning, which is why I feel the term is essentially medically misleading if not meaningless. In recent years, "bioidentical" has been used to refer to made-to-order (a.k.a. custom-compounded) hormone treatments that pharmacies create for a particular woman. Over the years, celebrity promoters (like actress Suzanne Somers) and some websites have claimed that custom-compounded hormone therapy is safer and more *natural* than hormones made by drug companies.

But custom-compounded estrogen and progesterone formulations are not approved by the Food and Drug Administration (FDA) because they haven't been tested for safety, efficacy, absorbability, potency, purity, or to see if they actually contain the prescribed amounts of hormones. In other words, you really don't know what you're getting with the formulations, and each time you pick up a new dose, it could be different even with the exact same prescription. As NAMS notes, "There is no scientific evidence that these compounded medications are safer or more effective than government-approved hormones." Also, custom-compounded hormones are typically more expensive than FDA-approved versions of HT.

The truth is, there are many well-tested, FDA-approved hormone therapy products that meet the original definition of "bioidentical" and are commercially available from pharmacies—but they're not custom-compounded. I prescribe FDA-approved bioidenticals every day because they have a nice safety profile, they come in many different forms (oral, transdermal, and so on), and they work. Patients often prefer this formulation because they know that other types of estrogen are animal-based (mostly from horses' urine) and that creates an "ick" factor for some women; to others, it feels like animal cruelty. I also use conjugated equine estrogens because sometimes that's the only thing insurance will cover. And I do have a few patients who use specialty custom-compounded hormone therapy because they have allergies to ingredients that are in commercially prepared estrogen products, which is a legitimate approach in my view. There is also a bioidentical progesterone in oral form that I often use (Prometrium), which has been found to be a bit safer than some other progesterones made in a lab. Unfortunately, custom-compounded progesterone is not absorbed well through the skin, which means it may not be doing its intended job of protecting the uterus; this is why many menopause experts, including me, are wary of custom-compounded progesterone creams. In general, my advice is to spend less time worrying about what's "bioidentical" and to focus more on the preparation that's likely to be right for you. Ideally, you want to make sure the HT preparation is FDA-approved and not custom-compounded.

A couple of years ago, Missy, fifty-seven, a lawyer, came to me because she was having a similar flavor of bothersome symptoms from head to toe—dry skin, dry eyes, and vaginal dryness. Her vaginal tissue was so dry that she was avoiding sex with her partner, and when she did have it, she would bleed the next day and feel sore for three more days. Many of her friends were on bioidentical hormone therapy and were encouraging her to try it. Missy was really confused about the differences between bioidentical creams and over-the-counter creams to treat vaginal dryness; she also wondered if she should consider systemic hormone therapy of some form.

After discussing the differences between the various approaches and formulations, the risk-to-benefit ratios, the costs, and safety profiles, she decided that she did not really need systemic hormone therapy, that vaginal dryness was her priority for obtaining relief. So I put her on a vaginal estrogen cream that she used twice a week, and within twelve weeks, it helped. When she came back to see me, Missy said it was a miracle and it restored her and her wife's sex life.

The Other Hormonal Change

Let's not forget about another sex hormone that can be relevant to the menopausal experience—testosterone. While it's usually thought of as a male hormone, women have testosterone, too: It's produced mostly by the ovaries and the adrenal glands—and it contributes to libido and estrogen production and helps maintain bone and muscle mass.[9] Testosterone levels peak in a woman's twenties and decline slowly after that until they're at half their peak levels by menopause. After estrogen production stops, the ovaries continue to produce some testosterone and so do the adrenal glands; however, women who

experience surgical menopause after having their
ovaries removed sometimes experience a sharper
drop in their testosterone levels.[10]

While some studies have shown a beneficial
effect of testosterone therapy (from creams, gels,
patches, pills, or injections) on women's low sex drive,
it's not FDA-approved for this purpose. Even so, the
International Menopause Society and the North
American Menopause Society agree with the global
consensus position statement endorsed by the world's
leading endocrinology, menopause, and reproductive
societies supporting the use of low-dose transdermal
testosterone for low libido in women.[11] So sometimes
I do prescribe it for women who are distressed by
their low libido and who have a low blood level
of testosterone; if someone has low libido but
normal or elevated testosterone levels, it's probably
psychologically rather than hormonally based, and
I wouldn't recommend testosterone therapy. The
concern is that if testosterone levels get too high in
women, they can experience permanent hair loss,
deepening of the voice, enlargement of the clitoris,
acne, and facial hair—symptoms most women want to
avoid! Other effects from too much testosterone can
include bone loss, heart conditions, and possibly other
detrimental effects.

Also, women who can get pregnant—because they
still get their period, even if it's irregular—should not use
testosterone if they aren't using contraception because
it could cause abnormal genitalia in a female fetus. And
testosterone therapy should not be used as a means

of gaining muscle mass. I mention this because I have had women from the fitness industry attempt to get testosterone from me. (They didn't succeed.)

THE GOOD, THE BAD, AND THE TRICKY

On the positive side of the equation, systemic hormones are very effective for treating hot flashes, night sweats, and vaginal dryness, as well as sleep disturbances and irritability. They also can help with painful intercourse and ease overactive bladders, and may help with recurring urinary tract infections. In terms of long-term health perks, systemic hormone therapy protects your bones, reducing your risk of bone fractures later in life, and may help prevent type 2 diabetes. And if it's started within ten years of menopause, HT may lower your risk of heart disease and diabetes.

Now for the not-so-good news: Combination hormone therapy and estrogen alone can increase the risk of stroke—but that heightened risk can be mitigated by using transdermal estrogen, and with any formulation, any increased risk dissipates when a woman stops taking hormones. Also, there is an elevated risk of blood clots with oral HT—and the risk increases as women get older; with transdermal estrogen, however, the risk of blood clots may be lower at any age. As far as breast cancer goes (which tops the list of many women's health fears) the potential added risk of breast cancer from hormone therapy is actually lower than the increased risk of breast cancer that comes with obesity, smoking, drinking more than five alcoholic beverages per week, high blood pressure, or diabetes.[12] So it's important to keep these elements of risk in perspective.

Beyond these concerns, there are various contraindications[13] for the use of hormone therapy. I like to think of these in two categories, as absolute contraindications (as in: red light) or possible contraindications (as in: yellow light). Absolute contraindications (red light) for HT include active breast cancer or a personal history of estrogen-sensitive breast cancer, a pulmonary embolism (blood clot in the lung) or an unprovoked blood clot (one that wasn't caused by an accident or surgery), stroke, dementia, or a personal history or inherited high risk of thromboembolic (a.k.a. blood clotting) diseases. Possible contraindications (yellow light) include high triglyceride levels, migraine headaches, leiomyomas (a.k.a. fibroids), unexplained vaginal bleeding, liver disease, coronary heart disease, and a history of endometrial or ovarian cancer. When it comes to progesterone, women with a history of hormone-positive breast cancer shouldn't take it; also, some commercially available forms of oral micronized natural progesterone are made with peanut oil, which means they can't be used by women with a peanut allergy. Lastly, women with a history of seizure disorders shouldn't take Prometrium because the drug could lower the seizure threshold, meaning it can increase the risk of having a seizure.

The risks of HT vary depending on the type, dose, duration of use, route of administration, the timing of initiation, and whether a progestogen is used. With every woman, treatment should be individualized, based on all of these parameters, in order to maximize her benefits and minimize her risks; along the way, there should be periodic reevaluations of the benefits and risks of continuing HT or discontinuing it. For women who are fifty-nine and younger or within ten years of the onset of menopause—and who have no contraindications—the benefit-to-risk ratio is most favorable for treatment of bothersome vasomotor symptoms (like hot flashes and night sweats) and severe genitourinary syndrome (GSM) of menopause and for those who have an elevated risk for bone loss or fracture. For women who start HT more than ten or twenty years from the onset of menopause or who are age sixty or older, the benefit-to-risk ratio is less favorable because of the greater risks of coronary heart disease, stroke, venous thromboembolism, and dementia. While age alone may present a yellow light, that doesn't mean the window has slammed shut; individualization is essential for this issue, and women need to discuss their concerns with a knowledgeable health-care provider.

When Janice, fifty-one, came to see me, she was interested in hormone therapy because she was having severe night sweats that were not only drenching her but also interfering with her quality of sleep. But she didn't think she could take it safely because her father had had a blood clot, which was treated with anticoagulation therapy, and she was worried that she would follow in his footsteps. So we discussed the risks of HT and her personal medical history. It turned out that Janice had been on birth control pills for five years, and she had had two pregnancies that resulted in Cesarean sections—without ever having blood clots. I did test her for the most common genetic mutation for blood clotting, which is a factor V Leiden mutation, and she was negative for that.

All of this meant that since she tolerated these risky situations well, she would likely tolerate postmenopausal hormone therapy well. To decrease her risk for blood clots further, we decided to go with a transdermal patch; she felt comfortable with that decision after we reviewed the benefit-risk profile. To put her risk in perspective, we also discussed the fact that her father was a smoker and had high blood pressure as well as other reasons why he may have had a blood clot; she had none of these. She started using a transdermal estrogen and progesterone patch and it dramatically reduced her night sweats and awakenings from sleep. Her husband benefitted from these improvements, too.

As you can tell, the question of whether to use hormone therapy is complex for many different reasons. For one thing, there's a lot of pressure surrounding the issue, but it's time for people to stop judging or shaming women for either taking or not taking hormone therapy. *There's no place for that!* For another thing, it's not just a simple yes-or-no decision: A woman's symptoms, personal health risks, health status and history, and lifestyle habits need to be part of the equation. And there are issues related to timing, dosage, delivery system, and duration to consider. So it's a complex decision. Your physician is your partner in making it, not only because your doctor would be the one to prescribe hormones, but also because we in the medical profession are continuously learning more about the effects of hormone therapy on women's bodies as they go through this journey. I encourage you to take maximal advantage of the partnership with your physician throughout the menopausal transition. That way you can make the best health-related choices for *you*, every step of the way, so you can feel and function at your best.

Myths and Realities About Hormone Therapy

As with so many aspects of menopause, myths and misconceptions abound when it comes to hormone therapy. Here are three big ones that I want to dispel right now:

Myth: You can't use postmenopausal hormone therapy if you're in perimenopause.

Reality: Yes, you can.[14] It seems that many doctors get stuck on this issue, telling women that they cannot use hormone therapy unless it has been twelve months since their last period. But there's no reason to withhold hormone therapy until that end point. HT, when used in perimenopause, is meant to help reduce, alleviate, or control the symptoms of low estrogen states that can trigger menopausal symptoms. Many women have menopausal symptoms such as hot flashes, vaginal dryness, and severe mood changes while they are still getting their periods, and research suggests there is a tendency for women to have more years of menopausal symptoms when their symptoms start during perimenopause.

As an expert in menopause and hormonal care, I will tell you that perimenopause is much trickier to treat than menopause because during perimenopause a woman's body is still making hormones even as we are trying to control her symptoms. By contrast, after menopause, a woman is producing little to no estrogen so it's easier to control menopausal symptoms with hormone therapy.

It's important to remember that using hormone therapy is not contraception and isn't designed to prevent pregnancy, so if you're still getting your period and you don't want to get pregnant, you will want to use a contraceptive method. I have some women use a progesterone-releasing IUD and the postmenopausal estrogen patch as a one-two punch that covers birth control and menopausal symptoms. Here's an interesting twist: Using continuous oral contraceptives (traditional birth control pills) may control menopausal symptoms, too.

Myth: Your doctor should be "for" or "against" hormone therapy.

Reality: In the ideal world, your doctor would consult with you about your medical history and symptoms to determine whether hormone therapy is right for you by reviewing the risks and benefits of this treatment option. However, most doctors get very little training in treating menopause and even fewer doctors have seen hormone therapy prescribed or prescribed it themselves, especially if they were trained in the last ten to twenty years. Currently, hormone therapy is FDA-approved to treat severe hot flashes and severe genitourinary syndrome of menopause[15] (which includes vaginal dryness, burning and irritation, pain during sexual activity, and urinary frequency and urgency), as well as osteopenia (bone loss); it is the most effective medication available to help with those symptoms/conditions and should be considered as first-line treatment.

Moreover, most NAMS doctors stand in agreement[16] that the benefits of hormone therapy outweigh the risks in women who start HT within ten years of menopause and who have no known contraindications to using estrogen. Having said that, women still have the right to choose their treatments: If they cannot or don't want to use hormone therapy, then they can consider relying on lifestyle changes, over-the-counter supplements, or non-hormonal medications to manage their symptoms.

Myth: There's a time limit for using hormone therapy for menopausal symptoms.

Reality: Not necessarily. Both the American College of Obstetricians and Gynecologists (ACOG) and NAMS state[17] that there is no longer a red-light time limit on using hormone therapy for menopausal symptoms. Now, there's a yellow light, which requires shared decision-making about whether or not to move forward with HT or continue using HT after age sixty. The change in thinking happened because we now know that the risks don't necessarily add up in a cumulative fashion with each passing year. For example, the biggest risk of hormone therapy is the rare risk of a blood clot—which happens to one in one thousand women when using oral HT and one in two thousand when using transdermal HT[18]—and the risk is highest in the first six months on hormone therapy, then it declines back to baseline.

At every age and with each year on hormone therapy, a woman and her doctor should come together to make a shared plan about her continuation or weaning off of hormone therapy. They should consider the woman's current symptoms and quality of life, and any new medical conditions that have arisen when determining if a woman should stay on HT or come off it. It's not just about celebrating a particular birthday.

4

What's Your Menopause Type?

The intensity of menopausal symptoms may depend partly on a woman's age and general health status, as well as many other factors. Unfortunately, it's impossible to predict a particular woman's menopausal experience ahead of time. (Wouldn't *that* be helpful?!) Part of the challenge is that individual women experience different clusters of symptoms, and there's just no way for women or their doctors to know who will experience which ones—at least not yet. That's the dream!

Given our current reality, this is where the menopause type quiz comes in. When I see patients in person or via telemedicine appointments, we go over similar questions in the course of our conversation. Since you and I can't do that, I have created this quiz for you. Answering the following questions will help you identify your personal menopause type based on your health history and how your current symptoms are affecting you. As you'll see, more than one response may resonate with you, so choose all the answers that apply to you. This is for your eyes only—unless you choose to share it with a family member, a friend, or your doctor—so don't hold back or judge your responses. Just answer the questions as truthfully as possible.

1. Did your periods end before age forty?
   Yes / No
   ANSWER KEY: If you chose yes, you have the Premature

Menopause Type. Make a note of it and keep reading because you could have another type as well.

2. Did you have a surgery that involved removing both of your ovaries or chemotherapy before you reached natural menopause?

ANSWER KEY: If you selected yes for either option, you have the Sudden Menopause Type. Make a note of it and keep reading because you could have another type as well.

3. Think about where your most annoying menopause-related symptoms are on your body. Are they mostly:
   a. *From the neck up (meaning in my head)*
   b. *Below the waist*
   c. *All over my body*
   d. *Nowhere*

ANSWER KEY: If you selected a, you likely have the Mind-Altering Menopause Type; b suggests you may have the Seemingly Never-Ending Menopause Type; c indicates that you have the Full-Throttle Menopause Type; and d means you have the Silent Menopause Type. Make a note of it and read on.

4. How long have these disruptive symptoms been going on?
   a. *Less than a year*
   b. *Two to five years*
   c. *Six to ten years*
   d. *Symptoms—what symptoms?*

ANSWER KEY: If you chose a or b, you could have either the Full-Throttle or the Mind-Altering Menopause Type. If you selected c, you may have the Seemingly Never-Ending Menopause Type; and d signals the Silent Menopause Type.

5. To what extent are your menopausal symptoms affecting the quality of your work, your relationships, or your recreational life?

   a. *Not at all*
   b. *A little bit now and then*
   c. *Quite a bit consistently (I think)*
   d. *Like a wrecking ball*

   ANSWER KEY: If you chose a, you have the Silent Menopause Type; b could signal the Seemingly Never-Ending Menopause Type; c may mean you have the Mind-Altering Menopause Type; and d indicates you have the Full-Throttle Menopause Type.

6. If your menopausal experience were a movie, which of the following would be the most appropriate title (never mind the actual plot of these flicks)?

   a. *Too Much, Too Soon*
   b. *A Shock to the System*
   c. *Altered States*
   d. *A Nightmare on Elm Street*
   e. *The NeverEnding Story*
   f. *Ghost*

   ANSWER KEY: If you chose a, you likely have the Premature Menopause Type; b could signal the Sudden Menopause Type; c may mean you have the Mind-Altering Menopause Type; d indicates you have the Full-Throttle Menopause Type; e suggests the Seemingly Never-Ending Menopause Type; and f indicates the Silent Menopause Type.

7. Based on your menopausal experience so far, what qualities would you most like to regain in your life?

   a. *A boost in energy and to feel like my real (biological) age again*
   b. *To tame the shock to my body and restore my vitality*

   c. *To calm the chaos in my body and mind and to feel less whip-lashed by symptoms*

   d. *A boost to my mood and improved clarity in my brain function*

   e. *Stress relief and an increase in stamina*

   f. *Feeling the same as I do now well into the future*

ANSWER KEY: If you chose a, you likely have the Premature Menopause Type; b could signal the Sudden Menopause Type; c may suggest the Full-Throttle Menopause Type; d may mean you have the Mind-Altering Menopause Type; e suggests the Seemingly Never-Ending Menopause Type; and f indicates the Silent Menopause Type.

IT'S TIME FOR SCORING

Review your responses and count up how many times you chose each type. This is where things get a bit tricky because quite often women don't fall exclusively into one menopause type or another. In other words, you can be more than one type—a hybrid or mixed breed, so to speak—depending on your answers. For example, if you answered yes to question 1, you definitely have the Premature Menopause Type but you could also have the Mind-Altering Menopause Type if you chose *a* for question 3. Similarly, if you answered yes to the second question, you have the Sudden Menopause Type but you could have another one as well, such as the Full-Throttle Type if you selected *c* for question 3. You get the picture!

There can be some overlap between the different types, or a woman can have predominant traits from one type but also some crossover elements from another type. That's why it's essential to accurately identify your hybrid menopause types. This is the best way to create a personalized plan of action that's likely to relieve *your* unique set of symptoms and protect your current and future health and well-being, as the chapters that follow will show. If you urgently need relief from certain symptoms, you might choose to prioritize the chapter or chapters that focus on your menopause type(s). But if you opt to read the book straight through, you'll glean helpful insights and advice that will deepen your understanding of the menopausal experience and guide you in treating your own symptoms and perhaps offer support to friends and family members.

Here are snapshots of each type:

The Premature Menopause Type, which occurs before age forty, can bring a rush of symptoms such as hot flashes, night sweats, mood swings, mental fogginess, and others. The symptoms aren't different from the other types; it's the timing that defines the Premature type.

The Sudden Menopause Type, which often results from surgery or chemotherapy (but can occur for other reasons, as you'll see in chapter 6), often feels like a shock to a woman's system with both its arrival and its intensity.

The Full-Throttle Menopause Type, which is marked by intense symptoms from pretty much every direction in your body and mind, can be overwhelming and sometimes debilitating.

The Mind-Altering Menopause Type, which mainly involves mood shifts (possibly including anxiety, depression, irritability, and/or mood swings) and cognitive changes such as brain fog, difficulty with concentration, and memory challenges.

The Seemingly Never-Ending Menopause Type, which is usually characterized by one or two symptoms (such as the occasional hot flash, persistent vaginal dryness, or low libido, or less common ones like dizziness or olfactory changes) that continue long after expected.

The Silent Menopause Type, where a woman is largely free of menopausal symptoms. Even so, it's important for her to pay attention to new health challenges and risks that emerge post-menopause due to the drop in reproductive hormones.

If you have any doubt about which menopause type(s) you have, please read all the chapters that could possibly apply to your experience. Also, consider perusing the others, because you may discover helpful diet, exercise, and psychological strategies that could help you on this journey. Without further ado, let's get down to the nitty-gritty with the chapters that follow.

Part II

DISCOVERING YOUR MENOPAUSAL ROAD MAP

5 | The Premature Menopause Type

Michele, twenty-six, a marketing assistant, came to see me after working with a reproductive endocrinologist who didn't properly address her concerns or help her obtain relief for the way she was feeling. During high school and college, Michele's periods had been infrequent and her periods came to a complete halt in her midtwenties. That's when she started having hot flashes, sleep disturbances, and vaginal dryness, and her libido did a disappearing act. After going through a battery of tests, Michele found out she was menopausal. She felt really dismissed by the reproductive endocrinologist who geared all her questions toward Michele's reproductive potential, rather than the way she was feeling. Michele, who lived with her boyfriend, wasn't interested in getting pregnant. What she wanted was relief from her symptoms. "I feel like I'm fifty-six, not twenty-six," she told me at our first office visit, "and I want to get my energy and sex drive back."

To treat her menopausal symptoms and protect her long-term health, I prescribed an oral combination of estrogen and testosterone in higher doses than I would give a symptomatic woman in her fifties. In Michele's case, it was important to replace the hormones that she should have been getting naturally at her age but wasn't. I also prescribed a vaginal estrogen to help with vaginal dryness and painful sex. Three months later, she came back, hugged me, and said, "You saved my life! I feel twenty-six again." (An interesting footnote: Michele's twin sister also experienced menopause at twenty-six and because she *did* want to have a baby, she got pregnant with the help of a donor egg and had a child.)

To put this in perspective: It isn't common for women to reach menopause in their twenties but it's also not unheard of. At first blush, the concept of "premature" or "early" menopause may feel subjective—if a woman feels too vibrant and youthful to have gone through menopause, for example. But it's not subjective: *Premature* menopause occurs before age forty, while *early* menopause occurs between the ages of forty and forty-five.

According to the latest research,[1] premature menopause occurs in 1.7 percent of women in the US, while early menopause affects 3.4 percent of women in the US; by contrast, in Korean women, the prevalence of premature menopause is 2.8 percent and early menopause occurs in 7.2 percent. These trends add to the picture created by previously identified ethnic differences,[2] in which African American and Hispanic women were found to have a higher prevalence of premature menopause than Caucasian women.

I do wonder if these percentages are underestimated because women often aren't identified as having premature or early menopause. In the electronic medical records, there's an actual diagnostic code a doctor can note for premature or early menopause, just like there is for hypertension—but this info is often missing from women's charts. So I do think there's an underdiagnosis of premature and early menopause. In my clinic, I see many women of different races or ethnicities who have premature or early menopause, which isn't surprising given that treating menopause is my specialty. Sadly, many women come from outside my regional area because they feel their medical concerns and mental health struggles weren't taken seriously or treated adequately by health care professionals where they live. Many women simply get a pat on the back and a comment like, "Well, you no longer need to buy tampons" or another version of a *well, that's over* moment. No significance is made of the diagnosis; it gets brushed over. But it shouldn't because this diagnosis carries significant health concerns.

Besides being highly disruptive to women's lives, premature or early menopause brings a host of new health risks that don't usually affect relatively young women. With the loss of estrogen at a younger age, women with premature or early menopause face a higher risk of heart disease, angina (atypical chest pain), osteoporosis, sexual dysfunction, mood disorders, and some neurologic diseases such as dementia. In fact, a 2019 study[3] found that, compared with women who had menopause at age fifty or fifty-one, those who reached menopause before age forty had a 55 percent higher risk of having a nonfatal cardiac event, such as a heart attack or angina, before the age of sixty. And women whose premature menopause is caused by an autoimmune disease have an increased risk of developing adrenal insufficiency, hypothyroidism, diabetes mellitus, myasthenia gravis, rheumatoid arthritis, and systemic lupus erythematosus.[4]

Premature or early menopause can happen for a variety of reasons, including premature ovarian insufficiency (or POI, when a woman's ovaries simply quit working normally far ahead of schedule), the presence of underlying autoimmune conditions (such as rheumatoid arthritis, lupus, scleroderma, pernicious anemia, celiac disease, inflammatory bowel disease like Crohn's disease or ulcerative colitis, or autoimmune thyroid disorders such as Hashimoto's or Graves' disease), chromosomal abnormalities like Fragile X syndrome or Turner syndrome, mumps, genetic factors (including a family history of premature ovarian insufficiency), chemotherapy or pelvic radiation treatments for cancer, or surgical removal of both ovaries before age forty. In rare instances, heavy smoking and possibly drug use can bring on premature menopause as well. And a recent study[5] found that being a child of a multiple pregnancy, being underweight, or never having children are also risk factors for premature or early menopause.

But the truth is: Some causes remain unknown. We just don't know why they happen.

Regardless of the suspected cause, often there's no mystery to whether a woman has gone through premature menopause because her periods will have stopped at least a year before her fortieth birthday—it's that simple. But in some instances, women can begin having perimenopausal symptoms such as hot flashes, night sweats/cold flashes, vaginal dryness or pain with sex, urinary urgency, an increase in urinary tract infections, difficulty sleeping, mood changes, libido changes, and brain fog, along with very occasional periods—at which point they may benefit from having their ovarian function tested. Sometimes blood levels of follicle-stimulating hormone (FSH), which stimulates the ovaries to produce estrogen, and anti-mullerian hormone (AMH), which is produced by cells in the small follicles in the ovaries, are measured to gauge how well a woman's ovaries are functioning and to determine whether she is nearing menopause.

In my experience, there is some benefit to having these lab tests but it's not as helpful as many women believe. These test results provide only a snapshot of what's happening at a particular time—that is, the minute your blood is drawn—and menopause is diagnosed retrospectively, a year after a woman's last period. It's more useful to look at trends over time in FSH levels, which increase as a woman gets closer to menopause, and estradiol levels, which decrease when a woman gets closer to menopause. Of course, when a woman's periods stop before age forty or forty-five, pregnancy needs to be ruled out and other possible causes of missed periods such as certain thyroid disorders and polycystic ovarian syndrome, or PCOS, should be checked for as well.

When a woman experiences early or premature menopause, she may get a surprising and often abrupt rush of symptoms such as hot flashes, night sweats, mood swings, mental fogginess, vaginal dryness, and decreased sex drive—the usual symptoms of menopause. It's not the symptoms that are unique to premature or early menopause. It's the timing.

Psychologically, a woman who goes through menopause before age forty may feel older than her years, which can affect her quality of life. While her friends are having babies, she may be struggling with drenching hot flashes, moodiness, and other unpleasant symptoms that can make her feel socially and emotionally out of sync with her peers. Research[6] from Australia found that experiencing menopause before age forty "resulted in multiple disruptions in the women's lives" and the women reported that "many aspects of their lives now seemed to be 'out of synchrony.'" A study in the UK[7] found that women who experienced menopause before age forty reported high levels of depression and perceived stress and low self-esteem compared to the general population.

And if a woman experiences premature menopause when she's still interested in having children, that can feel like a serious betrayal by her body. She can feel blindsided and devastated to learn that her plans for creating a family have been turned upside down. She can feel out of place among friends who are still complaining of periods or discussing ovulation kits or the best sex positions for getting pregnant. The effects can spill over into her work life, creating a sense of uncertainty or a lower threshold to burnout.

This happened to Jessica, a freelance copywriter who found out that she had premature ovarian insufficiency at age thirty-nine. At the time, her daughter, Ella, was eighteen months old and Jessica was hoping to have a second child. After six months of trying, she hadn't been able to get pregnant so she went to see a reproductive endocrinologist who ran tests and diagnosed Jessica with premature ovarian insufficiency. That's when she realized her period hadn't returned after she'd stopped breastfeeding Ella. She had been attributing her disturbed sleep and night sweats to postpartum hormonal changes—suddenly she saw them through a different lens. Jessica felt crushed that having another baby wasn't in the cards for her anymore. She found playdates with other kids and their moms and dads difficult and teared up every time she saw siblings playing together in the park.

Jessica and her husband discussed various kinds of assisted reproductive technology, but she didn't want to go that route. When she came to see me, her grief was significant, so I recommended therapy first. Later, we discussed her symptoms—exhaustion, feeling hot all the time, joint aches and pains, brain fog, and very low libido—and how we might treat them. She decided to use movement (running, in particular) as her mood-enhancing medication. She'd had a blood clot when she was on birth control pills, so we decided to treat her remaining symptoms without hormone replacement therapy; instead, to help with her sex drive, we used a non-hormonal medication called Addyi (flibanserin), which is FDA-approved for low libido in premenopausal women and works by increasing dopamine in the brain, so it also is great for mood and sleep when taken at bedtime. Since she had a mild case of overactive bladder after the birth of her daughter, she chose to start taking oxybutynin, a medication approved to treat overactive bladder that also has good efficacy for reducing hot flashes. Once she began sleeping through the night more consistently, her brain fog and exhaustion improved. She also did pelvic floor therapy and used a daily vaginal moisturizer containing hyaluronic acid and vaginal estrogen twice a week (vaginal estrogen isn't absorbed systemically, so it wasn't contraindicated for her, given her blood clot history). Her mood stabilized, her sex life improved, and she began feeling more like her usual self.

MAKING TREATMENT DECISIONS

Because of the health risks associated with the early loss of estrogen, treatment for the Premature Menopause Type typically centers around hormone replacement therapy—namely, significant doses of estrogen and progesterone (if the woman still has her uterus) and possibly testosterone—to replace what a woman isn't getting but should be getting naturally at her age. Simply put, a woman who has gone through menopause before the age of forty needs estrogen to protect the health of her heart, bones, vagina, bladder, and brain—this is really a medical necessity. Without estrogen, she will face a higher risk of heart disease, osteopenia or osteoporosis, vaginal dryness or pain with intercourse, urinary incontinence, and impairments in memory and cognition—any of which can make her feel older than she is, given that these conditions typically occur among older women. Research[8] has also found that women with premature or early menopause have a higher risk of developing anxiety and depressive symptoms over the long term—but that taking estrogen decreases these mental health risks.

Keep in mind that most of the research on the use of hormone therapy is based on natural menopause and extrapolations are made from that and applied to premature or early menopause. But the physiological effects, risks, benefits, and outcomes of hormone replacement therapy are very different for women who have experienced premature or early menopause than they are for women who experience natural menopause at the usual time (around age fifty-one). In my clinic, I make a point of telling women who've experienced premature or early menopause this, and that the benefits of taking hormone *replacement* therapy (HRT) significantly outweigh the risks for most women with this type of menopause. Without HRT, these women have higher risks of developing heart disease, bone loss, dementia, and a worsening quality of life. Don't get me wrong: Hormone therapy is safe for many women who experience natural menopause but for them it's an option, rather than a necessity like it is for women who've experienced the change long before the average age.

When it comes to HRT, women who have experienced

premature or early menopause often need a slightly higher dose of estrogen than women who experience natural menopause.

What we're trying to do is physiologically replicate estrogen levels that would be normal at age thirty-six or forty if a woman hadn't gone through menopause; this is not only to treat menopausal symptoms but to reduce the risk of a woman developing heart disease, osteoporosis, dementia, pelvic floor disorders, and other conditions that stem from the loss of estrogen. By contrast, with hormone therapy (HT), we're administering a low dose of estrogen to address symptoms related to menopause—and it typically takes less estrogen to get the job done. My preferred way of prescribing estrogen is as a once-daily regimen, to keep things simple.

If a woman still has her uterus, she needs progesterone to protect it from uterine hyperplasia, a buildup of the uterine lining, which increases the risk of precancerous or cancerous cells developing. The risk of uterine cancer or precancer can increase from the effects of unopposed estrogen (meaning estrogen without progesterone) in women who have an intact uterus. If a woman starts getting her period again after starting estrogen therapy—which is not that uncommon among women with premature ovarian insufficiency— then I would recommend a progesterone-releasing IUD to protect against pregnancy and to serve as the progesterone part of HT. (As a side benefit, the progesterone that's released directly into the uterus thins the lining enough to significantly decrease menstrual bleeding, and when it's used for five years, it's been shown to reduce the risk of uterine cancer.) If the idea of an IUD is unappealing, she can use a long-acting progesterone like Nexplanon, or take progesterone nightly in oral form.

Meanwhile, testosterone supplementation may help protect a woman's libido, muscle mass, and energy if she experiences premature or early menopause. Contrary to popular belief, testosterone is not just a male hormone—women make it and need it, too.

It's just that women need only about one-tenth the amount that men do, and women stop making most of the testosterone their bodies naturally produce after menopause. If you think about it from an evolutionary biology perspective, this makes sense: Testosterone has various functions in the female body, but the main one is to support libido, and biologically speaking, the purpose of a woman's sex drive is to reproduce; so if a woman can no longer reproduce because she's postmenopausal, she doesn't *need* to have a thriving libido, from that vantage point. But as we all know, sex isn't just a utilitarian activity in the race to reproduce; it can be a highly pleasurable one, too—so many women want to protect their sex drives and sexual functionality at any age. And that's where testosterone supplementation comes in after menopause.

The North American Menopause Society[9] supports the use of testosterone-containing products to treat low libido (a.k.a. low sexual desire) after menopause, even though testosterone treatments are not approved by the Food and Drug Administration for use in women. Nevertheless, physicians (including me!) sometimes prescribe it for that purpose in an off-label capacity. Unfortunately, research on the physiological impacts of testosterone on the female body is sparse, but we've had glimmers of insights from a few studies. And I can tell you from my clinical experience, that when used correctly, testosterone replacement has benefits for libido and sometimes also for energy and cognition in postmenopausal women who have low testosterone levels.

As a case in point, consider Carrie, a thirty-year-old nurse from Alaska, who flew to Boston to see me with her husband because she wasn't getting relief for her crushing fatigue, insomnia, weight gain, mild hot flashes, and nonexistent libido. She hadn't had a period in fourteen months and she felt as though she was being treated like a medical mystery in Alaska because her healthcare providers couldn't figure out what was going on or how to help her. As we sat in my office reviewing her medical information and lab test results, we mapped out a treatment plan that covered her physical health (with a high-dose estrogen patch, daily application of a low-dose topical testosterone cream, and insertion of a progesterone-releasing IUD to protect her uterus), her mental health (including her frustration and disappointment about not being able to have another baby as a sibling for her four-year-old daughter), and her sexual health.

She went home to Alaska and began her treatment. Within ten weeks, she was sleeping well and having fewer hot flashes. She had gained the energy she expected to have at thirty and enjoyed the return of her libido. She also lost the twenty pounds she'd gained during her transition to menopause and went back to exercising and lifting heavy weights before her shifts. And as a health-care professional, she felt more confident in her ability to care for patients. She was so pleased with the improvements that she said she'd be happy to fly to Boston every year to see me because she felt so well cared for. (Luckily, I got a license to practice telehealth in Alaska.)

BASELINE TREATMENT PLANS FOR THE PREMATURE MENOPAUSE TYPE

What follows are two baseline treatment plans for women who have premature or early menopause. The first treatment plan focuses on the use of hormone replacement therapy (HRT), which as you've seen is really the gold standard for this type, given that these women have lost estrogen much earlier than the average age for menopause (fifty-one). This reality makes treating the Premature Menopause Type unique. But some women can't use estrogen replacement therapy—perhaps because they have a history of an estrogen-responsive cancer, an unprovoked blood clot, a heart attack, or stroke—or they have strong feelings about *not* taking hormones, so the second plan addresses how to treat premature menopause without hormones.

With either treatment plan, if you have additional symptoms that aren't relieved by these recommended approaches, you can choose from the extensive menu of symptom-oriented solutions in chapter 12 to ease what's still bothering you.

Plan A: Using Hormone Replacement Therapy

If a woman can take oral estrogen, I like to start her with 1 milligram oral estradiol once daily and increase her dosage to the maximum of 4 milligrams daily over a period of many months—it's a thoughtful and calculated process. The goal is for the woman to have blood levels of estrogen between 40 and 120 pg/mL, though women with premature menopause who take estrogen are likely to have estrogen levels on the higher end of the spectrum (often between 70 and 120 pg/mL) simply because they're taking higher doses; this allows them to get closer to the levels they would normally have at their age if they hadn't reached menopause early. Also, this higher estrogen level is often needed to help control their symptoms. While a woman's heart, brain, and bones may be protected with a lower blood level of estrogen, when women with the Premature Menopause Type have their estrogen get too low (say, 40 to 50 pg/mL) they end up experiencing hot flashes like crazy or other symptoms like joint pains or intense fatigue.

I also have most women with premature or early menopause use vaginal estrogen cream at night, two to three times per week, to prevent vaginal atrophy, dryness, or pain with intercourse. Eventually, they can drop it if the systemic estrogen dose they're taking is high enough to control these symptoms. The goal with vaginal estrogen cream is to prevent vaginal atrophy, as well as any atrophy of tissue in the labia or clitoris—both of which are rich in nerve endings that help with sexual pleasure, arousal, and orgasm—as well as protect these women from recurrent urinary tract infections (UTIs).

If a woman with premature or early menopause still has her uterus and is taking estrogen, I would also have her take 100 milligrams of oral progesterone in the form of micronized natural progesterone (Prometrium) at bedtime nightly and increase it to 200 milligrams if she's using greater than 1.5 milligrams of oral estradiol daily. Progesterone is necessary to protect the uterus from experiencing overgrowth of the lining and possibly from the development of uterine cancer while taking estrogen replacement. Of course, if a woman no longer has her uterus, she doesn't need progesterone because she can't get cancer in an organ that has been removed. But you do need to take progesterone even if you had a uterine ablation or uterine artery embolization to protect the uterus because it's still there. Alternatively, you can use a progesterone-releasing IUD, which can stay in place for seven years; this offers the added benefit of not needing to titrate the dose of progesterone if a woman changes her estrogen dosage.

In women with pre-existing medical conditions like high blood pressure, diabetes, high cholesterol, or migraines, I prescribe transdermal estrogen—either as a patch that delivers the hormone through the skin or a gel containing estrogen that's absorbed by the skin. I like to start these women with a 0.05 milligram transdermal estrogen patch, worn on the belly, twice weekly (meaning, a woman has to change it after three and a half days), or an application of a 0.5 milligram gel (Divigel) nightly to the thighs or behind the knees. Then, I add 100 milligrams oral progesterone (Prometrium); this can be increased to 200 milligrams as her dose of estrogen increases.

Once we get their estrogen (and if needed, progesterone) dosage right, I discuss testosterone replacement with my patients, to prevent loss of energy and libido. This can be handled by applying topical testosterone at levels that are appropriate for a woman to help her achieve systemic levels of testosterone that are between 30 and 60 ng/dL. If a woman still needs birth control, I highly recommend the non-hormonal IUD (Paragard) or the progesterone-releasing IUD (such as Mirena) with the addition of testosterone because women with premature ovarian insufficiency can still ovulate, however infrequently; testosterone is teratogenic to a fetus so it's crucial to use contraception while taking testosterone replacement therapy. The female body typically has plenty of testosterone until menopause, so if a woman goes through premature menopause, it's worth discussing replacing this hormone so she can maintain a sense of youthful vitality.

Plan B: Treating Premature Menopausal Issues without Hormones

As previously mentioned, most women with premature menopause should use HRT unless they have a clear contraindication such as estrogen-positive breast cancer, a history of an unprovoked blood clot, or heart attack or stroke. It's really the gold standard of treatment for premature menopause. Even the Food and Drug Administration[10] supports the use of HRT formulations "that most closely mimic normal ovarian hormone production and continuing HRT until the normal age of natural menopause" in women with premature ovarian insufficiency; the goal is to decrease their risk of developing various health problems such as decreased bone mineral density, cognitive decline, increased risks of cardiovascular disease, type 2 diabetes, and autoimmune disease.

If a woman with premature menopause *can't* use HRT—or is strongly opposed to using it—there are other options besides just having to grin and bear unpleasant menopausal symptoms. My recommendation is for all women in this category to use a vaginal moisturizer (such as FemmePharma's Mia Vita) every day and a lubricant (such as Slippery Stuff or überlube) during intercourse—simply because the vaginal and labial tissues become drier after menopause. Depending on the menopausal symptoms a woman with premature menopause is most bothered by, here are some other possible treatments:

- If she has low libido, sleep troubles, and mood issues, she can take Addyi (a.k.a. flibanserin), an FDA-approved medication that's available by prescription for hypoactive sexual desire disorder (including low libido) in premenopausal women but is often used in postmenopausal women, too. The drug increases dopamine in the brain, which has a mood-enhancing effect, and when it's taken at night, it can produce a sense of relaxation that sets the stage for better sleep.

- If she has moderate to severe depression or anxiety, she might benefit from taking an antidepressant such as Paxil, Celexa, Lexapro, or Pristiq. At low doses, these have the added benefit of blunting hot flashes. If intense anxiety, rather than depression, is the primary mood symptom, Zoloft or Lexapro may be beneficial. With all of these antidepressants, it's helpful to know if a family member has benefitted from one or another because often there are genetic patterns in terms of the efficacy of psychiatric medications; otherwise, finding the right medication is a matter of trial and error.

- If insomnia or sleep disturbances are her primary complaint, a sedating antidepressant called trazodone may help. It is non-addictive and can be taken on an as-needed basis. I strongly urge women to avoid benzodiazepines like Ativan, clonidine, and Xanax because these are addictive; my feeling is they should really be used only in emergency or severe situations.

- If she has osteopenia—bone density that is lower than normal but not low enough to be considered osteoporosis—she can take 35 milligrams of Fosamax (alendronate sodium) once a week. While Fosamax is usually used to treat osteoporosis, when you have osteopenia at age thirty-seven or forty and cannot take estrogen, I believe bone loss should be treated. This is a much lower dose than is used for osteoporosis.

LIFESTYLE INTERVENTIONS

Whether you use HRT or another medication, there are important lifestyle-related interventions that can help you feel better now and reduce your risk of developing long-term health problems after menopause. It should go without saying but I'll say it anyway: Avoid smoking and exposure to secondhand smoke (a.k.a. passive smoking)—it's toxic to just about every organ in the body.

Here are lifestyle modifications I recommend for women with premature or early menopause, given that they have a higher risk of developing heart disease and osteoporosis, in particular, due to the early loss of estrogen:

Dietary Directives

Consume a mostly plant-based diet with about 50 percent of your calories coming from carbohydrates, adequate protein (at least 20 grams at breakfast, lunch, and dinner), and the right number of calories (1,500 to 2,000 calories per day, depending on your activity level) to help you maintain a healthy weight and restore or preserve your energy and vitality. This dietary approach, which is similar to the Mediterranean diet, can also reduce your lifetime risk of developing heart disease, type 2 diabetes, and osteoporosis. Carbohydrates are the macronutrient the body prefers as a source of energy, and eating enough carbohydrates prevents your body from burning up protein for energy; this means protein can serve as the raw material that builds and repairs cells and tissues in the body, which is its intended purpose.

Sticking with a plant-based diet—including fruits, vegetables, whole grains, legumes, nuts, and seeds—will also ensure you get plenty of fiber. Many people think of dietary fiber as being important for digestion, especially regular bowel movements, which is true. But it also helps regulate blood sugar levels, nourishes beneficial bacteria in the gut (which will send signals to the brain that help regulate mood), and helps you stay satiated and energized. The recommendation is to consume 25 to 30 grams of fiber daily.

Replace saturated fats—found in meats, full-fat dairy products, butter, and tropical oils—in your diet with unsaturated fats such as olive and canola oils, avocados, nuts, seeds, and fatty fish like salmon. Consuming excessive amounts of saturated fat contributes to clogged arteries, which can impair blood flow to the brain, heart, and extremities. By contrast, eating healthy, unsaturated fats can protect your heart and brain health, reduce inflammation, and do other good deeds throughout the body.

To keep your energy levels high, make an effort to consume foods that are rich in:

- **B vitamins** (think: fortified breakfast cereals, yogurt, chicken, avocado, sunflower seeds, and salmon), which help your body convert the food you eat into glucose, which in turn gives you energy;
- **magnesium** (almonds, cashews, and peanuts, chia and pumpkin seeds, edamame and black beans, yogurt, quinoa, and fortified breakfast cereals), which promotes blood flow to the muscles and brain;

- **zinc** (crab, oatmeal, chickpeas, cashews, yogurt, and pumpkin seeds), which is necessary for energy and metabolism; and
- **iron** (found in fortified breakfast cereals and other grains, lean meat, poultry, seafood, tofu, legumes, and dark green, leafy vegetables), which is also involved in energy production. Once you're postmenopausal and no longer losing blood through a monthly period, your body's need for iron declines and it's easy to get enough from food. To improve the absorption of the non-heme iron found in plant foods, consume iron-rich foods with things that are rich in vitamin C. Good pairings include spinach salad with red pepper slices, black beans with tomatoes, and fortified cereal with sliced strawberries.

To keep up your energy, plan on having three meals and one to two snacks during the day. Going too long between eating can give you a sag attack or make you feel down or irritable, which can trigger spur-of-the-moment snacking on sweets, chips, or other foods that are handy but don't offer much in the way of nutrition. Plan your snacks ahead of time—ideally, a combination of protein and carbohydrates—in a 200-calorie portion. While there's nothing wrong with consuming moderate amounts of caffeine, it's a mistake to rely on caffeine to pep you up; excessive amounts can send your mood on a roller-coaster ride and interfere with your sleep. Also, limit your alcohol intake (to one drink per day) to reduce the frequency and severity of hot flashes, and drink plenty of water throughout the day to maintain your energy; even a mild case of dehydration can cause fatigue.

Here's what a day's meal plan might look like:

Breakfast: 1 cup plain Greek or Icelandic yogurt with ½ cup berries; 1 to 2 slices whole-wheat toast topped with 1 to 2 tablespoons peanut butter or almond butter

Lunch: Salad made with 2 cups leafy greens, cherry tomatoes, sliced carrots, slices of red or green pepper, cucumber, 4 ounces canned drained tuna or salmon, ¼ avocado, 1 tablespoon olive oil and Balsamic vinegar; 2-ounce whole-wheat roll

Dinner: 4 ounces grilled chicken or fish; 1 cup cooked brown rice, whole-wheat couscous, or quinoa with 1 to 2 teaspoons olive oil; 1½ cups steamed or roasted broccoli, asparagus, or cauliflower

Snacks: 2 tablespoons hummus with a handful of sugar snap peas or carrots; ¼ cup homemade trail mix with dried cherries, dried apricots, almonds or walnuts

As far as dietary supplements go, I suggest taking vitamin D (800 to 1,000 IU) daily because it's difficult to get enough from food alone. If your calcium intake from food is falling short of 1,200 milligrams per day, consider taking a calcium supplement, no more than 500 milligrams at a time. If you're a vegan or vegetarian, it can be hard to get enough vitamin B12, which helps transform the food you eat into energy that every cell in your body can utilize; in that case, a B12 supplement may be in order. Also, if you suffer from insomnia, taking 250 to 500 milligrams of magnesium oxide or 5 milligrams of melatonin an hour before bedtime may help.

Exercise Rx

When it comes to physical activity, I believe in doing things you enjoy, whether that's walking or jogging, playing tennis or golf, cycling, swimming, dancing, or something else. Having said that, it's super important for women with premature menopause to check the following boxes on a regular basis: doing weight-bearing exercise (to protect bone mass), aerobic exercise (for heart and lung health), and strength training (to build and preserve muscle mass and bone density and boost your metabolism).

Besides protecting your long-term health, exercising regularly can help mitigate many menopausal challenges. For example, performing aerobic or strength-training exercise can boost your mood, help with body temperature regulation, set the stage for better sleep, and assist with weight management. Regular yoga or Pilates sessions can increase your attention and focus and calm your nervous system, while also improving your physical strength, coordination, and flexibility.

Fortunately, several forms of exercise check more than one movement-related box—for example, walking and jogging are both weight-bearing and aerobic. Also, high-intensity interval training (HIIT) can give you a major bang for your effort: By alternating short bouts of intense exercise with less-intense periods, you can rev your metabolic rate and burn more calories, promote muscle mass and fat loss, and lower your blood pressure, blood sugar, and resting heart rate, among other perks. And it only takes twenty to thirty minutes! You'll find a sample body-weight HIIT workout in the appendix, as well as guidance for how to turn any aerobic activity into a HIIT session. HIIT workouts can be done in group settings or solo at gyms or at home (you can find plenty of HIIT workouts online).

My recommendation is for women with premature menopause to do twenty to thirty minutes of aerobic exercise four or more times per week, plus resistance training (whether it's using your body weight, dumbbells, resistance bands, or something else) two or three times per week. Don't forget to incorporate stretching sessions into your exercise life to keep your muscles flexible.

Testing, Testing

After menopause, every woman should be screened for certain medical conditions—such as osteoporosis, diabetes, high blood pressure, and cholesterol abnormalities—that become more common after the end of their reproductive years. In addition, it's a good idea for women with premature menopause to get screened for common autoimmune conditions: Specifically, I recommend getting screened for antibodies for thyroid conditions, celiac disease, and pernicious anemia, which can be done with a simple blood test.

Here's the reasoning: As previously mentioned, premature ovarian insufficiency is often thought to be autoimmune in nature and where there's one autoimmune disease, there often lurks another. The sooner we identify the presence of an autoimmune disease, the better we can treat it and the better a woman will feel.

Improving Your Headspace

When you're diagnosed with early or premature menopause, it can feel like biology played a cruel trick on you. And if you were still planning your family or intending to add to it, discovering that your reproductive system has permanently shut down may be seriously disappointing. It can feel like a major loss. In some instances, women with premature ovarian failure may be able to conceive a pregnancy with assisted reproductive technology (ART) or egg donation; if that's a goal, it's important to get a prompt referral to a reproductive endocrinologist and infertility specialist so you can assess the viability of your remaining eggs and your options.

When women are struggling with the emotional aftershocks of premature menopause, I often recommend therapy with a licensed social worker or psychologist so they can talk about what they may have lost or how unfair it feels to reach menopause so young. There are also great support groups such as EarlyMenopause.com and the Daisy Network (daisynetwork.org), which is based in the UK but is primarily online. Even using social media and searching under hashtags such as #earlymenopause or #prematuremenopause can help you find support groups that may be close enough that you could attend in person.

Make sure you connect with support groups that are comprised of women who have experienced *early* menopause; attending a group with women who are dealing with menopause in their fifties could make you feel more isolated in your experience. This is a case where it's wise to stick with your type, as in: women who've had premature or early menopause. There are also podcast episodes about early and premature menopause, some of which have great insider tips for how to deal with it; plus, hearing other women talk about their own experiences can make you feel like you're not alone and give you a sense of hope and connection to others who are in the same boat.

Social Dilemmas

Sometimes women with premature menopause feel out of step with their peers socially and emotionally. After all, if friends are talking about how to get their bodies baby-ready or what to buy for a layette, it can be hard to relate if you're dealing with intense hot flashes or wild mood swings from menopause. One thing that can help is to try to meet people or join groups where you have a common interest, whether it's a book or photography club, a hiking or tennis group, or a volunteer organization; similarly, you could take a drawing or painting class or learn a new language. By spending time with people who have similar interests, regardless of their reproductive status, you'll find a sense of community, support, and connection that can be highly gratifying.

When you're ready, it also can be helpful to talk to close friends and older family members about what you're going through—in some instances, you might be surprised that they are more supportive and interested than you may think. Menopause has remained a conversational taboo for far too long—it's time for all women to open up the dialogue! But don't just rely on other people. It's important to come to your own emotional rescue as well.

To that end, make it a priority to get plenty of good-quality sleep every night; doing so can enhance the way you feel and function—and regulate your moods. The same is true of exercising regularly—and if you do it with a workout buddy or an exercise class, these connections can help you avoid feeling isolated.

To help yourself feel energized and upbeat regularly, I also recommend using the following strategies:

- **Put color on your side.** If being around certain colors seems to pep you up or calm you down, it's not your imagination: Research has found that different hues really can affect your mood. So if you want to pump up your energy or get excited, put on a red or yellow shirt or scarf, or don a pair of sunglasses with yellow-tinted lenses. If you want to cultivate calm, look at something blue or green, perhaps by taking a walk outside and gazing at the sky or trees.

- **Write your heart out.** Whether you put pen to paper or type on a computer, writing about upsetting experiences or emotionally charged issues in your life can be good for your health and emotional well-being. This is called expressive writing, and research[11] has found that it improves symptoms from a variety of stressful health conditions and reduces anxiety and negative thinking by essentially "offloading" worries from your mind. All it takes is fifteen minutes a day—and there's no need to be concerned about spelling, punctuation, grammar, or other writing conventions. (This is for your eyes only!)

- **Expose yourself to sunlight.** Taking a walk in the sunshine first thing in the morning or having breakfast while sitting next to a sunny window can help jumpstart your energy and alertness for the day. Sunlight is basically your brain's wake-up call. Similarly, getting a dose of sunlight during the day can help reinvigorate you. If that's not possible, consider buying a commercial light box that emits 10,000 lux— the brightness that simulates what you'd see on a naturally sunny day. Using these has even been found to ease depression and seasonal affective disorder.

- **Count your blessings.** When you focus on what you're grateful for in your life, it's like turning on a positivity switch in your brain: Instead of letting the stresses and strains in your life take center stage, the good things in life take over, which boosts your mood and your mind-set. Make a point of spending a few minutes every evening jotting down three to five specific things you appreciated that day—it could be a compliment a colleague gave you, feeling strong during your workout, catching up with an old friend by phone, or noticing new flowers blooming in your yard. Do this on a daily basis and soon you'll naturally stay more attuned to what's good in your life.

- **Consider using a standing desk.** Besides being beneficial for your posture—helping you avoid "tech neck" and low back pain—research has found that alternating between sitting and standing at a desk can help with blood sugar regulation, as well as increasing muscle activity and fat oxidation and calorie burning. Some people also find that using a standing desk for at least part of the day boosts their stamina and focus.

- **Modify your breathing.** You probably know that engaging in certain breathing patterns can calm you down—well, the opposite is true as well. To boost your energy and alertness, try this yoga-inspired breathing pattern: Inhale for a count of two, then exhale for a count of two; inhale for a count of two, then exhale for a count of three; inhale for a count of two, then exhale for a count of four; inhale for a count of two, then exhale for a count of five. Repeat the pattern a few times then return to your normal breathing pattern. The oxygen flow in your blood will have improved and you'll likely feel invigorated and more focused.

- **Put together motivating playlists.** As any athlete can tell you, music has the power to pump you up for competition. Even if you're not into sports, research[12] has found that your favorite tunes can increase energy levels, improve your mood, harness your focus, and delay physical and mental fatigue. So put together a few playlists with your favorite songs, new or old, for different purposes—to boost your alertness and focus, to rev up your energy and motivation, and to help you calm down after an intense activity.

- **Spend time in nature.** Whether you take a walk in the woods or a park, use your senses to soak up the sights, sounds, smells, tastes, and tactile sensations. Research[13] has found that be-

yond the soothing sights in nature, a variety of influences—
such as the inhalation of phytoncides (compounds emitted
by plants), negative air ions, and microbes—can have a beneficial effect on your health and well-being. In fact, spending
just twenty minutes a day outside has been found to significantly boost people's vitality levels and energy, according to
a series of studies[14] from the University of Rochester.

Women with premature menopause can personalize treatment
of their symptoms by consulting the DIY menu of remedies in
chapter 12. There, you'll find just about every menopausal symptom known to womankind along with evidence-based approaches
that can help relieve them. By customizing your treatment plan
based on your most bothersome or persistent symptoms, you can
restore your physical and emotional equilibrium and get back to
feeling like yourself again. The goal here is to help you feel as
vibrant and youthful as your actual age, rather than your menopausal status.

6

The Sudden Menopause Type

Jennifer, a trial attorney, says that while she "always knew meno-pause was on the menu," its abrupt arrival came as a shock. She was forty-five and had had a baby just four years earlier, when suddenly she was beset with tsunamis of hot flashes, heart pal-pitations, and sleep disturbances due to drenching night sweats. During the day, she felt exhausted and irritable and struggled to get things done. "It seemed like anger, frustration, and shame were ruling my life," she said in retrospect. While in court, she would break into a "shockingly profuse sweat that was impossible to hide or control." Every evening, she'd arrive home feeling wiped out and she'd struggle to avoid being cranky and short-tempered with her family. On the weekends, during playdates with her young daughter's friends and their moms, she felt old amidst her peers, some of whom were pregnant again. In short, she said, "I felt trapped in a body that was betraying me."

By the time she came to see me, Jennifer had tried various over-the-counter supplements and Chinese herbs but nothing had eased her symptoms. She didn't want to take hormone therapy because she was worried about cancer risk given that a couple of women in her family had had breast cancer. While certain forms of hormone therapy could have been safe options for her, I wanted to honor her wishes so we avoided it entirely. After a thorough medical history, a physical examination, and blood tests, we discovered that her sud-den menopause was related to diminished ovarian reserve (DOR), in which the ovaries lose their reproductive capacity ahead of schedule. As it happens, DOR ran in her family.

There are other reasons why a woman may experience the Sudden Menopause Type. These include having chemotherapy or radiation treatments for cancer, which can cause ovarian failure/dysfunction, or surgical loss of both ovaries during procedures related to ectopic pregnancy, endometriosis, ovarian cyst removal, or ovarian cancer. Sometimes the onset of sudden menopause happens when women decide to have both of their ovaries removed in order to reduce their risk of breast and ovarian cancer if they have BRCA1 or BRCA2 gene mutations, or other high-risk gene mutations, or Lynch syndrome. (In these instances, the result is often referred to as "risk-reducing surgical menopause.")

But as it did with Jennifer, sometimes menopause comes on suddenly for reasons other than surgery or medical treatments. I once treated a patient who went into menopause at age forty-seven after a serious car accident. *Really!* The physical and emotional stress of the accident threw her into hormonal havoc that caused her ovaries to shut down.

In each of these instances, the onset of menopause is abrupt and a woman doesn't go through perimenopause, the usual, gradual transition when hormone levels wax and wane, leading up to her final period. Instead, menopause is suddenly foisted upon her and the abrupt loss of hormones often causes more intense symptoms than those that occur with a gradual downshifting to natural menopause. Sometimes sudden menopause has a particularly intense psychological component, too, because women who experience it may have recently learned that they have cancer or a high risk of cancer, or have undergone harsh treatment for cancer—all of these scenarios can be incredibly stressful, physically and emotionally. In these instances, these women may find themselves second-guessing their decisions about treatment or preventive actions or engaging in "What if?" thinking, as they imagine unfortunate outcomes, all of which can ratchet up angst and worry.

More often than not, experiencing sudden menopause can feel like a shock to the system. Because of their abrupt and intense onset, the symptoms can be jarring physically and psychologically, which can lead women to feel at odds with their bodies. When a woman experiences sudden menopause, she may get a surprising, and often rapid, flood of symptoms such as hot flashes, night sweats, mood swings, mental fogginess, vaginal dryness, and decreased sex drive. (In fact, loss of libido is often more pronounced after surgical menopause than it is with natural menopause.)[1] Any or all of these symptoms can affect her quality of life, including her sexual desire and functionality due to vaginal atrophy. Let's be honest: Vaginal atrophy is a horrible term because it sounds like a disease, but it really refers to the fact that the vaginal tissues become thinner and drier due to the loss of estrogen that comes with menopause. Not only can this make intercourse painful, but it can also lead to bothersome symptoms in the urinary tract. And if a woman with sudden menopause has undergone chemotherapy or radiation or taken other medications (such as aromatase inhibitors or selective estrogen receptor modulators/SERMS, like tamoxifen) to treat her cancer, those treatments may have further altered the pH level of the vagina, which can exacerbate these symptoms. It's a distressing double whammy!

A Mouthful of a Name for a Common Condition

With a phenomenon called the "genitourinary syndrome of menopause" (GSM for short),[2] a variety of changes and symptoms can occur to the vaginal and vulvar tissue, as well as to the urinary tract. The pH level of the vaginal tissue increases, and the tissue itself becomes thin, dry, and less elastic due to decreased secretions, which can lead to tearing and bleeding during sex. Besides leading to thinning and dryness in the vagina, these changes also affect the labia and clitoris, which can make sex less pleasurable. (I've had some patients report feeling "completely numb" down there or like their labia has shrunk after they experienced sudden menopause.) What's more, tissue in the urethra and the base of the bladder also becomes thinner, making women more susceptible to urinary tract infections (UTIs) or what feels like a UTI—because the acidic urine irritates the dry urethra—even when they don't test positive for one.

Ready for some more unfortunate news? Unlike menopausal symptoms (like hot flashes) that generally improve over time, genitourinary symptoms often worsen because of the continuous lack of estrogen and other changes related to aging. The good news: There are a variety of treatment options, from non-hormonal remedies (such as vaginal lubricants and moisturizers) to vaginal estrogen treatments to other prescription therapies (such as a drug called ospemifene/Osphena or a vaginal insert of low-dose dehydroepiandrosterone, or DHEA, such as prasterone). There is help; it's a matter of knowing where to look for it. Fortunately, I do.

As is true for any woman who reaches the north side of menopause, the risks of heart disease, osteoporosis, and cognitive decline begin to increase due to the loss of estrogen. In fact, changes

in cognitive function are an often overlooked long-term consequence of menopause, especially with surgical menopause that occurs before the age of natural menopause. Research has found that
women who undergo surgical menopause often underperform on
memory tasks and have reductions in their cognitive function, especially if the surgical menopause occurs at younger ages.[3] (Remember: Depending upon the age when the surgery occurs, there
can be an overlap between early menopause, surgical, and sudden
menopause.) When estrogen replacement is given, these risks are
mitigated—but hormone therapy may not be an option for all
women with the Sudden Menopause Type. This is an issue these
women should explore with their physicians, because it involves
weighing potential health risks (such as a slightly increased risk of
cancer) with quality-of-life issues.

MAKING TREATMENT DECISIONS

For sudden or surgical menopause when the uterus and ovaries
are removed for reasons that are not related to cancer (such as abnormal uterine bleeding, endometriosis that spread to the ovaries,
adenomyosis, or recurrent ovarian cysts), estrogen replacement
therapy on its own has the greatest benefits and the fewest risks.
Taking a low dose of estrogen can address symptoms related to
sudden menopause—such as hot flashes, night sweats/cold flashes,
vaginal dryness or pain with sex, urinary urgency, an increase in
urinary tract infections, difficulty sleeping, mood changes, libido
changes, and brain fog—and reduce a woman's risk of developing
heart disease, osteoporosis, dementia, pelvic floor disorders, and
other conditions that stem from the loss of estrogen. (Interest-
ingly, the Women's Health Initiative found that women who had a
hysterectomy and took estrogen without progesterone had a statis-

tically decreased risk of developing breast cancer.) If a woman still has her uterus, she needs progesterone to protect it from uterine hyperplasia, a buildup of the uterine lining, which increases the risk of precancerous or cancerous cells developing. Simply put, the risk of uterine cancer or precancer can increase from the effects of unopposed estrogen (meaning, estrogen without progesterone) in women who have an intact uterus.

If a woman has experienced sudden menopause because of a gynecologic cancer or breast cancer, figuring out whether hormone therapy is an option needs to be addressed on an individual basis. It's not necessarily an across-the-board "no." For example, in women who've had surgically treated, early-stage endometrial cancer and experienced surgical menopause, the North American Menopause Society[4] holds the position that use of hormone therapy may be considered; by contrast, non-hormonal therapies are advised for women with more advanced or higher-risk endometrial cancer. And the use of systemic hormone therapy in women who've had breast cancer is generally not advised. At this point, not enough is known about the long-term risks in women who've been treated for ovarian cancer.

The point is: On this issue, too, there isn't a one-size-fits-all answer. It really needs to be handled with a careful and calculated discussion of the potential risks versus benefits for each woman's immediate and long-term health and well-being.

By the time Melanie came to see me at age forty-three, she had had a double mastectomy four years earlier because she was found to have a BRCA2 gene mutation, which increased her risk for breast and ovarian cancer. The mother of two kids, ages six and seven, and a social worker, she was planning to have her ovaries removed to further reduce her risk. But she was worried that by removing her ovaries to reduce her risk for cancer, she would be "trading one risk for another" because her risks of developing heart disease and bone loss would go up. So we had a long discussion about the pros and cons of surgically inducing menopause before the age of forty-five.

Ultimately, because Melanie hadn't had cancer and she was concerned about the elevated risk of heart disease from having early menopause, she decided to use an estrogen patch (to protect her heart health and bone health) and have a progesterone-releasing IUD (to protect her uterus) placed during her surgery to remove her ovaries.

When she came to see me after her surgery, she said that she hadn't missed a beat because she started her patch two days after the surgery. That's right—she completely sidestepped menopausal symptoms, thanks to smart planning. She actually mentioned that she felt "even better than before" because the decision-making and surgery were now over. Menopause had happened and she was okay. She was actually feeling quite strong and proud of herself because by initiating a treatment plan before symptoms appeared, she didn't need to suffer.

BASELINE TREATMENT PLANS FOR THE SUDDEN MENOPAUSE TYPE

What follows are two baseline treatment plans for women who have the Sudden Menopause Type. The first treatment plan focuses on the use of hormone therapy (HT); the second plan addresses how to treat surgical or sudden menopause without hormones. Whichever treatment plan you choose, you'll also find recommendations for lifestyle modifications that are suitable for all women with the Sudden Menopause Type. Keep in mind that if you have additional symptoms that aren't relieved by these recommended approaches, you can choose from the extensive menu of symptom-oriented solutions in chapter 12 to ease what's still bothering you.

Plan A: Using Hormone Therapy

For women with sudden menopause who want to use hormone therapy and don't have any contraindications to HT, I recommend the use of transdermal estrogen—namely, applying Divigel (estradiol gel) to the upper thigh every morning after taking a shower or wearing a transdermal patch, to treat hot flashes and night sweats. The estrogen is also likely to help with vaginal dryness, brain fog, and joint aches and pains. The goal is for the woman to have blood levels of estrogen between 40 and 70 pg/mL, though they could be higher if she's on the younger side (as in under age forty-five).

There are two primary reasons I prefer transdermal estrogen for women with sudden menopause: Many of these women are recovering from surgery, and transdermal estrogen has been shown to have a lower risk of blood clots compared to oral estrogen formulations. Second, for women who have high-risk genetic mutations for breast cancer, there's some data that transdermal estrogen confers a slightly lower risk for breast changes.

If a woman with sudden menopause still has her uterus and is taking estrogen, she needs to take 100 milligrams of oral progesterone in the form of micronized natural progesterone (Prometrium) at bedtime nightly; this should be increased to 200 milligrams if she's using greater than 0.5 milligrams of Divigel daily or a 0.05 milligram estradiol patch. Progesterone is needed to protect the uterus from experiencing overgrowth of the lining and possibly the development of uterine cancer while taking estrogen therapy. Of course, if a woman no longer has her uterus, she doesn't need progesterone because she can't get cancer in an organ that has been removed. Alternatively, using a progesterone-releasing IUD, which can stay in place for seven years, offers the added benefit of not needing to titrate the dose of progesterone if a woman changes her estrogen dosage. An extra bonus: If a woman is considering having an IUD inserted, she can often do it at the time of whatever surgery she's having.

In addition, I recommend using vaginal prasterone, a form of DHEA, as a nightly suppository. (I find that women are more compliant with a nightly regimen than a twice-per-week one.) Because vaginal dryness and discomfort can be such a challenge in women with sudden or surgical menopause, we really want to protect the vaginal tissue. Once inside the cells, the prasterone is converted into estrogens and androgens, which are beneficial for the genital tissue in someone who was essentially shocked into menopause. These hormones don't travel systemically throughout the body.

Plan B: Treating Sudden Menopausal Issues without Hormones

For some women with the Sudden Menopause Type, there are clear contraindications to using systemic hormone therapy (if they've had an estrogen-positive breast cancer, for example), while for others, it's a gray area. And others may simply not want to use hormone therapy for reasons that are personal. Fortunately, for all of these women, there are other medications we can use to address unpleasant menopausal symptoms—in other words, there's no reason to suffer silently or needlessly! My recommendation is for all women in this category to use non-hormonal hyaluronic acid suppositories (such as SweetSpot Labs Rescue Balm, Mia Vita from FemmePharma, or a product from Rosebud Woman) every night to help with vaginal dryness and irritation. My patients have found that doing this has a very positive effect, and studies[5] have, too. By contrast, lubricants (such as Slippery Stuff or überlube) are meant to reduce friction during intercourse, so they are not for everyday use like vaginal moisturizers are—but they can make a difference, too.

Depending on the symptoms a woman with sudden menopause is most bothered by, here are some other possible treatments:

- To treat mood changes and hot flashes, Lexapro is a selective serotonin reuptake inhibitor (SSRI) antidepressant that can blunt hot flashes. When it's taken at night, it can help with mood (both depression and anxiety) and sometimes trouble with sleeping. Other options include the antidepressants Celexa and Paxil.
- Some women who have the Sudden Menopause Type may be taking tamoxifen (a hormonal therapy that's used to treat breast cancer), which interacts with many SSRIs. Lexapro, Effexor, and Pristiq are less problematic than many others when used in conjunction with tamoxifen.
- Another possibility if the woman is not taking tamoxifen is the SSRI Brisdelle (7.5 milligrams), which is the only non-hormonal medication that's approved by the FDA to treat hot flashes. It can be used with aromatase inhibitors, a class of drugs used to treat breast cancer in postmenopausal women.
- If a woman doesn't want to take an SSRI—perhaps because she tried them before and they didn't help or she had a bad reaction to them—she can consider alternatives for hot flash relief such as: taking 100 to 300 milligrams at night of gabapentin, an anti-seizure drug that's often used for nerve pain, or 5 milligrams of oxybutynin, which is typically used for overactive bladder, once or twice a day. While these medications may seem off-target for menopausal symptoms, I have seen great success with these drugs for reducing the frequency and/or intensity of women's hot flashes.
- If she has low libido, sleep troubles, and mood issues, a woman can take Addyi (a.k.a. flibanserin), an FDA-approved medication that's available by prescription for hypoactive

sexual desire disorder (including low libido) in premenopausal women, but is often used in postmenopausal women,
too. The drug increases dopamine in the brain, which has a
mood-enhancing effect, and when it's taken at night, it can
produce a sense of relaxation that sets the stage for better
sleep.

Another Promising Treatment on the Horizon

A novel, non-hormonal medication called fezolinetant
that's being investigated as a treatment for moderate
to severe hot flashes is showing great promise.[6] Some
data suggests that it can start to improve symptoms
after one to two weeks. Fezolinetant works in the
hypothalamus in the brain to reduce core body
temperature and the frequency and severity of
vasomotor symptoms, including hot flashes, that are
associated with menopause; as an extra perk, the drug
also appears to help with sleep disturbances.

A twelve-week study showed that the drug has
efficacy that's similar to hormone therapy. Given that
many women who experience sudden menopause
can't use hormone therapy, I see this as an especially
valuable development for them. I suspect it will be
FDA-approved and available on the market sometime
in 2023.

Because Jennifer, the trial attorney, didn't want to take hormone therapy due to her fears about cancer, I had her start taking
Brisdelle to treat her debilitating hot flashes and sleep disturbances.

I also advised her to join a support group for women going through menopause. She learned paced breathing techniques to quell her hot flashes and started doing twenty-minute high-intensity interval workouts to boost her energy. With the help of these strategies, a B vitamin complex, vitamin D supplements, and some extra support from her husband, Jennifer began feeling more like her usual self within a couple of months.

LIFESTYLE INTERVENTIONS

Whether you use HT or another medication, there are also important lifestyle-related interventions that can help you feel better now and reduce your risk of developing long-term health problems after menopause. It's a given that you should avoid smoking and exposure to secondhand smoke (a.k.a. passive smoking)—because it's toxic to just about every organ in the body; if you smoke, you need to quit. It's that simple.

What follows are lifestyle modifications I recommend for women with sudden menopause. These are designed to help women with the Sudden Menopause Type regain their physical and emotional equilibrium.

Dietary Directives

As a starting point, stick with a primarily plant-based meal plan that includes at least 20 grams of protein at every meal and the right number of calories (1,500 to 2,000 calories per day, depending on your activity level). Fill half your plate with fruits and vegetables, one-quarter with lean protein-rich foods, and one-quarter with whole grains at every meal. In addition to ensuring that your diet checks all the boxes for your body's basic health needs, it's a good idea to choose foods that will calm the shock to your system from sudden menopause and ease inflammation from surgeries or other medical treatments you may have had.

Consume a rainbow of colorful fruits and vegetables (think: berries, leafy green vegetables, carrots, peppers, broccoli, cauliflower, grapes, and the like) and you'll naturally treat your body to antioxidant-rich foods that have anti-inflammatory properties and other health-promoting perks that help restore balance in the body. Seasoning your food with herbs and spices that have anti-inflammatory properties—such as turmeric, cinnamon, cloves, oregano, rosemary, and ginger—does double duty by giving your taste buds a treat and helping you reduce your sodium intake.

Eating a variety of protein-rich foods from plant and animal sources in the right amounts throughout the day will supply your body with the essential amino acids it needs to repair damaged tissues and build new ones. This is easy to do if you include three to four ounces of cooked boneless poultry or seafood, one cup tofu, one cup Greek or Icelandic yogurt, or three-quarters of a cup low-fat cottage cheese in each meal. Consume fish or seafood at least twice a week, or take omega-3 supplements and consume foods with added omega-3 fatty acids—such as fortified eggs, milk, soy milk, and yogurt—because omega-3 fatty acids tame inflammation and help reduce your risk of developing heart disease, stroke, vascular dementia, or cognitive decline as you get older.[7] Cold-water fish—such as salmon, sardines, lake trout, mackerel, black cod, and tuna—are especially rich in omega-3 fatty acids; walnuts, chia seeds, flaxseed, soybean oil, and canola oil also contain omega-3s.[8]

Replace saturated fats—found in meats, full-fat dairy products, butter, and tropical oils—in your diet with unsaturated fats such as olive and canola oils, avocados, nuts, seeds, and fatty fish like salmon. Consuming excessive amounts of saturated fat contributes to clogged arteries, which can impair blood flow to the brain, heart, and extremities, whereas healthy, unsaturated fats can protect your heart and brain health and reduce inflammation throughout your body.

Estrogen and other sex hormones play a role in insulin resistance, and the abrupt drop in estrogen that occurs with sudden menopause may further compromise the body's ability to deal with large amounts of carbohydrates. So it's important to focus on consuming foods that are rich in fiber, such as whole grains (like oatmeal, quinoa, and brown rice), vegetables, legumes, and nuts and seeds, and to avoid or limit foods with added sugars, including honey and maple syrup, and baked goods to help with blood sugar regulation.

To help tame the sudden storm that hit your body, make an effort to consume foods that are rich in these mighty minerals:

- **Magnesium** (in almonds, peanuts, chia and pumpkin seeds, quinoa, black beans, yogurt, avocados, and fortified breakfast cereals), which helps regulate blood pressure, restore proper fluid balance, and promote a sensation of calm;
- **Calcium** (in milk, yogurt, cheese, fortified soy milk, and fortified orange juice), which helps regulate blood pressure and balance fluids in the body, in addition to protecting bones;
- **Potassium** (in potatoes, legumes, butternut squash, yogurt, milk, seafood, bananas, and orange juice), which supports blood pressure regulation, fluid balance in the body, muscle contractions, and nerve signals.

To help you reconnect with your body and feel like yourself again, practice mindful eating. Sometimes described as "the art of presence while you eat,"[9] mindful eating involves bringing your full attention into your eating experiences, not only in terms of the foods you choose to eat but also in the very act of eating them. It's a matter of tuning in to the sensory experience of eating, the tastes, textures, and aromas of your food, on a moment-to-moment basis. It's a matter of eating slowly, savoring the flavors, and staying attuned to your body's signals of hunger and satiety while you're eating. The idea is to do this without judging what you're eating or trying to restrict how much you eat—but by practicing mindful eating, people often end up eating enough but not too much. The keys are to eat at a table when you're not distracted (no multitasking!), to chew your food slowly and thoroughly, and to truly focus on how it tastes.

Here's what a day's meal plan might look like:

Breakfast: Cinnamon Apple Oatmeal: microwave ½ cup dry oats with 1 cup of 1 percent (low-fat) milk. Stir in chopped apple pieces and ¼ to ½ teaspoon ground cinnamon; 1 egg, hard-cooked or scrambled in 1 teaspoon olive oil

Lunch: Veggie Wrap: ¼ cup hummus spread on a medium whole-wheat tortilla, with sliced cucumber, sliced green bell pepper, sprouts, and 1 ounce Havarti cheese

Dinner: Shrimp Stir-Fry: 4 ounces cooked shrimp, 1½ cups mixed vegetables such as broccoli florets, sliced carrots, and red bell pepper seasoned with low-sodium soy sauce. Serve with 1 cup cooked brown rice.

Snacks: 1 cup canned, drained pineapple chunks (or fresh) mixed with 1 cup plain fat-free Greek or Icelandic yogurt; ½ cup no-salt-added cottage cheese and 6 whole-wheat crackers

As far as dietary supplements go, I suggest taking vitamin D (800 to 1,000 IU) daily because it's difficult to get enough vitamin D from food alone. If your calcium intake from food is falling short of 1,200 milligrams per day, consider taking a calcium supplement, no more than 500 milligrams at a time. If you're a vegan or vegetarian, it can be hard to get enough vitamin B12, which helps transform the food you eat into energy that every cell in your body can utilize; in that case, a B12 supplement may be in order. Also, taking a probiotic supplement[10]—the most common ones include various strains of Lactobacillus and Bifidobacterium—may help enhance your immune function so that you can stay healthy after having an intense medical treatment.

If you're taking medication to treat cancer or prevent a recurrence, be sure to check with your oncologist before taking supplements. Some herbal supplements and vitamin supplements can interact or interfere with prescription drugs or treatments. And the last thing you want to do is compromise the effectiveness of a medical treatment by taking a supplement.

Exercise Rx

As far as physical activity goes, my recommendations depend largely on your current health status, including whether you recently had surgery, chemotherapy, or are taking other powerful medications. If you've had surgery, it's important to build up your strength, stamina, and conditioning slowly—over the course of months, not weeks. My suggestion is to start with walking and functional fitness exercises, using your own body weight—moves such as lunges, squats, wall push-ups, wall sits, push-ups (starting on your knees), planks, and the like. These moves will strengthen your body in ways that will make it easier and more comfortable to perform everyday activities like showering, blow-drying your hair, cleaning, cooking, and more.

Doing mind-body exercises like yoga, Pilates, or tai chi is also beneficial: While you're strengthening your muscles and improving your flexibility, balance, and coordination with these exercise modalities, you'll also be engaging your mind. With each of these, there's a focus on concentration, precision, breathing, rhythm, and flow—all of which will help you feel centered in your body and calm the nervous system.

As your strength and stamina increase, you may want to combine exercises that will boost your aerobic capacity and strengthen your muscles: Choose activities that are low impact such as cycling, swimming, water aerobics, or using the rowing machine, stationary bicycle, or elliptical machine. These will help you avoid jolting or jarring your body while you exercise. If you add strength training to the equation—by lifting weights, using weight machines, or exercise bands—you'll build and preserve muscle mass and bone density and boost your metabolism, which will help with weight control.

By the time Candace, thirty-six, a stay-at-home mother with two young sons, came to see me, she had been diagnosed with a BRCA1 gene mutation and treated for early-stage breast cancer, which was estrogen-receptor positive. As a result of her mastectomy, the chemotherapy, and use of the drug Lupron to shut down her ovaries, her periods had stopped. Even so, it was recommended that she have her ovaries removed to reduce her risk of ovarian cancer. Still reeling from everything that had happened to her body in the previous three years, Candace wanted to know how she would feel after undergoing surgical menopause. In particular, she was worried about her sexual health.

Given her diagnosis, she wasn't interested in hormone therapy but she wanted to be proactive about her health and well-being. Before she had her ovaries removed, we discussed the importance of vaginal health and I told her that a vaginal estrogen could be safe for her, despite her medical history. Ultimately, she decided to use vaginal DHEA (prasterone) instead, starting a few weeks after the surgery.

When she came to see me ten weeks after the surgery, she was feeling sluggish, slow, depressed, weak, and tired. We focused on changing her diet to include more protein and fats to keep her blood sugar on an even keel and help boost her energy. She also started doing at-home workouts in her basement using the Tonal system (an adaptive strength-training system that includes on-screen workouts). She hired a babysitter on Sundays so that she would have uninterrupted time to cook and prepare meals, which helped her feel ready for the week ahead. At our last meeting, we discussed adding Wellbutrin to her regimen because this antidepressant could help increase her libido, which was on the downslide. These measures helped her feel better and more in control of the changes she was going through.

Improving Your Headspace

As you've seen, experiencing sudden menopause can be a serious jolt to your body and mind. Between the abruptness of the onset of symptoms, their intensity, and the sudden loss of your reproductive years, you may be reeling emotionally as well as physically. That's why it's important to tame the turmoil by eating well, exercising regularly, staying well hydrated, and making it a priority to get plenty of good-quality sleep on a nightly basis. To help yourself feel calmer and more balanced from the inside out, I also recommend using the following strategies:

- **Join a support group.** If you're experiencing sudden menopause because you were treated for a female cancer or you had a hysterectomy because you're at high risk for breast or ovarian cancer due to your family history or genetic factors, I strongly suggest finding a support group that caters to women in your situation. Many women who are experiencing sudden menopause find it helpful to connect with other women in the same boat; in a support group, you can talk honestly about what's happening to you and how you're feeling, which can bring a sense of relief and help you know that you are not alone. Some good organizations to start with: FORCE (FacingOurRisk.org); the National Ovarian Cancer Coalition (Ovarian.org); Susan G. Komen (Komen.org); and Young Survival Coalition (YoungSurvival.org).

- **Practice self-compassion.** Acknowledge that you're going through a difficult experience, and that you're not feeling or functioning at your best. Be kind and understanding toward yourself, providing the same support that you would give to a close friend. Validate your feelings, and comfort and reassure yourself by reminding yourself that this difficult period will pass. By showing yourself the same consideration and care that you would give to a friend, you'll feel better—and you'll be your own ally.

- **Stay focused on what you *can* control.** Yes, the shock to your body from sudden menopause may feel unsettling and out of your control, but there are plenty of things in your life that are within your control. Concentrate your attention and efforts on where you can wield influence—your diet and exercise habits, your organizational skills, how you manage your time and spending habits, and the like—and you'll feel empowered (not to mention less overwhelmed and disheartened by changes that you *can't* control).

- **Engage in guided imagery.** When you're feeling out of sorts, close your eyes and imagine that you're in a beautiful, serene, safe place in nature—perhaps a lush, colorful garden, a mountain vista, or the seashore. Use all your senses to conjure up how it looks, sounds, smells, tastes, and feels. Spend a few minutes allowing yourself to experience how restorative it feels to be there. When you open your eyes, try to hold on to that peaceful feeling for as long as you can.

- **Scan your body for tension.** Give yourself a time-out occasionally during the day and take a few moments to do a body scan to assess where you're carrying tension in your body, then to consciously let it go: Start at your head and work your way down, checking in with your forehead, your neck, jaw, shoulders, back, arms and hands, legs and feet; along the way, note any points of tension, then let it go by intentionally relaxing those muscles as you think about them beginning to feel heavy and warm.

- **Follow your breath.** Sit comfortably in a quiet place that's free of distractions and focus on your breathing: Slowly inhale through your nose for three seconds then exhale through your mouth for three seconds. Continue this for three to five minutes. By counting and controlling your inhalations and exhalations,[11] you will naturally calm yourself and ground yourself, both in your body and in the present moment.

- **Adopt a power pose.** It's no secret that the way you hold your body can affect how you feel and function. Research[12] has found that when people assume an open or expansive stance, allowing themselves to take up space around them, they subsequently feel more confident and powerful than when they assume a contracted posture. This form of nonverbal behavior has been found to help people perform better in interview situations and boost their confidence in their decision-making abilities.[13] What's more, adopting an upright posture, rather than a stooped one, increases positive emotions such as optimism, vigor, and happiness.[14] You can put these findings to good use in your everyday life. Striking a power pose is a way to embody strength, confidence, and influence; practice it regularly—and you'll start to feel that way naturally.

- **Engage in intentional acts of body kindness.** As you experience sudden menopause, it's important to remember that your body is essentially your home. It's where you live; it's your vehicle for moving through the world; it's what allows you to hug or snuggle with your loved ones, and do so much more in life. So make a point to nurture it and engage in caring choices for your body every chance you get. How? By resting when you're tired, stretching when you're tense, treating your skin to a soothing lotion when it's dry, using a deep conditioner for your frazzled hair, and complimenting yourself when you look in the mirror. These little "treats" will help you embrace your body as it is now—and take pride of ownership in it.

In addition to taking these steps, women who experience sudden menopause can personalize treatment of their symptoms by consulting the DIY menu of remedies in chapter 12. There, you'll find just about every menopausal symptom ever experienced along with evidence-based approaches that can help relieve them. By customizing your treatment plan, based on your most disruptive symptoms, you can reset your physical and emotional equilibrium. Ultimately, the goal is to help you get through this chapter of your life as steadily and comfortably as possible. You can do that—I promise.

7

The Full-Throttle Menopause Type

A few years ago, Kathryn, fifty-two, a public relations executive with four kids, came to see me, complaining that she felt as though her body had launched a full-scale rebellion after her periods had ended eighteen months earlier. Not only was she suffering from frequent hot flashes and night sweats, but she was experiencing sleep disturbances, significant hair loss, and intense fatigue, and her libido had done a disappearing act. Kathryn had been having one to two glasses of wine at night and using sleeping medications to try to self-medicate herself to sleep, but that wasn't working; she would often wake up feeling foggy-headed and tired. She was being treated for high blood pressure so while she was interested in trying herbal preparations to ease her symptoms, she was (rightfully) concerned that they might interact dangerously with the hypertension medications she was prescribed.

During our initial appointment, we discussed her priorities for getting relief from her myriad symptoms. Usually, I have women who have the Full-Throttle Menopause Type, as Kathryn did, keep a journal to track their most bothersome symptoms over time. But Kathryn had such a clear sense of what she wanted to focus on that we launched into action immediately. We decided to put her libido issues on the back burner so that we could focus on helping her feel better during the days and nights. To help her get some prompt relief from vasomotor symptoms such as hot flashes and night sweats (which are related to the dilation or constriction of blood vessels), I prescribed a low-dose estrogen patch, which she began wearing that very evening, and a nightly progesterone capsule. To improve her body-temperature regulation and her blood pressure, I urged her to engage in brisk walking or yoga every day and to ditch the alcohol and sleeping pills and stick with a regular sleep-wake schedule instead. She began taking biotin supplements to improve her hair health (and help her hold on to it) and iron and zinc supplements to boost her energy. Week by week, she began feeling more vibrant and balanced. When I saw her again eight weeks later, she looked fresh and bright-eyed and acted much livelier.

As Kathryn discovered, women who have the Full-Throttle Menopause Type experience *terrible* symptoms from nearly every conceivable angle—hot flashes, night sweats, sleep disturbances, sexual dysfunction, weight gain, hair loss, skin changes, joint pain, and more. This unpleasant collection of symptoms often stems from natural, not surgical, menopause but that's of little consolation because it can be absolutely overwhelming and sometimes downright debilitating. Many of these women seem to have a harsh onset of symptoms, leaving them feeling like they were run over by a truck. Many of these women feel like their lives are spiraling out of control because the symptoms are so intense and they feel terrible. Some of these women have said things to me like, "I no longer feel like myself!" or "I feel like I'm having an out-of-body experience and it's a bad one!" or "If this is my new normal, I will risk anything to feel better!"

Why do some women experience the Full-Throttle Menopause Type while others don't? We don't have a precise answer but there are theories: One is that the drop in estrogen levels that occurs during menopause causes the body's thermostat (a.k.a. the hypothalamus in the brain) to become more sensitive to slight changes in body temperature,[1] which can trigger a hot flash; women with the Full-Throttle type may have an extra-sensitive thermostat that can lead to hot flashes just from having someone breathe on them (or even sit next to them). Another theory is that there may be a genetic predisposition to developing an even more narrow thermo-regulatory zone during menopause, which can lead to more hot flashes and night sweats. When it comes to experiencing intense mood changes during menopause, we do know that women who had postpartum depression or severe PMS are more likely to ex-perience mood disorders in perimenopause and after menopause. (For more on this, read chapter 8.)

As is the case for any woman who becomes menopausal, the risks of heart disease, osteoporosis, and cognitive decline begin to increase with the Full-Throttle type due to the loss of estrogen. In the more immediate timespan, quality-of-life issues become para-mount because a woman who is experiencing Full-Throttle meno-pause may feel like her body is launching a full-scale mutiny. She may feel like she's going out of her mind with frustration and she may find it difficult to focus, function, or fulfill her usual respon-sibilities. The intensity and diversity of these symptoms can take a toll on a woman's mood, increasing her risk of depression. Intense symptoms can also have a negative effect on her friendships and intimate relationships, including her marriage, because she may be inclined to withdraw from others. It's a rough experience, from every angle.

Something that's often overlooked is the fact that these intense symptoms can compromise a woman's work productivity and job performance. In fact, some data[2] suggests that women with un-treated menopausal symptoms leave the work force and retire sooner than women whose symptoms are either treated or silent. Tracy, fifty-four, an accountant at a prestigious international company, had become so sleep-deprived due to her relentless night sweats that she had extreme brain fog, difficulty concentrating, and depression.

Her symptoms were so bad and she was so afraid of making a huge mistake that would cost her company millions of dollars that she handed in her resignation before she came to see me. (Spoiler alert: Within three months of going on HT, her symptoms had subsided significantly and she went back to work at a lower-stress job.)

It's super important to recognize the Full-Throttle Menopause Type for what it is, because when it's not recognized women may seek care from many different doctors, hoping that at least one of them will identify the *mysterious* cause for what's making them feel so terrible. It's not unusual for women to start with their primary care physician or gynecologist, who may refer them to a psychiatrist, a sleep doctor, an endocrinologist, and maybe a rheumatologist. If women go hopping from doctor to doctor to address their various symptoms, health-care costs and frustration can mount significantly as they go down various rabbit holes seeking relief that is seemingly elusive. Once a woman realizes that her varied symptoms all may stem from the same thing (menopause), she can get on the path that will send her in the right direction for easing her symptoms.

If there's a silver lining for this menopause type, it's this: It's often easier to treat than some of the others because while there's a full crescendo of intense symptoms with Full-Throttle menopause, there's a decrescendo that often occurs with the right treatment. In fact, as quickly as these symptoms can come on with the Full-Throttle Menopause Type, they often resolve just as quickly with the appropriate interventions. So there's plenty of reason for hope—and inspiration for putting together a treatment plan that's likely to work for you.

MAKING TREATMENT DECISIONS

For women with the Full-Throttle Menopause Type, I have found that it makes the most sense to try to treat the most severe symptom first, which in this case is often hot flashes and night sweats. Women with this menopause type also report trouble with cognition, brain fog, fatigue, low libido, and other symptoms—but treating vasomotor symptoms first often gives us a significant leg up in addressing the others. By contrast, if we were to treat her (lack of) libido issues first and she ends up continuing to have intense hot flashes that interfere with her sleep, it's unlikely that her libido is going to make a comeback if she's feeling exhausted and edgy. So it's important to prioritize the most severe (or disruptive) or frequently bothersome symptom, then once a woman obtains some relief on that front, we can address her other complaints.

Hormone therapy (HT)—estrogen and progesterone (if you still have a uterus)—is the most effective treatment for moderate to severe vasomotor symptoms such as hot flashes and night sweats. Most menopause experts agree—as does the North American Menopause Society (NAMS) and the International Menopause Society (IMS)—that hormone therapy should be considered for women with intense vasomotor symptoms who don't have any contraindications (such as a history of estrogen-positive breast cancer, an unprovoked blood clot, or heart attack or stroke) to HT. Here's the simple reason: When it comes to using HT, the benefits outweigh the risks for most healthy women with intense vasomotor symptoms who are younger than age sixty or who start HT within ten years of their final menstrual period.[3]

Still, it's important to give this decision careful consideration, weighing the risks and benefits of treating these symptoms with HT, as well as the potential risks of *not* treating them. For many women, menopausal symptoms last five to seven years so you'll want to consider what it might be like to live with these intense Full-Throttle symptoms for that long—if you choose *not* to treat them. The repercussions might include losing significant amounts of sleep or having poor quality sleep, either of which can lead to high blood pressure, poor blood sugar regulation, increased appetite, weight gain, a downturn in mood, and trouble concentrating. That laundry list of unfortunate consequences is just from insufficient sleep! If you opt out of treating, you might also end up with low libido, vaginal dryness and discomfort, brain fog, and other unwanted changes to your quality of life.

Don't get me wrong: I'm not suggesting that the only way to treat Full-Throttle menopause symptoms is with HT. That's not the case. But HT is likely to deliver the broadest impact in terms of relief. It's like one-stop shopping for relief from many menopausal symptoms. And here's something many women don't realize: You don't have to be all in or all out when it comes to HT. Many of my patients choose to use HT for one or two years, to help them over the menopausal hump, then come off it.

If a woman wants to try HT to ease her Full-Throttle symptoms, I consider her medical history and personal preferences when deciding between oral or transdermal formulations. For women who have a history of high blood pressure, diabetes, migraines, high cholesterol, or irregular heartbeat, I would go with a transdermal delivery system (either a patch or gel). Since transdermal delivery avoids being broken down in the liver (like the oral form is), there's less risk of interactions with other medications she may be taking and also a decreased risk of developing blood clots compared to the oral form. If a woman doesn't have any underlying health conditions and isn't taking regular medications, she may be able to choose between oral HT or transdermal formulations, based on her personal preferences. (For example, nurses who work the night shift often prefer to use the weekly patch because it's easy to apply and easy to keep track of.)

Erin, forty-nine, a physician assistant in orthopedic surgery, was experiencing up to thirty severe hot flashes per day and drenching night sweats, which disturbed her sleep. She was also experiencing cognitive changes that made her feel like she wasn't at the top of her game when talking to patients. Worse, her Full-

Throttle menopause was so intense that during surgery, hot flashes were causing her goggles to fog, impairing her ability to see clearly and assist safely. (I know—yikes!) She had tried almost every over-the-counter preparation but hadn't gotten relief from any of them that lasted more than a week.

After discussing her options, Erin decided to give hormone therapy a try. With the help of HT, as well as reducing her intake of caffeine and other stimulants, and performing light exercise (such as yoga or walking her dog) in the evening, her symptoms improved considerably within two months. When she came back to see me, she said she felt as though she'd gotten her life back: Gone were the intense hot flashes during surgery and the night sweats that had kept her up half the night. She felt confident, sharp, and clear-headed again, which came as a tremendous relief to her, physically and mentally.

For women who can't or don't want to take hormone therapy, other medications may help ease some of the Full-Throttle symptoms. Antidepressants from the selective serotonin reuptake inhibitor (SSRI) and serotonin and norepinephrine reuptake inhibitor (SNRI) classes can be used at low doses in an off-label capacity: These have efficacy in reducing hot flashes and improving sleep due to the increase in serotonin in your brain. (No, it's not that doctors think you are depressed!) In fact, research[4] has found that women who took a low dose of venlafaxine (Effexor), an SNRI, to treat menopausal hot flashes and night sweats experienced a significant reduction in their vasomotor symptoms after eight weeks, although those who took low-dose estradiol gained a slightly greater benefit. Other medications that can help with hot flashes and are used in an off-label capacity include gabapentin (an antiseizure drug that's often used for nerve pain), oxybutynin (which is typically used for overactive bladder), or clonidine (which is used to treat hypertension). When choosing a non-hormonal treatment, I try to see if women have any other medical issues that would help us pick the best option; for example, if a woman doesn't want to use HT and she is experiencing an increased need to urinate, along with intense hot flashes or night sweats, going with oxybutynin would make sense.

BASELINE TREATMENT PLANS FOR THE FULL-THROTTLE MENOPAUSE TYPE

What follows are two baseline treatment plans for women who have the Full-Throttle Menopause Type. The first treatment plan focuses on the use of hormone therapy (HT); the second plan addresses how to treat your symptoms without hormones. Whichever treatment plan you choose, you'll also find recommendations for lifestyle modifications that are suitable for all women with this type. Keep in mind that if you have additional symptoms that aren't relieved by these recommended interventions, you can choose from the extensive menu of symptom-oriented solutions in chapter 12 to ease what's still bothering you. The goal is to cater to your needs and make this plan work for you.

Plan A: Using Hormone Therapy

For women with Full-Throttle menopause who want to use hormone therapy and don't have any contraindications to doing so, there are a few options. When it comes to oral HT, there's oral estrogen (half a milligram twice daily to keep blood levels very steady) along with oral micronized natural progesterone (Prometrium) at bedtime; or, some women may want to take a combined tab of estradiol and norethindrone (a form of progesterone that's like the mini pill) nightly if a once-daily dose is preferable. If a woman wants to use transdermal HT, she could go with a 0.05 milligram twice-weekly or weekly estrogen patch or a half-milligram estradiol gel in the morning (if symptoms are worse during the day) or at night (if symptoms are worse at night) *and* 100 milligrams oral progesterone (Prometrium) at night. The goal is for a woman to end up with blood levels of estrogen between 40 and 70 pg/mL, whether she's using oral estrogen, the patch, or the gel. Fortunately, I find that women with the Full-Throttle type tend to improve fairly quickly with even low doses of estrogen.

A progesterone-releasing IUD is also an option for progesterone replacement but most women with the Full-Throttle type want relief right away and don't want to wait to schedule an IUD placement. Remember: Progesterone is needed to protect the uterus from experiencing overgrowth of the lining and possibly the development of uterine cancer while taking estrogen therapy—but if a woman no longer has her uterus, she doesn't need progesterone. Some women choose to start HT with just progesterone, which can be great for improving sleep and has some efficacy in reducing hot flashes, though not as much as using estrogen. (While this may be a bit confusing, it's important to note that you can take progesterone without estrogen, and you can take progesterone even if you don't have a uterus.) Still, this is an approach that can help women start to feel better while they are mulling over whether to use estrogen therapy or if they have a contraindication to using estrogen therapy. If they're using HT, I have my Full-Throttle patients come back to see me in eight to ten weeks so we can adjust dosages as necessary.

The Full-Throttle Menopause Type is often accompanied by severe vaginal dryness, so often at our first visit I will also add a local or topical vaginal estrogen. About 40 to 50 percent of women who are using systemic HT will also need vaginal estrogen because this sensitive tissue needs the most TLC at this point in life. The creams are very effective, but they are messy. The Estring—a set-it-and-forget-it vaginal ring that can stay in place for up to ninety days—can be really easy when women are dealing with treating hot flashes. With this approach, genitourinary symptoms can improve in about ten to twelve weeks. Sometimes we can stop using the local or topical vaginal estrogen as the systemic form of HT kicks in and does the trick, but approximately 50 percent of women will need both.

As an add-on, testosterone replacement may be an option for treating low libido but I always start my Full-Throttle patients with estrogen and progesterone (if they have a uterus) or just estrogen (if they don't). Often, estrogen therapy, even without testosterone, can help women with diminished libido—so they might find that they don't need testosterone. Also, we need to prioritize feeling better overall before we address sexual health. After all, no woman wants to have sex if she hasn't been sleeping and is sweating 24/7!

Plan B: Treating the Full-Throttle Menopause Type without Hormones

For women with the Full-Throttle type who have clear contraindications to using systemic hormone therapy or who simply don't want to use hormone therapy for reasons that are personal, there are other medications we can use to address intensely disruptive menopausal symptoms.

Depending on the symptoms a woman with Full-Throttle menopause is most bothered by, here are some other possible treatments:

- To treat hot flashes, antidepressants from the selective serotonin reuptake inhibitor (SSRI) and serotonin and norepinephrine reuptake inhibitor (SNRI) classes can be used at low doses in an off-label capacity. In particular, research[5] has shown that paroxetine (Paxil), escitalopram (Lexapro), citalopram (Celexa), desvenlafaxine (Pristiq), and venlafaxine (Effexor) can improve the frequency and severity of hot flashes. In addition, the SSRI Brisdelle is the only non-hormonal medication that's approved by the FDA specifically to treat hot flashes. If a woman doesn't want to take an antidepressant, alternatives for relieving hot flashes include gabapentin (an antiseizure drug that's often used for nerve pain) or oxybutynin (which is typically used for overactive bladder).

- If insomnia or other sleep disturbances are a problem, taking trazodone (a prescription antidepressant and sedative) at bedtime may help. The same is true of mirtazapine (Remeron), an antidepressant that can aid with sleep. Or, a nightly dose of progesterone (Prometrium) can set the stage for better sleep (if a woman is open to using progesterone without estrogen).

- To help with irritability, weight gain, and fatigue, the antidepressant bupropion (Wellbutrin) may be a good option. Bupropion increases levels of the neurotransmitter dopamine, which has a slightly stimulating effect, thus helping with fatigue and mood. It has also been found to reduce cravings for carbohydrates, which may be why it often results in a small amount of weight loss (most commonly five to ten pounds). Note: This antidepressant does *not* help with hot flashes and in some cases may make them worse.

- If low libido persists after treating the most bothersome symptoms, a woman can take Addyi (a.k.a. flibanserin), an FDA-approved oral medication that's available by prescription for hypoactive sexual desire disorder (including low libido) in premenopausal women, but is often used in postmenopausal women, too. The drug increases dopamine in the brain, which has a mood-enhancing effect, and when it's taken at night, it can produce a sense of relaxation that sets the stage for better sleep. Alternatively, she could use the injectable drug Vyleesi on an as-needed basis: Available by prescription, the medication was approved by the FDA[6] in 2019 to treat hypoactive sexual desire disorder (including low libido) in premenopausal women but can be often used in postmenopausal women, too.

When Carly, forty-nine, came to see me with symptoms of Full-Throttle menopause, her hot flashes were waking her up every hour on the hour throughout the night. She was exhausted, uncomfortable, irritable, and struggling to get things done. She would spend her days working as an administrative assistant relying on caffeine to keep her awake. By the time she got home from work she was too tired to exercise, so her once-regular fitness routine was kicked to the curb.

Because her sister had had blood clots and a stroke, Carly didn't want to use hormone therapy. She had tried taking over-the-counter black cohosh and CBD oil at night that worked for about six months but then the nighttime hot flashes came back with a vengeance. Our first step was to address her sleep difficulties, which we did by making sure her bedroom was cold—and by that I mean under sixty-five degrees—and very dark. She began taking 250 milligrams of magnesium before bedtime but it didn't help; next, we went with trazodone, which helped with her sleep but left her feeling really groggy in the morning (which can happen for some women). Because the nighttime symptoms were still so disruptive, we decided to put her on 100 milligrams of progesterone (Prometrium) at bedtime, which proved to be a game changer for Carly. While she would still would wake up once during the night, this was a significant improvement from waking up every hour—and she found that she could easily fall back to sleep. She also used an app that provided white noise to drown out unwanted sounds from outside her home, and to reduce her need to go to the bathroom during the night, she stopped drinking liquids around 7 P.M.

Shortly after she started sleeping through the night, she began to feel more energized and better able to cope with whatever came her way. As an added bonus, her clothes were fitting better because she had lost five pounds from sleeping better and switching to a more plant-based diet. And as her mood took a significant turn in the upward direction, she realized that she had stopped snapping at coworkers and felt focused and happy at work again. Carly 2.0 was a major upgrade.

LIFESTYLE INTERVENTIONS

Dietary Directives

While there isn't an eating plan that will magically ease your symptoms, you can take dietary steps to help calm the chaos in your body and mind. The first step is to reduce your intake of highly refined carbohydrates such as chips, cookies, and candy; besides helping with blood sugar regulation, ditching the starchy, low-nutrient carbs will help you achieve and maintain a healthy weight, which could in turn result in fewer hot flashes. Step two: Make a point of planning your daily meals, ensuring that they have adequate protein from a variety of plant and animal foods and fiber from whole grains, fruits, vegetables, legumes, nuts, and seeds. Loading up on these nutrients will help you stay satiated for longer and reduce cravings for refined carbohydrates and added sugars. An added bonus: Protein digestion requires more energy (meaning: more calories are burned), which may provide a slight edge when it comes to weight control.

Keep in mind that consuming either caffeine or alcohol (especially red wine) can trigger hot flashes in some women—and that may include you. What's more, either substance could prevent you from getting the deep sleep you need. So stick with a moderate intake of caffeine and alcohol, if you do consume them. Avoid consuming caffeine after early afternoon at the latest. And skip the nightcap: While having a glass of wine or brandy before bed may make you sleepy initially, after you fall asleep alcohol's sedating effects fade away, leaving you susceptible to sleep disruptions especially during the second half of the night.[7] If you want a beverage that will help lull you to sleep and allow you to stay asleep, consider having a cup of warm chamomile, passionflower, or valerian root tea.

Here's a look at some specific nutrients that may help with different symptoms you may be experiencing with the Full-Throttle Menopause Type:

- **Isoflavones from soy foods:** While these have estrogen-like properties (albeit weaker ones than the estrogen the body produces), consuming isoflavones may help calm hot flashes in some women. In fact, research[8] has found that consuming soy isoflavones—which are made up primarily of the compounds genistein and daidzein—can reduce menopausal hot flashes by 25 percent. My feeling is: This is an area where every bit of improvement helps! So consider adding more lightly processed or raw soy foods—such as tofu, miso, edamame, and tempeh—to your meals and snacks.
- **Tryptophan and melatonin:** You're undoubtedly aware that the hormone melatonin plays a crucial role in promoting sleep; it also can affect mood and other bodily functions. Something else you may have been unaware of: The amino acid tryptophan plays a role in making melatonin, as well as serotonin, a mood-boosting brain chemical. Tryptophan is an essential amino acid, which means the body can't produce it, so it needs to be obtained from foods like milk, tuna, turkey, chicken, fish, oats, nuts, and seeds. Melatonin

is also found in milk, oats, and nuts (especially pistachios), as well as tart cherries, grapes, eggs, kiwi, strawberries, peppers, and mushrooms.[9] Vitamin B6 is also important for melatonin production; good food sources include chickpeas, tuna, salmon, chicken, fortified cereals, and bananas.[10] If you like having an evening snack, combine foods that are rich in fiber, protein, and melatonin-enhancing nutrients— such as a half cup tart cherries mixed with half cup plain Greek or Icelandic yogurt, or a quarter cup whole-grain cereal mixed with two tablespoons raisins and two tablespoons pistachios.

Here's what a day's meal plan might look like:

Breakfast: 2 eggs scrambled in 1 teaspoon olive oil, 2-ounce whole-wheat roll, 1 cup sliced strawberries

Lunch: Tuna avocado sandwich with lettuce and sliced tomato on whole-grain bread: 4 ounces canned drained tuna, 2 teaspoons mayonnaise, ¼ sliced avocado

Dinner: Chicken (or turkey) grain bowl: 4 ounces cooked chicken cut into cubes or shredded, 1 cup cooked quinoa, rice, or farro; chopped tomato; ¼ cup frozen and thawed edamame; ½ cup frozen and thawed or fresh corn; ¼ cup shredded Monterey Jack cheese

Snacks: ¼ cup unsalted peanuts and 1 cup hot cocoa or chocolate milk made with unsweetened, fortified soy milk, 1 teaspoon cocoa powder, and sweetener of your choice; cherry freeze: 1 cup frozen sweet cherries blended with 1 cup plain fat-free Greek or Icelandic yogurt

As far as dietary supplements[a] go, here's what I recommend considering:

- Black cohosh supplements may help with hot flashes and night sweats. Made from the plant's roots and rhizomes (underground stems), these supplements come in forms such as powdered whole herb, liquid extracts, and dried extracts in pill form.[11] Do not use these if you have a liver disorder!
- Valerian root supplements can help with insomnia and hot flashes. One study[12] found that when menopausal women took 255 milligrams of valerian root capsules three times per day, the severity and frequency of their hot flashes decreased considerably after four weeks, compared to women who took a placebo preparation. Preparations of the valerian plant, which is native to Europe and Asia, are made from its roots, rhizomes, and stolons (horizontal stems). Dried valerian roots and stems are prepared as teas or tinctures or put into capsules or tablets.

Exercise Rx

Because intense aerobic exercise can rev up the nervous system, I tend to recommend that women with Full-Throttle menopause symptoms engage in calming exercises like yoga, Pilates, tai chi, or qigong (an ancient Chinese practice that combines slow, deliberate movements, meditation, and specific breathing patterns). All

---

[a]Keep in mind: Dietary supplements, including herbal supplements, are not regulated by the FDA. I am recommending certain supplements because I have seen some of my patients benefit from them. But it's crucial that you discuss using any dietary supplement with your doctor; sometimes certain supplements can have problematic interactions with medications and this is something you'll want to avoid.

of these can lower the heart rate and reduce stress in the body. What's more, a review of the medical literature on this subject published in a 2017 issue of *Complementary Therapies in Medicine*[13] found that doing yoga can reduce vasomotor symptoms (like hot flashes and night sweats) and psychological symptoms (like anxiety and mood disturbances) in perimenopausal and postmenopausal women. And research[14] shows that practicing tai chi or qigong reduces symptoms of anxiety and depression and has other beneficial effects on psychological well-being.

You can also engage in rhythmic, meditative forms of movement such as walking, swimming, gentle cycling on a stationary bicycle, or using the elliptical machine. The key is to focus your awareness on your body and pay attention to your breathing[15] as you move through these activities.

Once your symptoms start to improve, you can gradually add back more intense forms of exercise: My recommendation is to start with resistance training—whether you lift weights or use weight machines or exercise bands or your own body weight—to protect your muscle mass, bone mass, and metabolism, then to progress to forms of aerobic exercise that appeal to you. (You could also try the HIIT workout in the appendix.) By incorporating strength training and aerobic exercise, you'll check all the exercise-related boxes for protecting your heart, lung, bone, and brain health, which become increasing concerns after menopause.

Improving Your Headspace

As you've seen, the Full-Throttle Menopause Type can be a highly tumultuous experience that can upend nearly every aspect of a woman's life. Between the breadth and intensity of your symptoms, you may feel like you're coming unhinged emotionally as well as physically. To help yourself tame the turmoil from the inside out, I also recommend using the following strategies:

- **Correct your distorted thoughts.** When you're in the throes of a Full-Throttle menopause experience, you might find yourself having unhelpful thoughts like, *I can't stand the way I'm feeling!* or *I'm going out of my mind here!* These are forms of cognitive distortions, which can include all-or-nothing thinking (viewing a situation in absolute terms), catastrophizing (making a situation seem worse or more threatening than it really is), and overgeneralizing (viewing a single upsetting event as part of an ongoing pattern), among others. The trouble is, all of these thought patterns have the potential to make you feel even worse! That's why it's important to learn to question or talk back to these twisted thoughts in your head. Consider: Can you really *not* stand this? Or do you mean that you don't like it? Are you really going crazy? Or is it more likely that you're frustrated? If you get in the habit of giving your distorted thoughts a reality check and correcting them, you'll dial down a source of stress (your thinking style) naturally.

- **Learn paced breathing.** When it's performed twice a day, a technique called paced respiration—which involves slow, deliberate, diaphragmatic breathing—can reduce hot flashes by up to 52 percent, research[16] has found. (As an added bonus: It can also calm your mind.) With paced breathing,[17] the goal is to inhale slowly through your nose for two to four seconds then exhale slowly through your mouth for four to six seconds. Continue doing this for five, ten, or fifteen minutes at a time. The reasons it helps: The technique increases the flow of oxygen throughout your body, decreases the stress chemicals your body produces, and induces the relaxation response—a positive triple whammy!

- **Let your imagination help you.** Close your eyes and create a mental picture of what it would look and feel like to be calm and comfortable in your body and mind. Imagine how you would move through the world (with comfort and ease) and deal with difficult situations (letting them roll off the back of your stress-proof raincoat). Practice keeping that calm, cool, and collected image of yourself in mind as you go about your daily life. And give yourself periodic time-outs to revisit that image with your eyes closed.

- **Find flow.** If you've ever become so immersed in something enjoyable that you were doing—whether it's drawing, gardening, playing a musical instrument, coloring in an adult coloring book, or something else—that you lost track of time and what was going on around you, you're no stranger to "flow." Coined by psychologist Mihaly Csikszentmihalyi, the concept of "flow" describes an optimal experience where you become completely absorbed in what you are doing because it's challenging, enjoyable, and rewarding. Besides being inherently gratifying, being in a flow state can quiet your mind, enhance your focus, and stimulate the release of dopamine—all of which can help you feel good both physically and emotionally. That's because the flow state engages your parasympathetic nervous system, which helps you relax and recover, as well as the sympathetic nervous system, which helps you stay alert.[18]

- **Engage in mindfulness meditation.** This form of meditation centers on being present in the here and now by focusing on your breath. When thoughts come to mind, treat them as if they were clouds passing in the sky—notice them and let them go—as you bring your attention back to your breath. Besides having a calming effect on your body and mind, mindfulness meditation has been found to improve sleep and quality of life and reduce vasomotor symptoms in postmenopausal women, according to research in the journal *Menopause*.[19]

- **Spend time with supportive friends.** If you're feeling miserable with menopausal symptoms, you may not feel much

like socializing; in fact, many women end up isolating themselves when they're stressed out by Full-Throttle symptoms.
That's a mistake because research[20] has actually found that
menopausal symptoms decrease as social support increases—
and that having high levels of perceived social support is associated with a better quality of life among postmenopausal
women.[21] So make an effort to get together with friends,
even if it's just to take a walk or have coffee. It doesn't have
to involve getting all dressed up and going to a fancy restaurant; you can keep it low key.

- **Hypnotize yourself.** People have a lot of misconceptions
  about hypnosis (no, you won't start clucking like a chicken!).
  Hypnosis is really just a deeply focused state that allows you
  to be receptive to suggestions. As far as menopausal symptoms go, hypnosis has been found to help with sleep disturbances,[22] anxiety,[23] and hot flashes.[24] And you don't have
  to go to a hypnotherapist to reap these benefits: The Evia
  Menopause app incorporates hypnotherapy techniques to
  help you manage hot flashes. It's great because it's right on
  your phone, which means you can do a quick session any-
  time, anywhere.

- **Develop your own CTFO technique.** When you feel beset
  by a storm of intense emotions, find a way to come to your
  own rescue and hit the reset button. To do that you'll want
  to create your own CTFO (chill the f*ck out) mechanism:
  You might take a deep breath, hold it in, and stretch your
  body as if you just woke up, then let your breath out with
  a loud exhale, the way certified health coach Megan San-
  chez does.[25] You might close your eyes, breathe deeply, and
  silently repeat a mantra like, "This upsetting moment will
  pass," or simply, "I'm going to chill." Or, take five and dance
  to Taylor Swift's "Shake It Off," imagining that you're shaking off stress, negativity, and other bad feelings while you

shake your body. Interesting factoid[26]: When your dog does a whole-body shake for no apparent reason—meaning, he isn't wet—it's his way of shaking off stress and tension.

In addition to taking these steps, you can personalize treatment of your symptoms by consulting the DIY menu of remedies in chapter 12. There, you'll find just about every menopausal symptom under the sun (and moon), along with evidence-based approaches that can help relieve them. By taking charge of your symptoms and customizing your treatment plan, you can get a grip on the changes that are upsetting you most and calm your physical and emotional equilibrium. Ultimately, the goal is to help you get to the other side of this experience, feeling as strong, upbeat, and healthy as you can be.

8 |

The Mind-Altering Menopause Type

When Renée, fifty-six, a history professor at a large university, came to see me, she was not only miserable but incredibly worried about her professional future. After becoming menopausal five years earlier, she initially considered herself fortunate to have had few hot flashes or night sweats. But her luck didn't last: By the time she was fifty-three, her mood had taken a downturn and she struggled with motivation because she was having trouble concentrating and thinking clearly. There were times when she found herself stopping mid-sentence during her lectures because she couldn't come up with the right word or she forgot where she was going with a particular point. She fell behind on grading papers and writing articles for publication.

Single and without children, Renée's whole world revolved around her work and social life, which was largely connected to the university. Her mental challenges had become intense enough that her self-esteem took a hit and she became withdrawn from friends and colleagues. She was even considering early retirement because she was worried that she might be developing early dementia and felt so defeated by her symptoms.

After consulting a neurologist who sent her for an MRI and neurocognitive testing, Renée was relieved—make that *thrilled*—to learn that she wasn't showing any signs of dementia. But she wasn't willing to accept her brain fog as the new normal, which is why she came to see me. Thank goodness she did, because I quickly realized that her symptoms stemmed from having the Mind-Altering Menopause Type and we designed a treatment plan. Because she was afraid of making more mistakes at work, she scaled down her course load and work hours for a semester so she could focus on taking the steps that would likely help her. We started with lifestyle interventions, including a brisk walk every morning and daily meditation sessions; Renée also started doing cognitive behavioral therapy (CBT) to address her mood issues. Meanwhile, I prescribed atomoxetine (Strattera),[1] a non-stimulant, cognition-enhancing medication that's often used for attention deficit hyperactivity disorder (ADHD). It really helped her ability to concentrate and get back on track with her work. Within several months, she was feeling and functioning like her old self again and returned to full-time teaching the following semester.

As Renée discovered, the Mind-Altering Menopause Type isn't often recognized or discussed by women. This can be particularly frustrating because a woman with this type may experience life-altering mood changes—including anxiety, irritability, depression, and dramatic mood swings—as well as cognitive changes such as brain fog, difficulty with concentration or attention, and memory challenges.[2] Indeed, recent research suggests that while many mood and cognitive challenges can start in perimenopause, they continue into the postmenopausal stage for some women,[3] particularly in the areas of learning, memory, attention, and working memory. Similarly, some research has found that menopausal status may influence the type of mood issue women experience during the menopausal transition—for example, one study[4] found that there's a greater likelihood of symptoms of depression during perimenopause and symptoms of anxiety during postmenopause. And some women, particularly during perimenopause, experience labile moods—swings between feeling down, edgy, irritable, or anxious.

Because these mood and mind symptoms can impair a woman's ability to function at work, as well as take a toll on her overall quality of life, they can thwart her professional success and damage her personal relationships. Some women describe periods of "emotional fragility" and find themselves unexpectedly bursting into tears in response to a sappy commercial on TV. Others feel as though they've become an emotional sponge that soaks up whatever feelings are around them. Still others experience a Dr. Jekyll and Ms. Hyde pattern of mood swings that make them feel as though they're undergoing (rapid!) personality transformations that truly affect their relationships. Not surprisingly, research[5] has found that women with perimenopausal depression report a significantly decreased quality of life, as well as reductions in social support.

Making matters worse, these women often end up seeing many doctors—gynecologists, internists, neurologists, psychologists, and others—without getting a clear sense of what's going on. That's because few doctors connect these symptoms to menopause (it's not necessarily their fault; they haven't been trained to). Granted, research has found the majority of women will not experience severe depressive symptoms during the menopausal transition. But for women who have a history of major depression or postpartum depression or even intense PMS, the menopausal transition is a biologically vulnerable time for a recurrence of depression. Meanwhile, the latest research also suggests that women who've *never* been depressed have a risk of depression that's two to two and a half times higher during the menopausal transition. The common denominator: Some women's brains are simply more sensitive to hormonal changes than others', and mood changes can occur when female reproductive hormones go on a roller-coaster ride or drop dramatically.

CONSIDERING THE WHOLE PICTURE

Other risk factors for experiencing major depression during the menopausal transition include having a history of childhood maltreatment,[6] a family history of depression,[7] being unemployed, and having a chronic health condition like hypertension or obesity.[8] What's more, the timing of menopause can be a factor: Studies have found that women with early or premature menopause have a higher risk of developing depression during the menopausal experience; by contrast, women who have a longer reproductive lifespan (from the age at which they started menstruating to the age at which they become menopausal) and women who reach menopause at a later-than-average age (fifty-two or older) have a reduced risk of developing depression.[9,10]

It would be a mistake to overlook the fact that the relationship between depression and sleep disturbances can go both ways: Depressive symptoms and the maladaptive thinking patterns that often accompany them can contribute to insomnia, and sleep problems can make mood changes worse. Of course, sleep disturbances and insomnia can also take a toll on a woman's cognitive function during the day; it's nearly impossible to think clearly or remember names or what it is you should be doing at any given time when you're starved for sufficient good-quality sleep. This is one example of the menopausal domino effect, where physical symptoms such as hot flashes and night sweats can lead to sleep disturbances, which can in turn cause depressive symptoms, anxiety, difficulty concentrating, and other mood symptoms. (Fortunately, cognitive behavioral therapy for insomnia, CBT-I, can help on all of these fronts among postmenopausal women, according to research.[11])

Meanwhile, cognitive changes can occur during the menopausal transition, and some women are more susceptible to these than others. Researchers[12] have labeled this a "window of vulnerability" for cognitive difficulties, too. This is a complicated issue, and not completely understood, but this much is clear: Changes in reproductive hormones, particularly estradiol, can play a role in memory function, including attention, verbal, and working memory, at midlife—a constellation of symptoms that many women experience as "brain fog."

Cam was forty-eight when she first came to see me for depression and sleep disturbances that were related to perimenopausal hormone changes. She was still getting her period sporadically (as in: every few months), but the stability of her moods took a major hit. As a house painter, Cam was very busy during the spring and summer months and had lags in her work during the winter. In the previous two winters, she had fallen into a deep depression where she often had trouble getting out of bed. Her wife of five years had urged her to go for cognitive behavioral therapy (CBT), where she was diagnosed with seasonal affective disorder. Therapy helped a little bit but Cam was convinced that something else might be going on, too, which is why she came to see me.

After discussing her symptoms, her current health, and her health history, it became clear that Cam was experiencing a major depressive episode so I started her on a low dose of Wellbutrin, which helped considerably. She started exercising regularly and cooking meals for her wife and became generally more engaged with life. But she still felt anxious at night and would wake up worrying about things she knew were out of her control—so I added 100 milligrams of progesterone at bedtime, and watched to see how it would affect her mood. I also recommended that she use a light box, take a vitamin D supplement, and put herself on a more consistent sleep schedule. After using the combination of these interventions for several weeks, she began sleeping better, felt more relaxed overall, and had more energy during the day. The key was that she relied on strategies that catered to her unique constellation of symptoms from the Mind-Altering type.

The reality is, it's not just the hormonal havoc of the menopausal transition that can increase women's risk of having mood changes at midlife. It's important to recognize that at this point in life, women may be dealing with a variety of other challenges—such as being responsible for caring for or supporting their aging parents *and* their kids (yep, this is the sandwich generation), going through a separation or divorce, becoming empty nesters as their kids go off to college or to start their own independent lives, or gaining greater responsibilities at work (which can be a great thing, as well as a source of stress). The point is: At this stage of life, women may be experiencing a barrage of changes physiologically, personally, professionally, emotionally, and socially—and this can be a lot to handle, especially for those who are susceptible to depression or other mood disorders.

MAKING TREATMENT DECISIONS

While some studies have found that using hormone therapy (HT) may help with mood and brain fog symptoms, this isn't currently considered a first-line approach. Simply put, HT is not approved by the FDA to treat menopausal brain fog. As the International Menopause Society (IMS) notes, the effects of hormone therapy on cognition and brain function during the menopausal transition are complex, and "there is insufficient evidence to recommend its use for the treatment or prevention of cognitive dysfunction." That said, if a woman is experiencing distressing vasomotor symptoms—such as hot flashes or night sweats—along with mood and cognitive changes, she may be a candidate for HT.

You may have heard that the Women's Health Initiative Memory Study[13] (WHIMS) found that, contrary to expectations, the use of combined HT (conjugated estrogens plus medroxyprogesterone acetate) or estrogen only in women who'd had hysterectomies, among women ages sixty-five and older, did *not* protect them against cognitive decline or Alzheimer's disease; in fact, it increased the risk of dementia and cognitive decline. This was more than fifteen years ago and the study looked at the effects of starting this formulation of HT in women over age sixty-five. Fast forward to today: Now researchers are looking at the use of HT for what it's FDA-approved for—hot flashes and night sweats or genitourinary symptoms—in younger women and following them long term to see how they fare cognitively. The results are pending, but what I can tell you right now is that in my clinical practice, I see women feel cognitively sharper when they use HT after suffering from brain fog and hot flashes.

Also, when the estrogen component in hormone therapy is used in combination with antidepressants, such as selective serotonin reuptake inhibitors (SSRIs) or serotonin and norepinephrine reuptake inhibitors (SNRIs), I have seen a synergistic effect, in which the antidepressant is more effective in improving mood and mental well-being.[14] We don't know what the mechanism is behind this effect but the theory is that estrogen may enhance the antidepressant response to SSRIs in postmenopausal women who are depressed. In a small study[15] involving women with perimenopausal depression who were taking an antidepressant and experiencing hot flashes, night sweats, irregular periods, sleep disturbances, and/or memory difficulties, researchers investigated the effects of estrogen augmentation (with 0.625 milligrams per day of conjugated estrogen) on the women's moods and memory; the women's depressive disorders had been in partial remission, and the researchers found that using short-term, low-dose estrogen to augment their antidepressant medication significantly improved their moods, but not their memory.

The Hidden Risks of Disordered Eating and Negative Body Image at Midlife

Just as the menopausal transition is a window of vulnerability for depression, the same is true when it comes to eating disorders for some women. Research[16,17] has found that the menopausal transition is associated with an increased prevalence or exacerbation of eating disorders and negative body image. The theory is that this may be due to changes in hormonal function, body composition, and conceptions of what it means to be a woman, biologically speaking. This is a time in life when some women, particularly those who have appearance-related concerns due to aging or who engage in body comparisons with others, exercise greater dietary restraint.[18]

Some research has also found that women who are overweight (or have a high waist circumference) or who have depressive symptoms or a history of past depression or childhood abuse have higher rates of binge eating and/or preoccupation with eating, body shape, or weight.[19] It's important to recognize that age and reproductive status don't protect women from these issues.[20] Fortunately, help—in the form of different types of therapy—is available for body image and disordered eating problems at any stage of life. But first these need to be recognized for what they are.

BASELINE TREATMENT PLANS FOR THE
MIND-ALTERING MENOPAUSE TYPE

As a starting point, it's wise to have a complete physical with your doctor to rule out the possibility that a medical condition could be responsible for your mood changes. Hypothyroidism (a.k.a. an underactive thyroid gland), for example, becomes more common in women at midlife and it can cause persistent fatigue, sluggishness, and depression, among other symptoms, whereas anemia could trigger fatigue, sleep disturbances, difficulty concentrating, and other mind-related changes. Be sure to go over your medications with your doctor because some drugs or combinations of medications can cause symptoms of depression or anxiety.

And if you're experiencing severe memory loss—like forgetting how to get to your home after running errands or how to operate your phone—talk to your doctor about getting a neuropsychological evaluation to see how well your brain is working. For less severe brain fog—like forgetting what you need at the store or experiencing the tip-of-the-tongue phenomenon (where you can't think of a word or name you were about to say)—you don't need this.

If you have extreme depression, thoughts of self-harm, or suicidal ideation, it's important to get in touch with a psychiatrist or psychologist right away. These symptoms are not to be taken lightly. If you have thoughts of harming yourself, please call the Suicide & Crisis Lifeline at 988, which operates twenty-four hours a day, seven days a week. Also, for women who have more complex psychiatric conditions like bipolar disorder or schizophrenia, it's important to have a menopause doctor, your primary care doctor, *and* a skilled psychiatrist all working together because menopause can worsen these underlying conditions.

What follows are two baseline treatment plans for women who have the Mind-Altering Menopause Type. The first treatment plan focuses on the use of hormone therapy (HT), assuming a woman also has vasomotor symptoms such as hot flashes or night sweats or genitourinary symptoms; the second plan addresses how to treat your symptoms without hormones. Whichever treatment plan you choose, you'll also find recommendations for lifestyle modifications that are suitable for all women with this type. Keep in mind that if you have additional symptoms that aren't relieved by these recommended interventions, you can choose from the extensive menu of symptom-oriented solutions in chapter 12 to ease what's continuing to distress you. The goal is to address your needs and come up with a plan that works for you.

Plan A: Using Hormone Therapy

For women with the Mind-Altering Menopause Type who want to use hormone therapy and don't have any contraindications to HT, this may be an option—if they have vasomotor symptoms or genitourinary symptoms or osteopenia. As you've seen, these are the only symptoms that menopausal hormone therapy is currently approved for.

If you're considering HT, I tend to suggest something quick and easy such as the twice-weekly CombiPatch (a transdermal patch that combines estrogen and progestin) or a weekly patch called Climara Pro (which also contains estrogen and a progestin). These are very similar in terms of efficacy; often insurance coverage dictates which one I write a prescription for. If you don't have a uterus and don't need progesterone, I would recommend starting with a twice-weekly or weekly estradiol patch. If you have a uterus and want to use the estradiol patch, you can take 100 milligrams oral progesterone (Prometrium) at night. In my experience, patches work really well for mind and mood symptoms because the hormones are slowly released into the bloodstream and they are easy to incorporate into your lifestyle (no need to remember to take an oral medication every day).

For some women, the progesterone can actually increase mood symptoms, particularly irritability and depression. If that happens and a woman has a uterus, I will have her take progesterone cyclically (for the first twelve days of the month, which is the minimum amount required for uterine health), or recommend having a progesterone-releasing IUD placed; because the IUD doesn't release progesterone systemically, it usually avoids the mood issues that are caused or aggravated by oral progesterone.

If mind or mood symptoms persist despite using HT, we could add Wellbutrin (bupropion), an antidepressant that in my clinical experience seems to help with depression and can boost low energy. As an added benefit, Wellbutrin also decreases cravings for starchy carbohydrates so it can help with emotional eating or binge eating; often using Wellbutrin results in slight weight loss on the order of five to ten pounds.

I recommend that all women with the Mind-Altering Menopause Type consider cognitive behavioral therapy (CBT) when anxiety and depression are causing them to have more bad days and nights than good ones. You can ask your primary care physician for a referral or consult Psychology Today (PsychologyToday .com) to find a therapist in your area; this way, you can get a glimpse of what issues they specialize in and whether they accept your insurance. Also, telemedicine can work wonders and there are online companies like Talkspace (Talkspace.com), BetterHelp (BetterHelp.com), and Cerebral (Cerebral.com) that offer opportunities to engage in therapy online, from the comfort of home.

Plan B: Treating the Mind-Altering Menopause Type without Hormones

For women with the Mind-Altering type who don't have a clear reason to use HT (meaning, they don't have vasomotor symptoms, genitourinary symptoms, or osteopenia) or who can't or don't want to use HT, there are other medications we can use to address intensely disruptive menopausal symptoms. Depending on which symptoms are most distressing for a woman with this menopause type, here are some other possibilities:

- To treat depression, cognitive behavioral therapy and medication is the best form of treatment. When the medication kicks in, it often provides a psychological/emotional boost that can enhance a woman's ability to work through difficult issues in therapy and implement the CBT strategies that are discussed. There are several antidepressants from the SSRI class (including sertraline/Zoloft, citalopram/Celexa, and escitalopram/Lexapro), and SNRI class (such as venlafaxine/ Effexor and desvenlafaxine/Pristiq) that can be helpful for depression at this stage of life. Choosing an antidepressant that's likely to work for you requires a close discussion with your health-care provider. Keep in mind: The effects of antidepressants don't kick in right away—it takes four to six weeks for them to become fully effective—so you'll need to be patient. Also, some women need to try more than one antidepressant to find the one that works optimally for them. Finding the right one is often a trial-and-error process. You might have clues about the type of medication that could help you if family members have responded well to a particular drug because genetic factors can play a role here.

- For anxiety, I would most likely prescribe a low dose of citalopram (Celexa) or escitalopram (Lexapro). Other antidepressants may be helpful, too, especially if they're taken at night. The only antidepressant I would avoid for anxiety is Wellbutrin because its stimulating effects can ramp up anxiety for some women. I generally avoid regular use of benzodiazepines because they can be addictive and the longer they are used, the harder it is to come off them.

- If you have trouble with brain fog or lack of focus, the anti-depressant bupropion (Wellbutrin) may help. I would also recommend being evaluated for symptoms of ADHD (attention deficit hyperactivity disorder). I sometimes see women with undiagnosed or subclinical ADHD who have found ways to work around or compensate for it until this point in their lives—then, menopause kicks in and brings a next-level challenge that makes their symptoms more unmanageable. If bupropion doesn't help sufficiently, we might consider stepping up with a non-stimulant medication such as Strattera (atomoxetine). For women who have bonified ADHD, stimulants such as Concerta (methylphenidate) or Vyvanse (lisdexamfetamine dimesylate) may be an option.

When Mary, fifty-two, came to see me, she told me that the last year of her life had been in complete upheaval. She works as a nurse serving the underserved population of the greater Boston area, including people with high rates of alcoholism, drug use, and drug abuse. Often in her line of work, she would confiscate controlled substances when people turned them over to her in her role as a mental health provider. Needless to say, her work is stressful, and it began to take a toll on her well-being.

Out of the blue, she had developed a fear of flying (which prevented her from going to a close friend's wedding) and she developed severe depressive symptoms after her period ended permanently. Her health-care provider had started her on an antidepressant, which helped a little but not much. That's when she came to see me for her personal mash-up of depression and anxiety that kicked into high gear after menopause. Married and without children, Mary told me that she was so depressed that at times she wanted to quit her job. Also, she was overeating because her emotions were spiraling and she was frustrated with this pattern.

Because she was already on an SSRI antidepressant, I decided to put her on the weekly Climara Pro patch for HT. I also suggested she go for CBT and learn biofeedback or self-hypnosis to help her calm down in any given moment (and distract her from using food to soothe her emotions) and adopt a more regular exercise regimen to boost her spirits. She took my advice to heart. When she bounced into my office three months later, she was feeling much better and said she felt like she had gotten her life back. The day after she left my office, she was due to fly on a trip to Mexico with her husband, and she wasn't the least bit worried about getting on a plane.

LIFESTYLE INTERVENTIONS

Dietary Directives

The connection between food and mood run deep, and while there isn't a particular style of eating that will relieve mood disturbances or brain fog, you can choose foods that may have a calming effect and/or improve your ability to focus. From a high-altitude perspective, it's important to consume primarily plant-based foods (many of which support the production of serotonin), as well as adequate protein (which is key to the production of dopamine, which plays a role in learning, cognition, and memory) and healthy fats (which are important for optimal brain function).

Be careful about relying on caffeine to improve your focus or alcohol to soothe your spirits: Too much of either can worsen depression or anxiety and interfere with good-quality sleep. So instead of reaching for a cocktail, beer, or glass of wine to unwind at night, try having a cup of warm herbal tea (such as chamomile, passionflower, or valerian root) to help promote better sleep, which will contribute to sharper thinking and memory performance.

Although consuming alcohol can have a relaxing effect at first and can even make you feel drowsy, it can prevent you from getting the deep sleep you want and need. Limit your caffeine intake to the early part of the day to prevent it from impairing your *zzz*'s, too.

Here's a look at some specific nutrients that may help with different symptoms you may be experiencing with the Mind-Altering Menopause Type:

- **Isoflavones:** These have estrogen-like properties (albeit weaker ones than the estrogen the body produces). Isoflavones in plant foods—including soy foods, chickpeas, fava beans, pistachios, peanuts, and other fruits, legumes, and nuts— support the production of serotonin, which has a calming effect on your mind.
- **Tryptophan:** The essential amino acid tryptophan is involved in the production of serotonin. The body can't produce tryptophan so it needs to be obtained from foods like milk, tuna, turkey, chicken, fish, oats, nuts and seeds, pineapple, bananas, kiwi fruit, and tomatoes.
- **Tyrosine:** A nonessential amino acid, tyrosine can improve alertness, attention, and concentration, and because it is turned into dopamine and other neurotransmitters, it may help relieve depression. Good dietary sources of tyrosine include soy products, chicken, turkey, fish, peanuts, almonds, avocados, bananas, milk, cheese, yogurt, lima beans, pumpkin seeds, and sesame seeds.
- **Magnesium:** This mighty mineral can help reduce stress and may promote a better night's sleep. Good dietary sources of magnesium include almonds, cashews, peanuts, chia and pumpkin seeds, edamame, black beans, yogurt, quinoa, and fortified breakfast cereals.

- **Omega-3 fatty acids:** A higher fish intake has been associated with a reduced risk of depression in both men and women—and there's no mystery as to why: Fish and seafood are good sources of omega-3 fatty acids. The omega-3 fatty acid docosahexaenoic acid (DHA) is a major component of brain cell membranes, and DHA along with eicosapentaenoic acid (EPA) have a wide variety of beneficial effects on neuronal functioning and inflammation and may help prevent vascular dementia and age-related cognitive decline.[21] What's more, a study in a 2021 issue of *Nutrition Research and Practice*[22] found that postmenopausal women with the highest omega-3 fatty acid intake from food had a lower prevalence of depression than women with the lowest intake.

- **Choline:** An essential nutrient, choline is needed to make the neurotransmitter acetylcholine, which is essential for memory and other brain functions as well as mood regulation.[23] Choline is present in eggs, lean meat, poultry, fish, beans, and quinoa—choline content is directly associated with the protein content in foods.

- **Lutein:** A potent carotenoid (antioxidant), lutein has beneficial effects on brain health during learning and while performing cognitive tasks as people get older.[24] Egg yolks are rich in highly bioavailable lutein, and leafy greens (such as kale and spinach), corn, bell peppers, and pistachios are also good sources of lutein.

Here's what a day's meal plan might look like:

Breakfast: Wild Blueberry Overnight Oats: Mix together ½ cup old-fashioned rolled oats, ½ cup unsweetened fortified soy milk, ¼ cup plain nonfat Greek yogurt, sweetener of your choice, and ½ teaspoon chia seeds. Place in a sealed container and refrigerate overnight. To serve, top with 1 cup wild blueberries (fresh or frozen and thawed).

Lunch: Salad made with 2 cups baby spinach, ½ cup canned mandarin oranges (drained), 2 chopped hard-cooked eggs, ½ cucumber peeled and chopped, ¼ cup feta cheese, and diced red onion, if desired. Top with ¼ cup lightly roasted soybeans, 1 tablespoon olive oil, and balsamic vinegar. Enjoy with 2 ounces crusty whole-grain bread.

Dinner: Baked fish in foil: 4 ounces haddock, cod, or other white fish, 2 tablespoons panko bread crumbs, 2 teaspoons olive oil, 1 cup canned drained tomatoes, and fresh parsley, as desired; 1 cup roasted cauliflower; 1 cup cooked brown rice, quinoa, or farro with 2 teaspoons olive oil.

Snacks: Smoothie made with 1 small banana, 1 cup unsweetened fortified soy milk, 1 teaspoon unsweetened cocoa powder, and 2 ice cubes; herbal tea and ¼ cup shelled pistachios

As far as dietary supplements go, I suggest taking vitamin D (800 to 1,000 IU) daily because it's difficult to get enough from food alone. If your calcium intake from food is falling short of 1,200 milligrams per day, consider taking a calcium supplement, a maximum of 500 milligrams at a time (your body can't absorb more than that).

Adaptogens—the New Kids on the Block

One of the latest buzzwords in the wellness world, adaptogens are a class of non-toxic plants—particularly herbs and roots—that are believed to provide the body with what it needs to handle physical and mental stress better. They have long been used in Chinese and Ayurvedic healing traditions, and while each adaptogen is believed to act a bit differently, they're all thought to recalibrate the body's stress response. Among the most well-researched adaptogens are:

- ashwagandha, an Ayurvedic herb that has been used to treat stress, anxiety, fatigue, sleep disturbances, and concentration difficulties
- Asian ginseng, which is often used to replenish energy, boost mood, and improve mental performance
- rhodiola, an herb that has been used to ease stress and relieve general fatigue, anxiety, headache, and depression

These days you can find adaptogens in supplements, powdered form, or in teas, tonics, and extracts, online or in health food or vitamin stores. Keep in mind that adaptogens aren't regulated by the Food and Drug Administration so it's a matter of "buyer beware" with these products, just as it is with other supplements. Some adaptogens can have problematic effects on blood sugar, blood pressure, or thyroid hormone levels, so if you have any chronic health condition or take medication on a regular basis, consult your doctor before taking adaptogens.

Exercise Rx

When it comes to physical activity and your mind, the best form of exercise is the one you'll actually do consistently. That said, there is substantial evidence that moderate-intensity aerobic exercise helps to mitigate symptoms of depression, partly by decreasing levels of pro-inflammatory cytokines[25] but also by increasing volume[26] in key areas of the brain including the hippocampus, the prefrontal cortex, and the anterior cingulate. In fact, engaging in regular aerobic exercise has been found to improve major depressive disorder as much as antidepressants do—and it has similar remission rates after one year; there's also some evidence that exercise may augment the benefits of antidepressant use[27] in a one-two punch fashion. What's more, research[28] has found that women who engage in regular physical activity at midlife have better self-esteem, which may have a positive overall effect on their mental health.

In the short term, moderate-to high-intensity exercise stimulates the release of endorphins (the body's feel-good chemicals), which can put you in a good (or at least better) mood right after your workout. By contrast, low-intensity aerobic exercise triggers the release of neurotrophic (or growth) factors that cause nerve cells to grow and forge new connections even as people get older.[29] This improvement in brain function can be a boon for women experiencing menopausal brain fog, and it can lead to a more upbeat mood in everyone because when your cognitive functioning is sharper, you tend to feel better. Regular exercise has even been shown to protect against age-related cognitive decline.[30] Keep in mind, though, that consistency is the key to reaping these mind and mood benefits; one workout won't have a sustainable effect.

The best approach is to start with physical activities, intensities, and durations that you are comfortable with and build up from there. If you include both moderate- to high-intensity activities (like Spinning or jogging) as well as lower-intensity activities (like walking), you'll maximize the release of different brain chemicals that can enhance your mood and mental functioning. And if you vary your activities, you'll keep your exercise life interesting and well-rounded for both your body and mind.

Research has found, for example, that performing water-based exercise[31] is associated with a decrease in depressive symptoms and improvements in quality of life after twelve weeks in women. A pedometer-based walking program has been found[32] to have a positive effect on depression, insomnia, and anxiety among postmenopausal women after eight weeks. Pilates training[33] led to significant improvements in sleep quality, anxiety, depression, and fatigue after twelve weeks among postmenopausal women. And postmenopausal women who participated in a hatha yoga practice for twelve weeks had a significant reduction in their stress levels and depressive symptoms and improvements in their quality of life.[34] You get the picture!

Many different physical activities can have positive effects on your mood and mind-set. My advice is to find one or two or three that appeal to you and to engage in some form of exercise at least five times per week.

Improving Your Headspace

As you've seen, the Mind-Altering Menopause Type can be a big bummer for your mood, your mind-set, and your memory. While you're addressing your symptoms from various avenues—such as medications, therapy, hormones, dietary changes, exercise, and making sleep a priority—you can take steps to harness the power of your mind and put it to good use to improve your mood and cognitive function. To that end, I recommend using the following strategies:

- **Join a mindfulness program.** Mindfulness-based stress reduction (MBSR) programs have been shown to help with a variety of physical and psychological conditions—and a study in a 2018 issue of *Scientific Reports*[35] found that MBSR can have a significant effect in reducing depression and anxiety associated with the menopausal transition. By combining mindfulness meditation, yoga, body scanning exercises, and cognitive strategies, MBSR can help you recognize your thoughts, feelings, and body sensations while developing a nonreactive awareness and acceptance of them. The net effect is to relieve the intensity of negative emotions. You can find MBSR programs online or at local health and wellness centers.

- **Put an end to rumination.** When you're feeling depressed or anxious, it's easy to fall into a pattern where you continuously mull over upsetting events or difficult challenges. You might think you're being proactive about solving your problems—but you could be engaging in a habit that can send you into a downward mood spiral. That's because rumination or overthinking "sustains or worsens sadness, fosters negatively biased thinking, impairs a person's ability to solve problems, saps motivation, and interferes with concentration and initiative," according to Sonja Lyubomirsky, PhD, a professor of psychology at the University of California, Riverside, and author of *The How of Happiness*. Research[36] has even found that depressive rumination takes a toll on cognitive processing speed and executive function. The keys to breaking a rumination habit are to recognize when you're doing it or distract yourself when you're inclined to do it; set a problem-solving time for later (say, fifteen to twenty minutes, but not before bed; then, swing into brainstorming mode during the appointed time (set an alarm to signal you to stop). With issues that can't be solved or improved, aim for a stance of acceptance.

- **Give yourself music therapy.** Recent research[37] shows that music therapy—intentionally listening to music at least three times per week—can help reduce depression and other menopausal symptoms after six weeks. The idea that listening to music can be therapeutic is hardly new; after all, it's known to stimulate the release of feel-good neurotransmitters (such as dopamine, serotonin, and endorphins) and the hormone oxytocin while decreasing the level of circulating stress hormones (such as cortisol). But this is one of the first studies to show that it can benefit women's mood symptoms during the menopausal transition. So turn on some tunes that appeal to you and let them wash over you.

- **Commune with nature.** Going for a walk on a nature trail or a hike in the woods is a good start but you can increase the mental health benefits if you fully engage your senses in the experience. How? By being mindful of the sights, sounds, aromas, and tactile sensations in your midst. This is a cornerstone of forest bathing (or *shinrin-yoku*), a Japanese walking practice that has been found to have a range of stress-reducing, health-promoting effects, including decreasing depression.[38] These perks aren't surprising given that you'll be able to look at greenery and fractals (patterns of repeated shapes of varying sizes that are abundant in nature), which send calming messages to the brain. You'll be able to smell phytoncides, which are aromatic, airborne particles emitted by plants and trees. And you'll hear soothing sounds of birds calling, the wind rustling through the trees, and perhaps the murmuring of a flowing stream. Let yourself soak in all that sensory stimuli.

- **Offload your to-do lists.** Instead of putting continuous pressure on your mind and memory to keep track of what you need to do, buy, or repair, write it down. Whether you prefer handwritten notes or lists on a digital device, you can take pressure off your overwhelmed mind by making lists and cheat sheets and relying on calendars and other scheduling aids to keep you on track. You'll be doing yourself a favor!

- **Minimize distractions.** Besides compromising your ability to perform and complete tasks, multitasking—handling multiple tasks simultaneously—decreases your awareness of your performance on those tasks (your metacognitive sensitivity, in technical terms).[39] This means you may not even know what you're not doing well when your attention is divided. That's why it's wise to try to minimize distractions and focus on doing one thing at a time if you're having memory or attention problems. Taking this approach will help improve your performance and productivity while easing the cognitive pressure you may be feeling.

- **Try tapping.** An emotional freedom technique that's sometimes referred to as psychological acupressure, tapping has been shown in scientific studies[40] to reduce anxiety, stress, posttraumatic stress disorder, depression, and cravings. By tapping your fingertips on your forehead or the side of your hand while breathing deeply, identifying the issue, and repeating an affirmation (such as "I am well" or "I am enough"), you can give yourself a mental time-out, distract yourself in a positive fashion, and stimulate the body's energy pathways (meridians) in a matter of minutes. (You can find tutorials for how to do it online.) Best of all, you can do tapping anywhere—the tools are always on hand (pun intended).

- **Use an app to soothe yourself.** These days, you can find an app for just about everything under the sun—including various aspects of psychological and emotional well-being. Whether you have an iPhone or an Android, you can find an app that will help you calm down and de-stress. Here are a few that I recommend: Calm (for promoting good sleep), Headspace (for learning mindfulness and reducing stress and anxiety), the Mindfulness App (which offers various guided meditations), and MyLife Meditation (which can help you manage your emotions in real time).

Here's something that's important to remember: The mood and cognitive effects you're experiencing with the Mind-Altering Menopause Type are likely to subside at least somewhat as your postmenopausal brain adjusts to having little to no estrogen around.[41] In fact, research[42] has found that for many women who struggle with cognitive performance during the menopausal transition, their verbal and working memory and information processing speed eventually improve to premenopausal levels over time. In other words, time may help relieve these challenges.

In the meantime, using the strategies described in this chapter as well as in the DIY menu of remedies in chapter 12 will help you personalize treatment of all your symptoms. Remember: The goal is to help you regain your physical, emotional, and mental equilibriums so that you can get back to feeling like yourself again. With some patience, flexibility, and creativity, I'm confident that we can get you there.

9

The Seemingly Never-Ending Menopause Type

For some women, one of the strategies that helps them navigate the bumpy road of menopause is the knowledge that it's really just a phase of life and eventually the disruptive symptoms will fade into the past. But . . . *what if they don't?* The reality is, some women have one or two symptoms such as the occasional hot flash, persistent vaginal dryness, or low libido, or less common ones like dizziness, olfactory changes (as in sensing bad odors), or their own changes in body odor that start at menopause and never seem to go away. Usually, these women assume these symptoms will dissipate, and the fact that they're not horribly bothersome makes them fall lower on their priority list of things to take care of. But even with just one or two unpleasant menopausal symptoms, women shouldn't feel embarrassed, silly, or like they're bothering their doctor by bringing them up. I firmly believe that every woman deserves to feel and function at her best, regardless of what's happening to her hormonally.

Consider Marian, who was sixty-four when she first came to my office. Menopausal at fifty, she suffered occasional hot flashes and vaginal dryness but as a working mother with three teenagers, she felt too busy to seek treatment. Eventually she tried over-the-counter menopausal dietary supplements and herbal remedies for her hot flashes, but they continued to come and go for many years. What bothered Marian the most were the persistent vaginal dryness and pain with intercourse she was experiencing, though she also had some urinary incontinence and frequent urinary tract infections (UTIs). These symptoms were so bad that she had been avoiding sex with her husband for a couple of years, which was disappointing and frustrating for both of them.

When Marian came to see me, we discussed her symptoms and preferences and decided to treat the dryness issue with a vaginal estrogen cream at night for two weeks; then, I had her taper down to a maintenance regimen, two or three times a week at night. She also started doing pelvic floor therapy to help with painful intercourse and she began using vaginal dilators to ever-so-gently expand her tight vaginal tissue and relax the pelvic floor muscles, in order to make intercourse more comfortable. To treat her hot flashes and incontinence, she began taking oxybutynin, an anti-cholinergic drug that's used to treat an overactive bladder. By taking these steps, four to six months later she was able to have pain-free sex again and reported a nearly 100 percent improvement in UTIs and a 75 percent improvement in hot flashes.

Lingering menopause symptoms can affect a woman's quality of life, her ability to function, and her state of mind. A 2015 study[1] that included more than seven thousand postmenopausal women from the US and Europe found that the presence of moderate to severe symptoms of vulvovaginal atrophy (now called the genitourinary syndrome of menopause, GSM)—specifically vaginal dryness, irritation, and pain during sexual intercourse—was associated with clinically meaningful decreases in quality of life, comparable to those seen with medical conditions such as arthritis, chronic obstructive pulmonary disease, asthma, and irritable bowel syndrome. Meanwhile, a study in a 2020 issue of the journal *Menopause*[2] found that women with vulvovaginal atrophy (a.k.a. GSM) have higher rates of depression and anxiety after menopause. The consequences can be significant.

What's more, the quality of a woman's sleep during the meno-pausal transition can have lasting effects on the quality of her slumber and her physical functionality after menopause and into older adulthood: A study in a 2021 issue of the journal *Sleep*[3] found that women with consistently high insomnia symptoms—including trouble falling asleep, frequent night-time awakenings, and/or early morning awakenings—had a slower gait speed while walking than those with few insomnia symptoms; that's a worrisome sign for their future health and functionality. Other research[4] has linked menopausal sleep disturbances with persistent insomnia and various physical impairments as well as cognitive and emotional impairments. The ripple effects are considerable!

Part of the issue is that some women with the Seemingly Never-Ending Menopause Type fall into the trap of thinking that nothing can be done about their enduring symptoms because they're just an inevitable part of aging. For example, a 2021 study[5] found that while genitourinary symptoms—such as vaginal dryness, irritation, itching, and dyspareunia (painful intercourse)—are quite prevalent among women during the menopausal transition, women are frequently unaware of their connection to menopause and their treatment options. (This is particularly unfortunate because unlike most menopausal symptoms, which naturally subside over time, these symptoms can persist throughout the rest of a woman's life unless she does something to address them.) And when women experience severe urogenital symptoms during or after the menopausal transition, they often have poorer sexual function—including challenges with lubrication, satisfaction, arousal, and orgasm, research has found.[6]

Another trap some women fall into is they assume that their menopausal symptoms will eventually stop (they have to, right?) so they try to grin and bear them. But then, years go by without any significant changes in those symptoms. It's important to remember that while the average length of menopausal symptoms is five to seven years, about 10 percent of women have symptoms that last longer than that.

To be honest, we don't have a full understanding about why some women experience lingering symptoms of menopause while others don't. It may be that some women's estrogen receptors just don't get the memo that they're no longer needed so these receptors continue to fire, looking for estrogen. There may also be a genetic component. And other risk factors are emerging through research. In a study[7] involving more than three thousand women, researchers from Wake Forest School of Medicine in Winston-Salem, North Carolina, found that women who begin experiencing hot flashes and night sweats during *perimenopause* were more likely to have these vasomotor symptoms frequently—and have them last for more than seven years (some lasted nearly twelve years!). This study also found that women who reported more stress and sensitivity to these vasomotor symptoms were more likely to have long-lasting effects, and the same was true of women who had more symptoms of depression and anxiety when these symptoms began. What's more, some evidence suggests that women who are current or former smokers or who are overweight are more likely to experience persistent or enduring vasomotor symptoms.

Yet another trap that women fall into is they don't get around to making an appointment for a doctor's visit for themselves because they're so busy taking care of everyone else in their lives while also juggling work and home responsibilities. Some of these women are dealing with caregiver strain from tending to older parents or other relatives, growing children (and their needs and activities), and sometimes their spouses; this web of caregiving can leave them feeling frayed at the edges and with little time or energy for self-care. (This phenomenon is often referred to as "role overload" or the "spillover effect.") Research[8] has found that sometimes it's the social circumstances of women's lives and their daily stress that have a more powerful effect on their health at midlife than the severity of their hot flashes.

There's also a subtype of the Seemingly Never-Ending Menopause Type that I call the Boomerang Type, where symptoms such as hot flashes, night sweats, and sleep disturbances might go away for a while then come back. Sometimes their return is seasonal; other times it seems random in terms of timing. We aren't sure why this happens. One theory is that the window for flexibility in body temperature regulation narrows when women lose estrogen at menopause but then the system may regain some flexibility—which might cause waves of menopausal symptoms to come and go. Or, the boomerang pattern might have to do with estrogen receptors getting retriggered, perhaps by changes in a woman's stress levels or sleep patterns. There is still much to be learned about this phenomenon.

DRILLING DOWN TO THE DETAILS

Let's take a closer look at some of the most common symptoms of the Seemingly Never-Ending Menopause Type. This is by no means a complete list of the symptoms that can stick around longer than women expect. These are simply the issues that I often see in my clinical practice.

Urinary incontinence: It can start with a drop or a trickle, perhaps when you cough, sneeze, laugh, or lift weights, or even while you're having sex. When a woman begins to leak urine frequently or severely enough for it to become a real nuisance, it's considered incontinence (a.k.a. loss of bladder control)—a problem that's surprisingly common, affecting more than 50 percent of women after menopause.[9]

There are two primary types of urinary incontinence: stress incontinence and urge incontinence.[10] Stress incontinence is characterized by urine leakage when there's increased abdominal pressure (from coughing, sneezing, bending over, and the like). Weight gain can worsen stress incontinence, and when women lose estrogen during the menopausal transition, there can be a weakening of the pelvic floor muscles that can increase the risk of urine leakage.

By contrast, urge incontinence reflects an involuntary loss of urine that can happen when a woman has that sudden gotta-go feeling and can't get to the bathroom fast enough; it occurs as a result of an imbalance between inhibitory and excitatory mechanisms in the detrusor muscle in the bladder wall, which contracts to push the urine out of the bladder and relaxes to keep it stored. Urge incontinence (a.k.a. overactive bladder)[11] can happen as a result of neurologic disorders or chronic irritation in the bladder (which can stem from trying to go to the bathroom when you don't really have to) but sometimes the causes are unclear.

For both types of incontinence, there are various treatment options—such as bladder training, pelvic floor muscle training (hello, Kegels!), biofeedback and pelvic stimulation, and medications—that can help. If you're not leaking consistently, I recommend bringing an extra pair of underwear with you because the purpose of underwear is to protect your pants; if you're wearing a pantyliner on a daily basis as a form of insurance, it's likely to irritate the labia. If you're leaking a fair amount of urine consistently, my recommendation is to see a urogynecologist who can help determine an appropriate treatment for your form of incontinence.

When Monica, sixty, a realtor, came to see me, she was having recurrent urinary tract infections, burning sensations with urination, and leaky bladder symptoms every time she walked into her house. As soon as she opened the front door, she had to run to the bathroom—sometimes she'd make it in time and sometimes she'd leak a little before she got there. This frustrated her to no end. She even avoided intercourse with her husband because she was afraid of leaking urine. Monica was wearing maxi pads every day because her underwear would be wet by the end of the day.

To treat her recurrent UTIs, I started her on Vagifem estradiol vaginal inserts nightly for two weeks, then dropped it down to twice a week. By decreasing the pH of the genitourinary region to a more acidic environment that's inhospitable to bacteria, the estrogen decreases the risk of UTIs. I discouraged her from wearing maxi pads and pantyliners regularly because trapping the moisture in these could create a breeding ground for yeast or bacterial infections, as well as irritating the labia and the urethra. To get her off her pads/liners, I recommended she buy some Dear Kate underwear (dearkates.com), which is made of moisture-wicking layers of fabric that protect women from leaks, stains, and odors. I also sent her to a pelvic floor physiotherapist to help her retrain her brain so she wouldn't leak at the sound of running water or other triggers. Within eight weeks, her symptoms of burning with urination had improved considerably and she began working with a urogynecologist—at my recommendation—to deal with what sounded to me like stress or mixed incontinence. I explained that just because she was leaking urine didn't mean that she had to accept it.

Sexual difficulties: If your libido does a disappearing (or diminishing) act and you have decreased thoughts or fantasies about sex and this bothers you, you may have developed hypoactive sexual desire disorder (HSDD), which occurs in approximately 12 percent of women ages forty-five to sixty-four.[12] One of the keys to making this diagnosis is: Low libido that doesn't cause considerable distress to you and/or your relationship doesn't make the cut; it has to bother you. In my clinical practice, many women who have these symptoms tell me that they either miss this sexual part of themselves or that it bothers their partner or their relationship so much that they want to do something about it.

Low libido can happen at this stage of life for a couple of

reasons. First, there's the loss of estrogen and testosterone as women go into menopause, which can dampen sexual desire. Second, there is some sort of evolutionary switch after you're no longer able to have children that can turn off or turn down sexual desire; it's no longer needed to propagate the species because a postmenopausal woman can't. Also, when a woman's life becomes overwhelmed with demands from numerous directions (work, multiple generations of the family, and so on), this can take a toll on her libido. Another factor that can contribute: When men experience erectile dysfunction, which becomes increasingly common with advancing age, it can lead to decreased sexual desire in women, research has found.[13] It really does take two to make things go right in the bedroom.

Here's the hitch: The longer you go without having sex and/or with having low sexual desire, the harder it can be for it to come back naturally. Fortunately, there are things we can do to help you get back that loving feeling.

After their kids had grown up and moved out of the house, Tia, sixty-six, came to me because her long-term partner was interested in rekindling their sex life. She realized it had been a long time since she found sex to be intriguing or pleasurable. And she told me that she wouldn't mind if she never had sex again, but that her partner might be pretty bummed about this. I asked some questions about the state of her relationship and she said she felt like she was in a loving, trusting partnership, so that wasn't the issue. Then, we discussed various strategies. I encouraged her to download the Rosy app (meetrosy.com), which addresses various aspects of women's sexual health, and to start reading some mild erotica to retrain her brain about sex—and remind her that it can be fun.

I also encouraged her to start with simple forms of touching like holding hands and accepting massages from her partner, because she realized it had been so long since they even embraced or had any foreplay. As they did this, she noticed that she started having some thoughts of sex. We then discussed that planning sex or planning to be intimate is often the better way to start back up again than to rely on spontaneity.

Things started to become more active in the bedroom but Tia was experiencing moderate pain with intercourse so I gave her vaginal Premarin cream to use twice weekly at night and a vaginal moisturizer to use on the other nights. With that, she was able to comfortably have penetrative sex—but she couldn't have an orgasm, which was a change from her younger days. After she tried using a couple of different sex toys without much success, I suggested she try using a topical, very low-dose testosterone preparation twice a week to improve blood flow to the labia and clitoris. This helped her orgasms, and while they weren't as powerful as when she was twenty-seven, she was happy to have this upgrade in sexual arousal and pleasure.

Genitourinary syndrome of menopause (GSM): With this phenomenon,[14] a variety of changes and symptoms can occur to the vaginal and vulvar tissue, as well as the urinary tract (including the bladder and urethra). Due to the loss of estrogen and the changes in the pH level of the tissue, which shuts down production of natural moisturizers and lubricants, the tissue itself becomes thin, dry, and less elastic after menopause. This can lead to tearing and bleeding during sex or to frequent urinary tract infections (UTIs). In some instances, a woman may feel like she has a UTI because the acidic urine irritates the dry urethra, even when she doesn't test positive for an infection.

In a tangentially related issue, some menopausal women find themselves getting up multiple times during the night to urinate, a condition called nocturia. This can happen as a result of the loss of estrogen and weakening of the pelvic floor. Besides being annoying and disruptive in their own right, these awakenings can cause some women to have trouble going back to sleep, which can lead to insufficient sleep or poor sleep over time, which can have unfortunate consequences for the way they feel and function during the day.

High pelvic tone: At first glance, this may sound like a good thing—after all, muscle tone is a highly coveted goal with strength training. In this case, however, high pelvic tone refers to a form of dysfunction that occurs when there is *too much* tension in the pelvic floor muscles. You want to be able to relax and tighten the muscles of the pelvic floor at will. High pelvic tone typically involves an unconscious tightening of these muscles, and it can affect a woman's sexual health, making it uncomfortable for her to have intercourse or even a pelvic exam. You might realize you have high pelvic tone if you notice that when you and your partner attempt to have intercourse or insert a sex toy, you feel as though you are squeezing your muscles to try to keep a penis or toy out of your vagina. Maybe you're doing this because you know it's going to hurt or maybe you're doing this without meaning to (which may be a sign of vaginismus, a condition involving the involuntary tensing or contracting of muscles around the vagina).

Kegels 101

In order to reap the pelvic floor–strengthening benefits from Kegel exercises, you need to do them correctly.[15] (Not everyone does.) In other words, you need to find the right muscles to contract and relax. One way to do this is to stop the stream of urine while you're peeing; if you can do that, you've identified the right muscles. (Don't do this on a regular basis, though, because it can lead to incomplete emptying of the bladder, which increases the risk of UTIs.)

The next step is to do Kegel exercises when your bladder is empty. You can do the exercises in any position—while lying down, sitting, or standing—by focusing on tightening only your pelvic floor muscles (not the muscles in your abdomen, thighs, or butt). Hold the contractions for two to three seconds then release; work up to doing at least three sets of ten to fifteen repetitions per day. (But don't overdo it: These muscles can suffer from overtraining and fatigue just like other muscles.)

If you have trouble isolating the right muscles, ask your health-care provider for guidance; in some instances, vaginal cones, biofeedback, or pelvic floor physical therapy can help you perfect your technique.

MAKING TREATMENT DECISIONS

With lingering menopause symptoms, the treatment depends entirely on what the distressing symptoms are. If these never-ending symptoms include hot flashes, night sweats, or severe genitourinary problems, hormone therapy (HT) may be an option. It used to be that there was a time limit to taking hormone therapy but that's not entirely true anymore—now the issue of timing depends on when a woman starts using systemic hormone therapy. Currently, the prevailing viewpoint is that for optimal safety, HT can be started in healthy symptomatic women who are within ten years of menopause or younger than age sixty and do not have contraindications to using HT,[16] according to the North American Menopause Society (NAMS). What this means in practical terms is that: If systemic hormone therapy is initiated within the ten-year window, there isn't an absolute time limit as long as your medical doctor clears you to continue taking HT.

As far as the Seemingly Never-Ending Menopause Type goes,

extending the use of HT "with the lowest effective dose is acceptable under some circumstances such as for the woman who has persistent bothersome menopausal symptoms," according to a NAMS position statement. "Use of HT should be individualized and not discontinued solely based on a woman's age." This really is an issue where shared decision-making comes into play.

In my own clinical practice, I treat some women who want to wean themselves off HT, in which case we can either slowly reduce their dosage or stop cold turkey. The truth is, if hot flashes are going to return after going off HT, it doesn't matter if you wean down slowly or go off HT suddenly. If I'm given a choice, I do sometimes lean toward the weaning-down approach because this way we can find out if they will feel well at a lower dose. If hot flashes return, we can decide whether to try to control them by going back on the previous HT dose or with lifestyle modifications or supplements if they're mild.

If a woman's lingering symptoms aren't in the vasomotor or genitourinary syndrome categories, there are oral medications we can consider using to treat her symptoms. In some instances various forms of therapy—such as biofeedback, pelvic floor physical therapy, and cognitive behavioral therapy for insomnia (CBT-I)[17]—may be beneficial. And lifestyle modifications can make a difference. The good news is: Help is available for menopausal symptoms that go on and on and on.

BASELINE TREATMENT PLANS FOR THE SEEMINGLY NEVER-ENDING MENOPAUSE TYPE

What follows are two baseline treatment plans for women who have the Seemingly Never-Ending Menopause Type. The first treatment plan focuses on the use of hormone therapy (HT); the second plan addresses how to treat your symptoms without hormones. Whichever treatment plan you choose, you'll also find recommendations for lifestyle modifications that are suitable for all women with this type. Keep in mind that if you have additional symptoms that aren't relieved by these recommended interventions, you can choose from the extensive menu of symptom-oriented solutions in chapter 12 to ease what's still bothering you. The goal is to make this plan work for you.

Plan A: Using Hormone Therapy

For women with seemingly never-ending hot flashes, night sweats, or severe genitourinary symptoms who want to use hormone therapy and don't have any contraindications to doing so, there are a few options. She can start with a weekly low-dose estrogen patch (0.025 or 0.0375 milligrams) and add 100 milligrams oral progesterone (Prometrium) at night if the woman has an intact uterus. This dose is lower than what we use for many other menopause types (Premature, Sudden, or Full-Throttle)—because often the severity of the symptoms is much less with this type; a little HT goes a long way in helping mild to moderate lingering symptoms. If a woman is more than ten years past menopause and her symptoms are severe, we can have a detailed discussion about the pros and cons of starting systemic HT now, based on her current health and medical history.

If symptoms are mostly related to vaginal atrophy or GSM (such as vaginal dryness and painful intercourse), I would consider local vaginal HT with the Estring, a vaginal ring that slowly releases a steady amount of estrogen into the vagina for three months. It is safe to use at any time and for any duration, as long as it is replaced every three months. One of the beauties of this approach is it's a set-it-and-forget-it method: It stays in place and doesn't need to be taken out for sex (though it can be) and the woman shouldn't feel it. If the Estring is not covered by insurance, or if a woman doesn't like this approach, then she can use a local estrogen suppository or cream nightly for two weeks and then two or three times a week at night for maintenance.

Another treatment option to consider is the Femring, a vaginal ring that releases estrogen over the course of three months; the difference is it releases a higher dose of estrogen than Estring so it is considered systemic HT, which means it can help with hot flashes, night sweats, and other systemic symptoms, too. If a woman is using Femring and she has a uterus, she will need to take 100 milligrams oral progesterone (Prometrium) at night to protect her uterus. If the lingering symptoms are hot flashes, night sweats, or severe GSM repercussions, the goal is for a woman to end up with blood levels of estrogen in the low 40s pg/mL.

For low libido, a woman could consider a very low-dose topical testosterone in the form of a cream or gel to be applied once daily if she has low testosterone levels. (Testosterone levels drop at menopause and it often ends up being too low for some women.) She doesn't need to be on estrogen or progesterone HT; she can just use testosterone for the sole purpose of treating low libido. The goal is to use a dose that's within the normal range for a woman and to keep her testosterone level within that normal range—but the upper end of normal—for a woman.

If a woman has trouble with sexual arousal or orgasm, I will sometimes add in a very low dose of a blend of compounded estradiol and testosterone in a cream that's applied daily to the labia and clitoris. If the problem is severe, I have women use a pea-sized amount nightly for two weeks, then taper down to every other day or twice weekly; if the symptoms are more mild, she can use it at night two to three times per week. With this treatment, there is no systemic increase in either estrogen or testosterone levels.

Plan B: Treating the Seemingly Never-Ending Menopause Type without Hormones

For women who don't have a clear reason to use hormone therapy or who have clear contraindications to using it, there are other medications that can address her bothersome lingering symptoms. Depending on the symptoms that are most distressing, here are some possible treatments:

- To treat severe, persistent hot flashes, if a woman is more than ten years past menopause, antidepressants from the selective serotonin reuptake inhibitor (SSRI) and serotonin and norepinephrine reuptake inhibitor (SNRI) classes can be used at low doses in an off-label capacity. In particular, research[18] has shown that paroxetine (Paxil), escitalopram (Lexapro), citalopram (Celexa), desvenlafaxine (Pristiq), and venlafaxine (Effexor) can reduce the frequency and severity of hot flashes. If a woman doesn't want to take an antidepressant, alternatives for relieving hot flashes include gabapentin (an anti-seizure drug that's often used for nerve pain), or oxybutynin (which is typically used for overactive bladder).
- If you're having severe symptoms of vaginal atrophy such as vaginal dryness and pain with intercourse, using a prescription non-hormonal oral medication called ospemifene (Osphena) might help. It's part of a class of drugs called selective estrogen receptor modulators (SERMs), which means it has estrogen-like effects on certain parts of the body but not others; as a result, it can help with changes in the vaginal tissue caused by menopause without affecting other parts of the body. As a side benefit, it can benefit bone health.[19] For vaginal dryness, I recommend that all women use a daily vaginal moisturizer (such as those from SweetSpot Labs or FemmePharma).

- For low libido, a woman can take Addyi (a.k.a. flibanserin), an oral medication that increases dopamine in the brain, which has a mood-enhancing effect and improves sexual functioning. Alternatively, the injectable drug Vyleesi can be used for low libido on an as-needed basis.

- If a woman has high pelvic tone or vaginismus, she may want to consider pelvic floor physical therapy (PFPT), which can help her learn to relax or better utilize the muscles of the pelvic floor. Sometimes it involves doing exercises for the core, including the low back and hip flexors; other times, using vaginal dilators—devices that can help relax the tense pelvic floor muscles—while doing specific exercises can help make intercourse more comfortable. Once these exercises are learned, women can do them on their own at home. (*Psst*: I really like the Milli vaginal trainer device—milliforher .com—because it can change sizes and vibrates for increased blood flow.) For pain with intercourse, over-the-counter lubricants (such as überlube or Slippery Stuff) are essential.

- If the need to urinate is sending you to the bathroom multiple times per night, make an effort to decrease how much liquid (especially alcohol and caffeine) you're drinking in the evenings. You also may want to talk to your doctor about whether an underlying medical condition (like diabetes) or a medication (such as a diuretic) that you're taking could be causing these nighttime awakenings.

Testing, Testing

With some symptoms that seem to be never-ending, I recommend that women have certain tests to see if something other than menopause could be causing the lingering distress. Being able to distinguish between possible causal factors will help guide the treatment. Here are my basic recommendations in this realm:

- Women with exceptionally long-lasting hot flashes should have an A1C and a TSH test to check for diabetes and a thyroid disorder, respectively. (Some symptoms of these medical conditions can mimic those seen in the menopausal transition.)
- For ongoing or recurrent pain with urination, I recommend women have a urine culture to see if it's due to a true bacterial urinary tract infection, which needs to be treated with antibiotics. If it's not, it's more likely to be related to the genitourinary syndrome of menopause (GSM), which warrants a different approach.
- For recurrent vaginitis, a woman should have vaginal cultures done to look for yeast and bacterial vaginosis, an infection that's caused by an overgrowth of bacteria naturally found in the vagina. If either of these is present, specific medications may be in order.
- If a woman has moderate to severe urinary incontinence, I would recommend seeing a urogynecologist for further testing and evaluation.

LIFESTYLE INTERVENTIONS

Dietary Directives

Because the lingering symptoms associated with the Seemingly Never-Ending Menopause Type are so varied, there isn't an eating plan that can address all of them. That said, making a point to consume adequate protein from a variety of plant and animal foods and fiber from whole grains, fruits, vegetables, legumes, nuts, and seeds will be beneficial for your overall health. This style of eating will also help you stay energized and satiated. In addition, protein digestion requires more energy, which may provide a slight edge when it comes to weight control. In the meantime, reduce your intake of highly refined carbohydrates, such as chips, cookies, and candy; besides helping with blood sugar regulation, ditching the starchy, low-nutrient carbs will help you achieve and maintain a healthy weight, which could in turn result in fewer hot flashes.

Keep in mind that alcohol and caffeine can trigger hot flashes in some women—so pay attention to whether they have this effect on you—and they can prevent you from getting the deep sleep you need. Stick with a moderate intake of caffeine and alcohol, if you do consume them. Avoid consuming caffeine after early afternoon at the latest—and skip the nightcap. If you want to have a beverage that will help you feel sleepy, try having a cup of warm chamomile, passionflower, or valerian root tea (or another non-caffeinated tea of your choosing).

Here are some specific nutrients that may help with different symptoms you may be experiencing with the Seemingly Never-Ending Menopause Type:

- **Isoflavones from soy foods:** These have estrogen-like properties, but they're much weaker than the estrogen the body produces—which means they may help calm hot flashes in some women. Soy isoflavones are made up primarily of the compounds genistein and daidzein. Good food sources include tofu, miso, edamame, and tempeh. Other (non-soy) isoflavones are found in chickpeas, fava beans, pistachios, peanuts, legumes, and nuts, while phytoestrogens (plant-based estrogens) are also present in plums, pears, apples, grapes, spinach, grains, garlic, and onions. An added perk: The isoflavones in plant foods also support the production of serotonin, a mood-boosting neurotransmitter (brain chemical).

- **Tryptophan, melatonin, and B6:** The amino acid tryptophan plays a role in making melatonin, a sleep-promoting hormone, as well as serotonin. Tryptophan is an essential amino acid, which means the body can't produce it—but you can get it from foods like milk, tuna, turkey, chicken, fish, oats, nuts, and seeds. Vitamin B6 is also important for melatonin production; good food sources include chickpeas, tuna, salmon, chicken, fortified cereals, and banana.[20] You can consume melatonin in milk, oats, and nuts (especially pistachios), as well as tart cherries, grapes, eggs, kiwi, strawberries, peppers, and mushrooms.[21]

Here's what a day's meal plan might look like:

Breakfast: 1 cup low-fat whole-grain cereal (not granola) with 1 cup unsweetened fortified soy milk, 1 banana

Lunch: Chicken and bean wrap: 1 medium 100 percent whole-wheat tortilla, 3 ounces cooked sliced chicken or turkey, ¼ cup canned, drained black beans, ¼ sliced red bell pepper, ¼ cup shredded cheddar cheese

Dinner: 4 ounces cooked pork tenderloin, 1½ cups steamed or roasted broccoli topped with 2 teaspoons sesame seeds, 2 ounces crusty whole-grain bread with 1 to 2 teaspoons olive oil

Snacks: ½ cup lightly salted roasted soybeans; 1 cup plain fat-free Greek or Icelandic yogurt and 1 cup fresh or frozen and thawed raspberries

As far as dietary supplements go, I suggest taking vitamin D (800 to 1,000 IU) daily because it's difficult to get enough from food alone. If your calcium intake from food is falling short of 1,200 milligrams per day, consider taking a calcium supplement, a maximum of 500 milligrams at a time (your body can't absorb more than that).

In addition, you may want to consider[b]:

- Black cohosh supplements if you have unrelenting hot flashes. Made from the plant's roots and rhizomes (underground stems), these supplements come in forms such as powdered whole herb, liquid extracts, and dried extracts in pill form.[22] Do not use these if you have a liver disorder!
- Equelle, a plant-based compound that mimics the effects of estrogen, which may help with hot flashes. Or Estroven, which contains herbs and soy isoflavones and claims to relieve a variety of menopausal symptoms.

---

[b]Dietary supplements, including herbal supplements, are not regulated by the FDA. I am recommending certain supplements because I have seen some of my patients benefit from them. But it's essential that you discuss using any dietary supplement with your doctor; sometimes certain supplements can have problematic interactions with medications and this is something you'll want to avoid.

Exercise Rx

Let's face it: The Seemingly Never-Ending Menopause Type is a test of your endurance. So the last thing you want your workout regimen to feel like is an endurance challenge—unless of course you happen to love doing marathons or triathlons, in which case, I say: More power to you! Otherwise, my advice is to choose forms of physical activity that you enjoy and that make you feel good. That could be moderate-intensity aerobic exercise in the form of brisk walking, cycling, swimming, aqua aerobics, or dancing—or more vigorous exercise such as Spinning or jogging.

It's important to engage in some form of aerobic exercise at least four times per week for the sake of your current and long-term heart and lung health. In addition, you should do resistance training—whether you lift weights or use weight machines or exercise bands or your own body weight—at least twice a week to protect your muscle mass, bone mass, and metabolism. (You could also try the HIIT workout in the appendix.)

Keep in mind that you also may benefit from doing gentle, calming exercises like yoga, Pilates, tai chi, or qigong (an ancient Chinese practice that combines slow, deliberate movements, meditation, and specific breathing patterns). These can help with balance, flexibility, posture, and strength—and because they're mind-body disciplines, they're a great way to distract yourself from your ongoing symptoms; they have also been shown to relieve psychological symptoms such as anxiety and depression. Believe it or not, Pilates has even been shown to improve sexual functioning in women.[23]

Improving Your Headspace

As you've seen, the Seemingly Never-Ending Menopause Type can challenge your patience and stamina, given that there's no clear end in sight. While you're addressing your lingering symptoms from various directions—such as medications, hormones, dietary changes, exercise, and making sleep a priority—you also can recruit your mind as your ally and put it to good use to improve your ability to cope with your symptoms. To that end, I recommend using the following strategies:

- **Practice acceptance.** Rather than resenting or chafing against your lingering symptoms, try to consciously accept that the situation is the way it is—for now, anyway—and acknowledge how it's affecting you. When you let yourself feel the way you feel and you accept those feelings without judging or reacting to them, you'll improve your ability to tolerate the discomfort and move through it. Don't get me wrong: I'm not saying to suck it up and deal with it; I'm trying to help you cultivate patience and acceptance as you pursue treatments that help you.

- **Cut yourself some slack.** As you continue to navigate this journey, it may help to make a concerted effort to keep your expectations of yourself realistic—and to lighten your load of responsibilities when you're not feeling well. Research[24] has found that exercising self-compassion—being kind, supportive, and understanding toward yourself during a difficult time (just as you would be toward a friend)—during menopause is associated with greater well-being among women at midlife.

- **Take breaks to recharge.** Periodically during the day, take ten or fifteen minutes to do something that grounds you or refreshes you. That could mean taking a walk outside, doing gentle stretching or deep-breathing exercises, listening to enjoyable music, or meditating. Give some thought to what helps *you* rejuvenate yourself or release your personal decompression valve, then dedicate time-outs to use those strategies. Think of this as a way to comfort yourself before you start feeling unsettled or exhausted.

- **Mine your personal history for lessons.** Think about difficult times or situations you've dealt with in the past, contemplate the specific approaches that helped you get through them, and consider whether some of those strategies might help you now. Maybe talking to a therapist or a trusted friend, getting extra sleep, or lightening your workload helped you navigate that unsettled period. Consider whether it's worth putting one or more of those strategies into practice again. By revisiting these past experiences, you'll also remind yourself that you're stronger and more resilient than you may realize.

- **Nurture your friendships.** You're probably familiar with the fight-or-flight response that comes from stress. Did you know that there's another stress response—called the "tend and befriend" response—that's more common among women? It's mediated by the release of oxytocin (often called the "cuddle hormone")[25] and various feel-good brain chemicals. You don't need to have a squad of friends to reap these benefits; having a few close friendships will help you navigate life's ups and downs, including menopause. The key is to cultivate those valuable friendships, maintain them, and turn to them when you need support, a dose of inspiration, or a healthy distraction.

- **Schedule time to watch something humorous.** We've all heard that laughter is good medicine. Well, get this: The physical and psychological benefits can appear before you even start to chuckle. Researchers[26] have shown that the anticipation of a mirthful laughter experience—such as planning to watch a funny video or movie later—triggers the release of endorphins (feel-good, pain-relieving chemicals) and human growth hormone (which helps with immune function), *and* it reduces circulating levels of three different stress hormones during the anticipation. That's right—the feel-good perks kick in immediately, long before the show begins.

- **Strike a ragdoll pose.** A cross between a muscle-relaxation technique and a deep-breathing exercise, the Robot Ragdoll technique involves tensing then relaxing your body in an effort to reset and rebalance it. Here's how to do it: Stand up straight and stiffen your body as if you were a robot—take a big breath in through your nose and hold it as you make all the muscles from your head to your toes really tight for five seconds. Then, release all the tension in your muscles and allow your body to go loose and floppy like a ragdoll, as you exhale slowly through your mouth. Repeat this pattern until you feel calmer and more relaxed.

- **Seek caregiving support.** If you're overwhelmed by the responsibility of caring for various family members, you may want to take steps to ease the stress from caring for aging relatives. Look for additional sources of emotional, financial, and practical support such as respite care, daycare, and social services.[27] Some good resources for these forms of help include: Eldercare Locator (Eldercare.acl.gov), the Family Caregiver Alliance (Caregiver.org), the Medicare Hotline (Medicare .gov), the National Alliance for Caregiving (Caregiving.org), and the Caregiver Action Network (Caregiveraction.org).

Rest assured: If you have additional menopausal symptoms that linger, you can personalize your treatment plan by consulting the DIY menu of remedies in chapter 12. There, you'll find just about every menopausal symptom ever experienced, along with evidence-based approaches that can help relieve them. By taking charge of all your symptoms, you can reclaim your physical and emotional well-being—and start to envision the end of this long chapter in your life. It really will come—and sooner if you use the advice in this book. Trust me!

10

The Silent Menopause Type

One of my patients, Susan, sixty-four, had an easy menopause for which she considered herself lucky. No hot flashes, no mood changes, and thanks to some assistance from coconut oil, sex was quite comfortable. She took great pride in her health and played tennis five times a week, maintained a slender body mass index (BMI) of twenty-one, and ate a mostly plant-based diet. For the most part, she stayed up to date with her checkups and screening tests. In short, everything was going swimmingly for Susan, a mother of adult twins and a grandmother of four—until one Thanksgiving: As the oven timer rang, she grabbed her mitts to remove the turkey and as she stood up with the turkey in hand, she felt a sharp pain in her back, heard a popping sound, and shrieked in distress.

A trip to the emergency room determined that the cause of the pain was a spinal compression fracture—and not just that, but a new diagnosis of osteoporosis based on the clinical finding of a fracture from a non-traumatic event. Susan was devastated—and mystified about how this could have happened to her. When I explained that the loss of estrogen at menopause also causes changes to a woman's bone density, she was flabbergasted that no one had counseled her about this. To protect her bones going forward, I started Susan on 2,000 units a day of vitamin D, and she chose to start a yearly intravenous (IV) infusion of a bisphosphonate for her osteoporosis. She also started doing physical therapy to help with her posture and to prevent future fractures, and we scheduled her for a follow-up bone density test.

Susan's case underscores that even women who sail through menopause without a hot flash or sleepless night need to change the way they tend to their health at this point in their lives. After all, changes that we can't feel or see happen to our bones, brains, vaginas, and heart health at midlife, partly due to the loss of natural estrogen, and these changes increase a woman's risk of developing various chronic health conditions and diseases.

Yet, because they feel fine, women who fit the silent menopause profile might turn a blind eye toward taking steps to prevent chronic health conditions—such as high blood pressure, cholesterol abnormalities, type 2 diabetes, heart disease, and osteoporosis—that become a greater risk after menopause. Research has found that the increased risk of cardiovascular disease that occurs in a woman's sixth decade of life stems from estrogen deprivation and from changes in her lipid profile, particularly to her total and LDL (artery-clogging) cholesterol levels. In 2020, for the first time ever, the American Heart Association even released a scientific statement noting that the menopausal transition itself should now be considered an independent risk factor for cardiovascular disease.

That's why women with the Silent Menopause Type need to focus on upgrading their lifestyle practices, and they need to make routine medical checkups a priority in order to catch possible health problems early when they can be most effectively treated or possibly even reversed. Even if you don't have menopausal symptoms, your risk of developing certain health conditions, such as cardiovascular disease (CVD, including heart disease and stroke), osteoporosis,[1] and urinary incontinence increase after menopause due to the loss of estrogen. Unbeknownst to you, the presence of estrogen had been quietly protecting various bodily systems, which is why certain health risks increase once estrogen does a disappearing act after menopause.

Hypertension,[2] which is a major risk factor for CVD, becomes more common among women after menopause. And cholesterol abnormalities—including elevated total cholesterol, increases in low-density lipoprotein (LDL, the artery-clogging form of cholesterol) and triglycerides (another type of fat in the blood), and a decrease in high-density lipoprotein (HDL, the "good" cholesterol)—become progressively likely. In fact, total cholesterol levels peak in women between the ages of fifty-five and sixty-five, which is about ten years later than they peak in men—and the loss of estrogen plays a role here, too, for women. Meanwhile, changes in insulin secretion and insulin sensitivity after menopause increase the risk of postmenopausal women developing type 2 diabetes.

Some of these changes also can increase a woman's risk of developing metabolic syndrome, a cluster of conditions that raises her risk of coronary heart disease, type 2 diabetes, stroke, and other serious health problems. To be diagnosed with metabolic syndrome, you need to have three or more of the following: high blood pressure (defined as 130 over 85 mm Hg or higher), elevated fasting blood sugar (100 mg/dL or higher), excess body fat around the waist (a waist circumference of greater than thirty-five inches for women), low levels of HDL (less than 50 mg/dL in women), or elevated triglycerides (150 mg/dL or higher).[3,4] Most of the factors associated with metabolic syndrome don't have symptoms—they're silent, in other words. This is why I advise women with the Silent Menopause Type to be sure to have annual physical examinations with their health-care provider and to have their blood pressure, cholesterol levels, and fasting blood sugar checked every year. Don't get me wrong: These silent conditions can happen with other menopause types, too. But if you have the Silent Menopause Type, you are at a higher risk for not having these screenings done regularly or being advised that the risks of these conditions increase after menopause even if you don't have menopausal symptoms.

High blood pressure should be treated when it is higher than 140 over 90 mm Hg on more than two occasions; however, I highly recommend relying on home blood pressure readings before starting a medication because many women get white-coat hypertension, higher blood pressure readings at a doctor's office because they feel stressed or anxious there. If you have prehypertension (120–139 over 80–89 mm Hg), which is a precursor or warning sign that you're at greater risk of developing full-blown hypertension, it's important to monitor your blood pressure closely and initiate lifestyle changes—such as sticking with a healthy diet, reducing your salt intake, drinking less alcohol, managing stress, and exercising regularly—to try to lower your blood pressure.

If your cholesterol levels are abnormal, you might automatically assume that you should start taking a lipid-lowering medication (a statin drug). But it depends on how high your total cholesterol is, how low your HDL cholesterol is, and other aspects of your health. The decision about whether or not to start a statin should be made by calculating your atherosclerotic cardiovascular disease (ASCVD) risk score, which establishes your ten-year risk of having a cardiovascular problem such as a heart attack or stroke. It takes into account your sex, age, race, total cholesterol, HDL (the "good") cholesterol, systolic blood pressure (the top number), and whether you have diabetes, are being treated for hypertension, or if you smoke. This score can help you and your doctor determine if you need a statin—the decision is not based just on your cholesterol levels. (You can calculate your ASCVD score if you go to this website: tools.acc.org/ldl/ascvd_risk_estimator/index.html#!/calulate/estimator/.)

To test you for type 2 diabetes, your physician might order a simple A1C blood test, which measures your average blood sugar level over the past two to three months. An A1C below 5.7 percent is considered normal; between 5.7 and 6.4 percent indicates you have prediabetes (a condition where blood sugar levels are higher than normal but not high enough to be considered type 2 diabetes); and a result of 6.5 percent or higher indicates you have diabetes. Alternatively, a fasting blood sugar test measures your current blood sugar after an overnight fast; a fasting blood sugar level of 99 mg/dL or lower is considered normal, 100 to 125 mg/dL indicates you have prediabetes, and 126 mg/dL or higher means you have diabetes.[5] Prediabetes is often a precursor to developing full-blown type 2 diabetes and on its own it increases your risk of developing heart disease and stroke; you can have prediabetes for years without symptoms. In fact, more than 80 percent of adults in the US who have prediabetes don't know they have it, according to the Centers for Disease Control and Prevention.[6] While type 2 diabetes is treated with medications and lifestyle changes (particularly to diet), prediabetes is typically addressed with lifestyle changes: If you're overweight and you lose 5 to 7 percent of your body weight, that can reduce your blood sugar level and your risk of developing type 2 diabetes; regular moderate-intensity physical activity—at least 150 minutes per week—can also make a difference.

Another silent risk that increases after menopause is osteoporosis. Without realizing it, women lose bone mass more rapidly after menopause due to decreased levels of estrogen. In fact, you may lose up to 25 percent of your bone density after menopause, at a rate of 1 to 2 percent per year. Osteopenia is a condition that involves a weakening of your bones and a loss of bone mineral density (BMD) because your body isn't making new bone as quickly as it's reabsorbing old bone—yep, your bones are constantly remodeling themselves—and it's a precursor to osteoporosis but it doesn't cause symptoms. The only way to test to find out if you have osteopenia or osteoporosis is to have your bone mineral density measured with a DXA scan, which uses an X-ray beam to measure calcified tissue in certain regions of the body; the result is expressed as a T-score, which reflects the difference between the patient's measured BMD and the mean value of BMD in healthy, young, matched controls.[7] The World Health Organization defines T-scores between –1 and –2.5 as osteopenic and scores below –2.5 as osteoporotic. I recommend that all women have a bone density test a few years after menopause, maybe earlier if they have risk factors for osteoporosis such as a family history of bone loss, a history of a non-traumatic fracture, gastrointestinal malabsorption issues, a thyroid or endocrine disorder, a history of amenorrhea (the absence of periods during your reproductive years) or an eating disorder or steroid use. Fortunately, there are lifestyle modifications you can make to prevent your bone loss from worsening. (You'll read more about this in the treatment section that follows.)

Snooze Control

Many people believe that sleep quality and sleep needs decrease as they get older. One of those beliefs is correct; the other is not. As people get older, decreases in deep sleep (stages 3 and 4) and rapid-eye movement (REM) sleep occur, while stages 1 and 2 (lighter stages of sleep) are increased,[8] which can set them up for more fragmented sleep. These are considered normal changes to what's called "sleep architecture" but there is not a decreased need for sleep in older adults.[9]

There are, however, sneaky sleep disorders that become more common as women get older and these could disrupt the quality of their sleep without their realizing it. In a study involving more than 6,100 women between the ages of forty-five and sixty, the Canadian Longitudinal Study of Aging[10] found that postmenopausal women are more likely to screen positive for obstructive sleep apnea (OSA), a disorder that's characterized by repetitive pauses in your breathing while you're asleep[11]; this can lead to loud snoring and frequent arousals from sleep. (Sometimes the sleeper is unaware of these but her bed partner is likely to notice them.) Besides leading to daytime fatigue and impaired attention, OSA is associated with an increased risk of developing insulin resistance, high blood pressure, heart disease, and stroke. In addition, research[12] has found that the menopausal transition increases the prevalence and severity of restless legs syndrome (RLS),[13] a condition that causes an intense, often irresistible, urge to move your legs during sleep. Making matters worse, the two disorders often coexist in the same person.[14]

The best way to have OSA diagnosed is with an overnight study at a sleep lab. The diagnosis of RLS is based on your symptoms. Both conditions can be treated with lifestyle measures, medical devices (such as a machine that delivers continuous positive airway pressure or dental appliances that can keep the airway open) for OSA, and medications for RLS. But first the proper diagnosis needs to be made. If you suffer from fragmented sleep or your partner tells you that you frequently snore loudly, briefly stop breathing, or move your legs while you're sleeping, see a sleep specialist.

MAKING TREATMENT DECISIONS

In recent years, I have had some menopausal women come to me wanting to use hormone therapy to prevent chronic diseases despite not having symptoms that warranted its use. This is how I usually handle this situation: I explain to them that hormone therapy is currently not approved by the Food and Drug Administration (FDA) or indicated for the primary prevention of chronic diseases; it is FDA-approved for hot flashes, night sweats, genitourinary symptoms of menopause, and osteopenia. (In situations like this, I do send these women for a bone density scan if they haven't had one already because many women do have osteopenia without knowing it; if they have it, they are a candidate for HT.)

Then, I discuss with them their reasons for wanting to use HT and what interventions they've considered or tried in the past. There may be situations—such as if a woman experiences pain during intercourse or vaginal dryness—where I will consider prescribing a low dose of an estrogen with progesterone (if they have their uterus) and monitor them closely. I do this because a) I want to help them feel better, and b) I'm concerned that if they're dead set on using HT and I don't help them, they may go to somebody who will prescribe something that may do more harm than good (such as pellet injections of hormones). I want women to feel like they have choices as they go through the menopausal transition so sometimes I'm willing to do this—but only if they don't have any contraindications to HT and if they commit to close monitoring by me. And I'm careful to dispel the notion that using HT at this stage of life could protect them from heart disease, dementia, or type 2 diabetes because we don't have randomized, controlled trials that show this is clearly the case.

Not long ago, Cara, fifty-three, a tall, slender long-distance runner (five-eleven, 145 pounds), mother of three, and entrepreneur, came to see me. Since becoming postmenopausal at age fifty, she had developed high cholesterol and went to see a cardiologist who put her on a statin medication to reduce it. The problem was, she started experiencing muscle pain and cramping in her legs, which forced her to curb her running schedule. She suspected these symptoms were from the statin (and they could have been) so she stopped taking it. The aches and pains eased somewhat, which allowed her to ramp up her running schedule again.

Because she had read that the loss of estrogen after menopause can cause elevations in cholesterol, she came to see me about the possibility of starting hormone therapy. I explained that HT is not FDA-approved for the prevention of cardiovascular disease or its risk factors (such as high cholesterol). I calculated her ASCVD score and it was in the range where she didn't *need* a statin to reduce her risk of heart disease. While her brother and father both had hypertension, Cara didn't have high blood pressure; in fact, she had no other risk factors for CVD.

Besides HT, we discussed other ways she could try to reduce her cholesterol through dietary measures as well as the option of trying a different statin drug if she wanted to use one (some are believed to be more likely to cause muscle symptoms than others[15]) and taking coenzyme Q10 supplements along with it; studies[16] have shown that coenzyme Q10 supplements ameliorate statin-associated muscle symptoms. She left my office saying that she would think about all this.

TREATMENT FOR THE SILENT MENOPAUSE TYPE

Given that the Silent Menopause Type is relatively symptom-free, there aren't specific treatment plans for this type. I would recommend treating specific symptoms as they emerge by using the extensive menu of symptom-oriented solutions in chapter 12. And

I do have recommendations for lifestyle modifications that are suitable for all women with this type, as you will see.

The reality is, hormone therapy isn't recommended for women who don't have disruptive symptoms of menopause, so it often isn't suitable for the Silent Menopause Type. Having said that, to preserve urogenital health, I sometimes will recommend that women with the Silent Menopause Type use low-dose vaginal estrogen—in the form of a cream, a tablet, or a ring—to help protect the integrity and moisture in those tissues and keep sexual intercourse pleasurable, not painful. While reports indicate that 50 percent of menopausal women experience symptoms of genitourinary syndrome—such as vaginal dryness and painful intercourse—every menopausal woman's body will experience changes in the genitourinary tract and the pelvic floor. To prevent these symptoms from occurring or to address recurrent urinary tract infections (UTIs), I prefer the low-dose, twice-weekly Vagifem or Yuvafem vaginal suppository at night, or a woman can use Estrace cream twice a week at night.

If a woman has osteopenia, there are three medication options to be discussed. The first is Fosamax (alendronate), which belongs to a drug class called bisphosphonates that are used for osteoporosis. Unfortunately, some women worry about extremely rare side effects from bisphosphonates such as osteonecrosis of the jaw, femur fractures, or inflammatory eye disease; in truth, the risk of having a fracture is significantly higher than having any of these, but these are among the reasons some women wish to avoid these drugs. The most common side effect is dyspepsia (indigestion) after taking them. Another medication option is an intravenous infusion of Reclast (zoledronic acid) that can be given once every two years for osteopenia: The infusion itself is about an hour from start to finish—and the most common side effect from this is a twenty-four-hour flu-like feeling that can occur after the first infusion, in particular.

For women with osteopenia who would rather consider HT

to improve their bone health, I will typically start them on a low-dose estradiol patch (0.025 to 0.0375 milligrams weekly), and progesterone is needed if she has an intact uterus. Estrogen works to stop bone from breaking down. Because the transdermal route has a lower risk for blood clots compared to oral preparations, and a woman with the Silent Menopause Type is likely to be symptom-free, this is my go-to option in this scenario.

If mild sexual challenges are present, we have a couple of options. If a woman has low sexual desire that isn't overly bothersome, the injectable drug Vyleesi, available by prescription, can be used for low libido on an as-needed basis. Or, if she has painful intercourse after menopause, prasterone (a form of DHEA, or dehydroepiandrosterone) can be used as a vaginal suppository at night; it provides a slight boost in estrogen and androgen levels, which may help with vulvovaginal atrophy and make sex more comfortable.

LIFESTYLE INTERVENTIONS

Dietary Directives

Given that you are fortunate enough not to be experiencing menopausal symptoms, the dietary advice I have for you relates to keeping this good trend going—and taking steps to protect yourself from chronic diseases that become more common after menopause. To that end, for your overall health, you won't go wrong with a Mediterranean-style diet. For your heart health, it's important to limit your intake of saturated fats (found in fatty meats, full-fat dairy products, butter, and tropical oils) and reduce your sodium intake (for the sake of your blood pressure); sodium is prominent in highly processed or packaged foods and restaurant fare. Replace saturated fats in your diet with heart-healthy (unsaturated) fats such as those found in olive and canola oils, avocados, nuts, seeds, and fatty fish like salmon. In particular, eating fish or seafood at least twice a week is heart-protective in several ways: The omega-3 fatty acids in fish and shellfish help reduce triglyceride levels and increase HDL levels; they play a role in decreasing platelet aggregation (thus reducing the risk of blood clot formation), and they reduce the risk of developing heart arrythmias.

Reduce your intake of refined carbohydrates—such as baked goods, ice cream, snack foods, and sugar-sweetened beverages—to help prevent insulin resistance, which increases your risk of developing type 2 diabetes and heart disease. Instead, focus on consuming high-fiber foods, such as whole grains, fruits, vegetables, legumes, nuts, and seeds; fiber helps prevent insulin resistance by slowing the release of glucose into the bloodstream and it helps promote better blood cholesterol levels.

Consume plenty of potassium by having five servings of fruits and vegetables per day. In particular, berries are loaded with phytochemicals called anthocyanins, which have antioxidant and anti-inflammatory properties that are beneficial for blood pressure and blood cholesterol levels.[17] By contrast, kale, spinach, bok choy, and other leafy greens supply nitrates[18] (beets do, too), compounds that are converted to nitric oxide and promote blood flow and normalize blood pressure, both of which reduce stress on the cardiovascular system; these veggies are also good sources of fiber and folate, which are beneficial for heart health, and leafy greens have vitamin K, which supports bone health.

After age fifty, women need to consume more protein to make and maintain muscle mass and produce bone cells. Depending on how much you weigh and how physically active you are, experts[19] recommend that women over fifty consume one to one and a half grams of protein per kilogram of body weight per day (remember: 1 kilogram equals 2.2 pounds). That means if you weigh 150 pounds, you need at least sixty-eight grams of protein each day.

Here are some specific nutrients that women with the Silent Menopause Type should pay attention to:

- **Calcium** (rich food sources include dairy foods, fortified orange juice, sardines and canned salmon with the bones, soybeans, and spinach) happens to be the most abundant mineral in the body; besides making up much of the structure of bones and teeth, calcium helps with proper blood vessel function, muscle function, nerve transmission, and fluid regulation.[20]

- **Magnesium** (abundant in almonds, cashews, and peanuts, chia and pumpkin seeds, edamame and black beans, yogurt, quinoa, and fortified breakfast cereals) promotes blood flow to the muscles and brain, helps with nerve transmission, and lends strength to the skeleton (BTW: bones contain about half the magnesium in the body).

- **B vitamins** (think: fortified breakfast cereals, yogurt, chicken, avocados, sunflower seeds, and salmon) help your body convert the food you eat into glucose, which in turn gives you energy; the B vitamins are also necessary for the production of neurotransmitters including serotonin and dopamine, and the transmission of messages between brain cells.

- **Vitamin D** (found in salmon, rainbow trout, sardines, mushrooms, fortified eggs, orange juice, and milk, as well as fortified soy, oat, and almond milks) promotes calcium absorption, bone growth, and bone remodeling, and reduces inflammation in the body.[21]

- **Vitamin K** (found primarily in green leafy vegetables, including broccoli and brussels sprouts) is essential for bone metabolism and proper blood clotting.[22]

- **Vitamin C** (plentiful in bell peppers, citrus fruits and juices, kiwi, broccoli, strawberries, and mango) may be best known as a promoter of immune function but it's also necessary to make collagen (part of bone tissue) and certain neurotransmitters, and for protein metabolism.[23]

To help you stay in tune with your body and manage your weight, practice mindful eating. Sometimes described as "the art of presence while you eat,"[24] mindful eating involves bringing your full attention into your eating experiences, not only in terms of the foods you choose to buy and eat but also in the act of eating them. The best ways to do this are to: always eat while sitting at a table (without the presence of screens) and to eat slowly, chew your food thoroughly, and focus on how each bite tastes and feels in your mouth. Mindful eating is a way of connecting with your body, and it can have a calming effect on your body and mind because it allows you to become immersed in the present moment. It takes practice to get it right so keep working on it.

Here's what a day's meal plan might look like:

Breakfast: Breakfast sandwich: toasted whole-wheat English muffin, 2 eggs, 1 slice (1 ounce) cheddar cheese, 1 orange

Lunch: 1 cup lentil soup; spinach salad made with 1 cup baby spinach leaves, ½ cup cherry tomatoes, ¼ cup chopped cucumber, and topped with 2 teaspoons olive oil and Balsamic vinegar and 2 teaspoons roasted pumpkin seeds; 2-ounce whole-wheat roll

Dinner: 4 ounces cooked salmon; 1 cup cooked brown rice, whole-wheat couscous, or quinoa with 1 to 2 teaspoons olive oil; 1 cup steamed or roasted broccoli, asparagus, or cauliflower

Snacks: ½ cup cottage cheese mixed with ⅛ teaspoon dried dill and pinch of garlic powder, and 1 cup pea pods or baby carrots; Blueberry smoothie: blend 1 cup frozen, thawed wild blueberries, 1 cup plain fat-free Greek or Icelandic yogurt, and ¼ cup 1 percent (low-fat) milk.

As far as supplements go, for women with this menopause type, I typically recommend taking supplements of vitamin D and calcium, omega-3 fatty acids, a B-complex (to boost energy), and magnesium (to promote sound sleep) at bedtime. Also, if they're taking a statin for cholesterol abnormalities, I advise women to take coenzyme Q10, an antioxidant that's naturally present in the body and plays a role in muscle cell energy production; coenzyme Q10 helps reduce the muscle and joint pains that are common side effects of some statin medications.

Exercise Rx

If you're already exercising regularly, keep doing what you're doing. But if you want to continue to improve your fitness level, you can increase the intensity or duration of your workouts by 10 percent per week, without risking injury or burnout. If you're not currently exercising, get moving! Find a physical activity you enjoy or just start walking regularly, and do it at least four times per week; start slowly and build up the amount of time you do it to at least thirty minutes.

If you prefer exercising alone, consider hiking, jogging or running, or swimming. If you want to make it social, try tennis, golf, or pickleball; join a running, cycling, or hiking group; or take an exercise class (such as Zumba, kickboxing, or Spinning) at a gym. Many of these forms of exercise (I'm talking about you, hiking, jogging, Zumba, kickboxing, tennis, and pickleball) are weight-bearing exercises, which means they're good for your bones. Whatever aerobic workouts you choose, be sure to add in strength-training workouts—whether it's using weights, machines, exercise bands, or your own body weight (with squats, lunges, push-ups, planks, and the like)—at least twice a week, to build and maintain your muscle and bone mass and strength.

Improving Your Headspace

Even though you seem to be sailing through the menopausal transition with few, if any, distressing symptoms, it's wise to bring your head into the equation to help ensure that this calm, cool, and collected pattern continues into the future. To help yourself feel balanced, centered, and upbeat, I recommend using the following strategies:

- **Reinvent self-care.** When people hear the term "self-care," they often think about spa days or taking a significant break from their day-to-day responsibilities. I prefer to think of self-care as things we can do in small increments every day to refresh and rejuvenate ourselves. This can be as simple as taking "me" time to read a book or listen to a podcast you're interested in, give yourself a facial or a manicure, go for a walk by yourself in nature—or anything else that soothes your heart, mind, and soul. For many women, the key to making room for this kind of self-care is to set boundaries with other people and be willing to say no to nonessential demands on your time and energy. Use it to invest in your own well-being—you deserve it!
- **Embrace a sense of purpose.** For many women, this stage of life presents a prime opportunity to infuse life with a new or updated sense of meaning or purpose. To create a vision for

what's meaningful to you, ask yourself: What matters most to me in life? What do I want to be remembered for? What issues or activities really make me feel excited or passionate? If you can articulate these desires to yourself, you can set specific goals to help yourself cultivate a sense of purpose, which will have beneficial effects on your mental and physical health. Research[25] has found that people in their sixties who have high purpose-in-life (PIL) levels have greater social support, resilience, health literacy, and better mental and physical health, all of which contribute to successful aging.

- **Listen to your body.** It's always sending you signals—the question is: Are you listening? To get in the habit of paying attention to your body's messages, give yourself a time-out periodically throughout the day and scan your body for signs of tension or discomfort.[26] Sit or lie down in a quiet place, close your eyes, and take a few deep breaths. Start with your feet and notice any sensations you feel, then notice how your legs feel. Move up to your abdomen and back and notice if they feel tense or tight; if they do, take a deep breath and try to soften them. Next, focus on your hands, your arms, your shoulders, neck, and jaw: Do they feel tight or relaxed? Can you soften or relax them? Try to become aware of every major part of your body, as best you can. Besides making an effort to relax them, consider what they're trying to tell you: Have you been sitting still too long? Is your posture suboptimal? Are you unwittingly tensing your muscles in response to stress? Once you know these answers, you can take steps to address the root causes of your body signals.

- **Find new ways to stay grounded.** When anxiety or stress start affecting you, try the 5, 4, 3, 2, 1 technique,[27] which uses your senses to help bring your attention back to the here and now and away from what's disturbing you. Here's how to do it: Sit comfortably and take a few deep breaths in through your nose, exhaling through your mouth. Then, look around you and notice five things you can see wherever you are; four things you can physically feel; three things you can hear; two things you can smell; and one thing you can taste. Finish the exercise with another deep breath—and go on with your day.

- **Take stock of your resources.** Before a challenging time arrives, sit down and make a list of people you could turn to in a pinch for support, assistance, and the like. Be sure to include family members, friends, colleagues, neighbors, and other acquaintances from your community. By doing this, you'll probably realize you have more people to turn to for emotional, practical, or financial support than you may have thought you did. And if you don't, it's a sign that it's time to make an effort to broaden your social network and cultivate new sources of support *before* you need it.

- **Consider what you appreciate about your body.** It's no secret that we live in a body-critical culture, where we often compare ourselves to others (especially on social media) or find fault with how we look. It's time to rewrite this play-book and express gratitude to your body for all the amazing things it does for you on a regular basis (hugging your loved ones, carrying heavy bags, cooking, gardening, taking you where you want to go, and so on), as well as the major gifts it has given you over the years (perhaps your children or an amazing adventure you went on).

- **Broaden your comfort zone.** When you're feeling fine and life feels relatively steady, it's easy to do the same things day after day, but eventually this can lead to feeling stuck in a rut. Since you have the benefit of being free of bothersome menopausal symptoms, why not expand your comfort zone and spark some personal growth in the process? You can do this by embracing new experiences or freshening up the usual ones. Consider signing up for a Color Run, a swing-dancing class, or a paddle-boarding adventure. Once a week, make a point to try a fruit or vegetable you've never had before—maybe a mangosteen, plumcot, or kohlrabi. If you're invited to play pickleball, go bird-watching, or go orienteering (if you don't know what it is, look it up), avoid your knee-jerk instinct to say, "No, thank you," and give it a try. Not only will your life feel fresher and more invigorating for the experience but you may even change the way you see yourself and the world in positive ways.

- **Volunteer to help others or the planet.** Sign up to mentor a student. Volunteer at a soup kitchen or a clothing drive for the poor. Or, volunteer in a local environmental restoration project. Regularly doing something to help others or the greater good gets you out of your head and helps you put your own challenges in perspective; it also can help you feel empowered. Studies have found that people who engage in more hours of volunteering report higher levels of well-being,[28] and as people get older, regular volunteering gives people a more positive self-perception of aging.[29]

While you may consider yourself lucky that the menopausal transition has been a breeze for you (as you should), don't let that stop you from staying alert to new symptoms that may emerge or being proactive about your mental and physical health going forward. If new symptoms arise, you'll find a vast array of remedies for just about every menopausal symptom in chapter 12. Turn to this treasure trove of strategies whenever you need it so you can take good care of yourself today, tomorrow, and for years to come. It's all part of your personalized treatment plan.

Part III

TREATMENTS TO TAME THE TUMULT

Prioritizing Relief and Your Safety

Consciously or not, we all have biases and preconceived notions about certain aspects of medical care, including some treatments. The journey through menopause is no exception. So before you create a personalized treatment regimen for *your* menopause type, it's wise to take stock of your preconceived ideas, personal preferences, and beliefs about different treatment options and give them a reality check. As a starting point, think about your assumptions or feelings about certain treatments—such as hormone therapy, the use of antidepressants, herbal preparations, or psychotherapy—and consider where they might have come from:

- Did you grow up in a family that valued stoicism and viewed therapy or the use of antidepressants for mood disturbances as a sign of weakness?
- Did catchy or alarming headlines in the media make you more or less inclined to try herbal preparations or [fill in the blank] to relieve your symptoms?
- How do you feel about alternative medicine, in general—are you open to it or skeptical?
- If a friend or family member took hormones during menopause and later developed, or even died from, breast cancer, did a causal connection take up residence in your mind?
- If you've heard that some doctors judge women for their

treatment decisions related to menopause, are you concerned that this might happen to you?

There are no right or wrong answers to these questions. The goal is to help you build self-awareness, to understand where some of your health-related attitudes come from. Once you have these insights, you can consider whether or not you want to continue to subscribe to those ideas or values as far as your menopausal symptoms go. Think of this as a way of helping you make more informed decisions for yourself from another perspective, in addition to having accurate health information.

Here are some other questions that are worth considering when it comes to your own menopausal experience:

- How intense or bothersome are your symptoms?
- Are they affecting your relationships, your work performance, your personal goals, and/or your quality of life?
- When was the last time you remember feeling like your best self and how badly do you want to reclaim that feeling?
- What are the downsides of trying to stick out your menopausal discomfort versus seeking treatment for your symptoms?
- Are you worried what friends or family members would think if you did take medicine or hormones or made lifestyle modifications in an effort to improve the way you feel and function?
- If you answered yes to the previous question, why do other people's opinions matter to you so much regarding how you handle your menopausal experience?

Once you have a greater awareness of these thoughts and beliefs, you'll be able to make more thoughtful decisions about what you're willing to do (or not) or take (or not) to try to obtain relief from your disruptive menopausal symptoms.

It's important for all menopausal women—regardless of their menopause type—to rank their most bothersome symptoms in order to set priorities for what they want to address. To make this exercise easier and more convenient, a checklist of common menopausal symptoms is provided below. Read through them and set priorities for seeking and obtaining relief from your most bothersome symptoms by ranking each one on a scale from 1 (mild) to 5 (debilitating); then, mark your top three symptoms that you'd like to focus on. This will put you in a better position to personalize your treatment plan in the next chapter.

Acne _____
Anxiety _____
Bloating _____
Brain fog _____
Breast tenderness _____
Burning mouth/gums _____
Decreased sexual sensation/arousal _____
Depressed moods _____
Difficulty concentrating or focusing _____
Dry skin _____
Fatigue _____
Frequent urinary tract infections _____
Hair loss _____
Hair thinning _____
Heart palpitations _____
Hot flashes _____
Insomnia _____
Joint aches and pains _____
Lack of motivation _____
Loss of sexual desire _____
Low energy _____
Mood swings _____

Nausea_____
Night sweats _____
Pain during sexual intercourse _____
Swelling in the extremities _____
Trouble staying asleep _____
Vaginal dryness _____
Vertigo _____
Weight gain _____

Talking to Your Family About Menopause

No matter how compassionate your partner and family members are naturally, they may not understand how menopause is affecting you. And, really, how could they? Every woman's experience is different, and there are so many myths and misconceptions about menopause out there. Plus, they're not inside your body or mind—and they're not mind readers.

To bring them up to speed on what you're experiencing and how they can be supportive, find a quiet time to have a conversation about it. You can be as detailed (or not) as you'd like to be about your symptoms and where you are in the menopausal transition. You could also show them key areas of this book if they want to know more about what happens physiologically during the menopausal transition. At the very least, explain how you're feeling and that menopause isn't something you "just go through," that the symptoms can last for a few years, and that you don't want to hear jokes about menopause. You might explain that you're experiencing brain fog or mood swings, headaches or weight gain, hot flashes or unusual fatigue—and that you don't feel like your usual self when you're in the midst of these symptoms.

Reassure them that if you're cranky or otherwise out of sorts, it has nothing to do with them—they shouldn't take it personally, in other words. Let them know what you're doing to try to alleviate your symptoms. And tell them how they can help—perhaps by giving you some extra time to yourself, helping out around the house more, or bringing you a glass of cold water when you're running hot. Make it clear that you're not looking for anyone to "fix" this—it simply can't be done—but that you're looking for support and understanding.

If you're experiencing sexual changes—such as discomfort or pain during intercourse or loss of libido—talk to your partner about them, emphasizing that these are due to the hormonal havoc you're experiencing, not your relationship. Then, discuss how you can approach these issues together; if you're seeing a doctor about these issues, you may want to let your partner know so that they realize how important this is to you. In the meantime, strive to preserve physical and emotional intimacy—perhaps by giving each other back rubs or foot massages and sharing your feelings—rather than focusing exclusively on your sex life.

If you're having sleep problems like insomnia or night sweats, brainstorm how you can address them together. Maybe it would help to spend some time relaxing together before turning in for the night. If night sweats or other temperature regulation issues are occurring, you can negotiate an appropriate room temperature and bed-covering setup that's likely to work for both of you. Or, one of you might opt to occasionally sleep in another room.

Be sure to let your family members have a chance to ask you questions about your menopausal experience. The goal here is to demystify what you're dealing with and to enlist support and sympathy from your loved ones. Remember, too, that when you talk to your kids about menopause, you're helping the next generation be better educated and more prepared than we are. Plus, in one way or another, you're all in this "change" together, and it's important for everyone to remember that this, too, will eventually pass.

When I see patients in my office, after we go over their medical history and I listen to their symptoms, I ask, "If I had a magic wand and could wave it and make your most distressing symptom disappear, what would it be?" Then, I give patients a few moments to answer. It's helpful to approach it this way because even if they've told me that they're having multiple symptoms, it's important for me to know which one is the most bothersome to them so we can really individualize their treatment plan. I ask the question this way because while a woman may have just told me that she has occasional mild hot flashes or night sweats, it may be that the brain fog or the pain she experiences during intercourse is truly the most bothersome. This is an area where it's a mistake for health-care providers to make assumptions.

It's also important to look for possible associations or ripple effects among various menopausal symptoms because sometimes they're there. For example, research[1] has found that chronic partial sleep loss leads to metabolic and hormone changes—including decreased glucose tolerance and decreased insulin sensitivity, increased evening levels of cortisol (a stress hormone), increased levels of ghrelin (a hormone that stimulates appetite), and decreased levels of leptin (a hormone that inhibits hunger and helps regulate food intake)—changes that can increase the risk of weight gain and obesity. Let's say a woman comes to me with a cluster of symptoms—such as loss of sexual desire, weight gain, mood swings, and fragmented sleep—that seem to be unrelated; if the first thing we target is the quality of her sleep and it improves, the other vexing symptoms may improve somewhat on their own. And even if they don't, being better rested will make it easier to treat the other symptoms because she will have a baseline state of feeling better.

That doesn't mean that you can't or shouldn't treat other symptoms that are bothering you. Sometimes it's easy and gratifying to reach for low-hanging fruit if you have dry skin or bloating, for example. If you can take effective steps to relieve these symptoms, which you'll find in the next chapter, you can gain a sense of empowerment that can motivate you to tackle the ones that may take longer to address. With this book, you're in the driver's seat of managing your menopausal transition, which is why I'm asking you to rank your symptoms, consider possible associations between seemingly unrelated ones, and set priorities for which ones to address first. Taking these preparatory steps will essentially give you a road map to follow.

Ultimately, the goal is to rewrite your menopause story with new ways to manage your experience and your expectations while shedding your fears and faulty judgments. Start with the baseline treatment plans including the lifestyle-related approaches in the chapters that apply to your menopause type(s); then, you can add strategies from chapter 12 to address your remaining bothersome symptoms. Think of this as a way to put together pieces of a puzzle to create a plan that works for you and to update it as you need to.

How to Talk to Your Doctor About Hormone Therapy

If the possibility of using hormone therapy (HT) is on your radar screen and you want to talk to your doctor about it, call your doctor's office to schedule a "problem-oriented visit" or a "hormone consultation,"[2] as opposed to a wellness visit, a diagnostic visit, or a preventive visit.

Who you decide to consult on this issue is really up to you: Your internist or family doctor may be just as equipped as your ob-gyn or an endocrinologist (if you have one) to talk to you about your menopausal experience. Yet because doctors have so many things to address in an annual examination or checkup, there really isn't time to give a discussion of HT the attention it deserves in that setting; that's why I recommend asking for a separate visit for the sole purpose of discussing your symptoms and the pros and cons of considering HT based on your health history, family medical history, and risk factors.

To organize your thoughts and prepare for the visit, I recommend creating a script or cheat sheet so you won't forget any key points in the stress of the moment. Start with your symptoms, saying something like: "For the past ___ months, I have had these symptoms: 1. ___; 2. ___; 3. ___ ." Then describe the severity of each symptom, how it affects the way you feel and function (be specific!), and what activities make the symptom better or worse. Be sure to mention specific treatments or interventions you've tried for each symptom and whether they've helped at all.

Remind your doctor about any chronic health conditions you have, medications you take regularly, and other essential facts about your family medical history and your personal medical history (whether you do or don't have a uterus, for example, or how you responded to hormonal contraceptives if you took them in the past).

Tell your doctor that you've been reading about the safety and efficacy of hormone therapy and that you'd like to discuss whether it might help you based on your symptoms and the information you've already shared. Then, mention which forms of HT (the pill, the patch, a gel, or cream) you're particularly interested in and why—and ask what your doctor thinks about all this for you, in particular. If your doctor is against using HT in your case, ask what they'd recommend instead to try to relieve the symptoms that are really bugging you. Emphasize that you'd like to engage in shared decision-making to come up with a treatment that's likely to help, not harm, you. If after having this conversation you don't feel like your personal preferences are being factored in or you're not resolving the issue the way you want to, it may be time to look for a new doctor, ask for a referral to a specialist, or seek a NAMS-certified practitioner on your own (see box on page 216).

How to Find a Menopause Specialist

You may know the differences between an MD, a DO, and a PhD—but do you know what an NCMP is? Many women don't. It's short for NAMS-certified menopause practitioner (NAMS stands for the North American Menopause Society), and it reflects specialized training that a health-care provider has undergone to treat menopause-related issues and has passed the NAMS certification exam. This is particularly helpful to know about, given that many clinicians don't have the knowledge or expertise to effectively manage menopausal issues. To find an NCMP near you, you can search the NAMS website by zip code at: portal .menopause.org/NAMS/NAMS/Directory/Menopause -Practitioner.aspx.

Don't get me wrong: If a doctor you know, like, and trust isn't on the list, that doesn't mean they won't do a good job of treating your menopausal symptoms. But if you're looking for a new health-care practitioner, this tool may help you find one who can help you with your menopausal experience.

12

Personalizing Your Treatment Plan

As you've seen, there isn't a one-size-fits-all approach to dealing with menopausal discomfort. There's no panacea that will work for every woman. The same thing is true for specific menopause types: While the baseline treatment plans in the previous chapters are a great starting point, even women who have the same menopause type(s) are likely to have their own unique constellation of symptoms. In other words, even the specific types don't follow cookie-cutter patterns. That's why it's important to personalize your treatment plan so you can get some relief from *all* the symptoms that are currently taking a toll on the way you feel and function—and to be prepared to address new symptoms that may emerge.

I can pretty much guarantee: At some point, new challenges and symptoms will arise on the sometimes rocky, winding journey through menopause so you might as well be prepared for them. Plus, having the wherewithal to personalize and modify your own treatment plan is empowering. It puts you in the driver's seat, which is where you belong on this journey.

Using the symptom checklist that you completed in the previous chapter, you can pick and choose remedies that cater to your particular menopausal symptoms, thus developing a customized plan of action that suits your current needs. The idea is to continue to follow the baseline plan for your menopause type if it's helping you to at least some extent, and to add remedies that address the symptoms that remain or that have recently emerged. That's where the following symptoms/solutions come in. Think of these as ways to supplement your basic approach, either on an as-needed basis or on an ongoing one, whichever makes the most sense for you.

ACNE: By the time you reach menopause, you may think that acne would be a distant dot in your rearview mirror. But menopausal acne is an actual thing[1]—and it may be due to hormonal imbalances, namely a higher ratio of androgens (male hormones) to estrogen as estrogen declines. In addition, stress, insulin resistance, lack of sleep, dietary changes, and other lifestyle changes may be contributing factors. To treat or reduce acne breakouts, try the following measures:

- Wash your face properly. Use a gentle cleanser that contains salicylic acid, benzoyl peroxide, or other antibacterial agents once or twice per day, as well as after exercising, and be sure to remove makeup before turning in for the night. Choose skin-care products wisely. If you're prone to breakouts, choose oil-free, non-comedogenic (non-pore-clogging) moisturizers, creams, and makeup.
- Try over-the-counter acne-fighting products. Toners or gels containing salicylic acid can help unclog pores while creams, gels, or lotions with benzoyl peroxide can reduce bacteria on the skin and dry up some oil from the skin's surface. Tread lightly with these, however, because postmenopausal skin is often drier and more prone to irritation.
- Don't annoy your skin. That means don't scrub or use excessively abrasive products because these practices can actually irritate the skin and trigger acne outbreaks. And don't pop

your pimples because this can lead to scarring, in which case you're trading one cosmetic problem for another.

- Look for dietary triggers. There aren't specific foods that can universally trigger acne flare-ups for women. But some women find that consuming lots of dairy products or refined carbohydrates (including sugar-laden foods) may contribute to breakouts. Your best bet is to pay attention to how your skin behaves in accordance with what you eat; if you notice your acne tends to flare up after eating a particular food, you may want to avoid or limit it in your diet.

- See a dermatologist. Doctors have a stronger arsenal of weapons to combat acne. These include topical antibiotics or oral antibiotics (such as tetracycline or doxycycline) which can kill the bacteria that contribute to acne; topical retinoids (such as tretinoin, tazarotene, and adapalene) that have anti-inflammatory properties and may improve cellular turnover and signs of aging on the skin; prescription hormonal therapy (such as the anti-androgen drug spironolactone and sometimes oral contraceptives); and lasers and light systems that reduce inflammation and sebaceous (oil) gland activity.

ANXIETY: Feeling like you're at the mercy of your body's menopausal changes can be nerve-racking in its own right. But if you're feeling truly anxious, it may be due to the fact that progesterone (a calming hormone) levels decline at menopause, often even before estrogen does. These changes can make you feel emotionally ill at ease or lead to frequent worry or nervousness; if, however, you feel intensely anxious 24/7 or have panic attacks, these may be signs of an anxiety disorder that warrants professional treatment. To tame run-of-the-mill anxiety, try these proven strategies:

- Get moving. Research[2] has found that aerobic exercise has a substantial effect in reducing anxiety among people who have anxiety disorders as well as those who simply have elevated anxiety. Whether you opt for a high-intensity workout (such as running or Spinning) or a gentler mind-body exercise such as yoga[3] or Pilates[4] is up to you.

- Give yourself breathing lessons. Doing any form of slow, deep breathing is likely to calm the sympathetic nervous system and reduce anxiety. One that's particularly effective at quelling anxiety is the 4, 7, 8 technique: Start by exhaling fully through your mouth as you make a whooshing sound; then slowly inhale through your nose to the count of four, hold that breath for a count of seven, then exhale fully through your mouth to a count of eight. Repeat this three more times. (Don't overdo it or you could get lightheaded.)

- Take a tea break. It may sound simplistic but having a cup of warm tea can soothe your jangled nerves. While green tea is often associated with having a calming effect, other brews—such as chamomile, rosemary, passionflower, lemon balm, and lavender teas—can have similarly soothing perks. Pick one that appeals to you but be mindful of the caffeine content so that you don't inadvertently rev yourself up.

- Treat yourself to a soothing scent. Inhaling the aromas of certain essential oils, especially lavender, has been found to alleviate anxiety according to a meta-analysis published in a 2020 issue of the *Journal of Affective Disorders*.[5] Not a fan of lavender? Damask rose,[6] bergamot, and lemon essential oils may also be used to relieve anxiety.[7]

- Use an app to calm yourself. Whether you have an iPhone or an Android, there's an app that will help you calm down and relieve your anxiety. A few that I recommend: Calm, Headspace, the Mindfulness App, and MyLife Meditation.

BLOATING/WATER RETENTION: You may be experiencing more bloating and water retention during the menopausal transition than you did in the past thanks to your wildly fluctuating then ebbing hormone levels. When your body experiences a surge of estrogen, you can end up retaining water, which can lead to belly bloating or swollen ankles. Also, if you're taking systemic hormone therapy, research suggests that the estrogen or progesterone supplementation may increase fluid retention. Fortunately, you can reduce bloating with some simple lifestyle adjustments:

- Drink more water. It may sound counterintuitive but you're more likely to experience water retention or bloating if you're dehydrated, even moderately. So drink up and try eating more foods with a high water content—like watermelon, cucumbers, and celery.
- Get your sweat on. One of the best ways to reduce water retention is with moderate to vigorous aerobic exercise, which will hasten the transport of water through your body.
- Elevate your legs. If you're prone to swelling in your ankles and calves, put your feet up periodically during the day to improve blood flow and decrease swelling. Wearing compression stockings or even tighter leggings also may help.
- Take a dip. Head to a pool—or even your bathtub if you don't have access to a pool—and immerse yourself in water. Research[8] has found that when pregnant women with edema (water retention) immersed themselves up to their armpits or did water aerobics in a pool for thirty minutes, they experienced a significant diuretic effect including reduced swelling due to water retention. The same principles and effects apply whether you're pregnant or postmenopausal—you'll lose the water retention. So take the plunge!

- Increase your intake of vitamin B6. Consider taking 50 milligrams of B6 (pyridoxine) up to three times per day because the water-soluble vitamin acts as a mild natural diuretic.
- Get your bowels moving. If you're constipated, you may be retaining water along with the rest of what isn't moving through you. So increase your fiber and water intake and consider taking a magnesium citrate supplement (250 to 500 milligrams once a day) to increase your gut motility.

BRAIN FOG: If you've been having trouble staying focused, thinking clearly, or recalling key words, you may be experiencing what's commonly referred to as menopausal brain fog. It's not a diagnosis but it is a real phenomenon. While the decline in estrogen is believed to play a role—given that estrogen protects the brain and enhances thinking and memory abilities[9]—sleep loss and stress may be contributing factors. Here are some strategies to help you cope:

- Ease the burden on your memory. Take notes and keep lists about things you want or need to do or buy, using a notepad or calendar or a digital device. And rely on calendars and other scheduling aids to keep you on track for where you're supposed to be and when.
- Practice mindfulness. In this instance, it's about being present-minded, fully in the here and now. That means slowing down and avoiding multitasking. It means doing one thing at a time and really focusing on what you're doing.
- Get some exercise. Besides boosting your mood, a bout of aerobic exercise can enhance your ability to focus and think clearly, thanks to improved circulation (which means more oxygen and nutrients are going to your brain) and the release of certain neurotransmitters (brain chemicals).

- Consume enough protein. It's essential for the production of dopamine, which plays a role in learning, cognition, and memory.
- Prioritize sleep. If you're not getting enough good-quality sleep on a regular basis, your brain won't function optimally—it's that simple.

BREAST TENDERNESS: You might think that breast tenderness or pain (a.k.a. mastalgia) would be a thing of the past once your periods are history but that's not necessarily the case for all women. Your first concern may be that it's a sign of cancer—you can go ahead and cross that off your worry list because breast cancer rarely hurts. It's more likely to stem from fluctuating estrogen levels—if you're perimenopausal or using hormone therapy—or a change in breast size, which can be caused by an increase in fat tissue, or fluid retention. In any case, here's what you can do to ease the discomfort:

- Wear a supportive, well-fitting bra. (Yes, it may be time to get professionally fitted again.) Make sure you wear a supportive sports bra when exercising, as well.
- Take an over-the-counter pain reliever such as acetaminophen or one of the non-steroidal anti-inflammatory drugs such as ibuprofen or naproxen.
- Consider cutting back on your intake of caffeine including chocolate. Some women's breasts are sensitive to the effects of caffeine and you may be one of them. Also, consider reducing your salt intake and make a concerted effort to drink more water. The reason: Mild dehydration actually causes fluid retention in the body, which can exacerbate breast pain.
- Give your sore breasts some TLC. If you can stand it, apply cold packs to your aching breasts as some women find this

provides relief. Anything frozen will do but bags of frozen peas are easy to mold to your breasts.

- Try an herbal supplement. Some women get relief from breast pain from taking evening primrose oil, which contains gamma-linolenic acid, an essential fatty acid. While the research supporting this effect is mixed, a 2020 study[10] found that women with mastalgia who took 1,300 milligrams of evening primrose oil twice a day gained significant pain relief—far more than a control group that took acetaminophen—after six weeks. It's a low-risk proposition because evening primrose oil doesn't cause side effects.

BURNING MOUTH/GUMS: There is actually something called burning mouth syndrome, which is characterized by burning, tender, tingling, or numbness sensations in the mouth—and it occurs particularly in postmenopausal women.[11] It isn't clear why this happens to some women, though it's recognized that anxiety, depression, and stress can exacerbate it, as can other forms of mouth irritation. Also, certain medications (like some anti-hypertension drugs) and nutrient deficiencies (such as low levels of vitamin B12, folate, zinc, or iron) may be associated with the syndrome.[12] The following measures may help at least somewhat:

- Get a soft toothbrush. And brush gently! Avoid toothpastes that contain abrasive chemicals (like the whitening variety) and mouthwash that contains alcohol.[13]
- Avoid foods that trigger flare-ups. Common ones include hot or spicy foods, alcoholic beverages, and citrus fruits and juices. If you notice that certain foods make your symptoms worse, steer clear of them. Be sure to stay well-hydrated.
- Try an over-the-counter numbing agent. Applying topical anesthetics (such as capsaicin gel or benzocaine) to areas of

burning in the mouth can reduce pain significantly.[14] (Be sure to choose formulas that are meant for the mouth.)

- Chill your mouth. Sipping a cold beverage, sucking on ice chips, or chewing sugarless gum may help ease the pain.
- See your dentist. It's important to rule out gum disease or an infection, which your dentist can do. In addition, he or she may be able to prescribe stronger medications to ease the burning sensations.

DECREASED SEXUAL SENSATION/AROUSAL: This can be part of the fallout from the genitourinary syndrome of menopause: When the pH level increases due to the drop in estrogen, the genital tissues lose hydration and blood flow and, hence, lubrication. As a result, some women don't feel much when they're touched in the vaginal or clitoral region. Or, they have trouble with orgasms. These are not trivial losses; they can take a toll on a woman's self-esteem and mood, as well as the intimacy in her romantic relationship. Here's what you can do about this:

- Engage in sensate focus. This technique, which was developed by Dr. William Masters and Virginia Johnson in the 1960s,[15] is used to improve intimacy and communication related to sex between partners. Sex therapists often recommend it when couples are addressing issues related to arousal, orgasmic, and erectile dysfunction. Rather than being goal-oriented, the idea is to perform a series of touching exercises that focus on the sensory aspects of touch like pressure and texture so that couples can relax and tune in to the sensual experience without having preconceived ideas of what *should* happen. As partners take turns being the toucher and the recipient of the touching, the exercises progress from non-genital touching to genital touching to mutual touching. (You can learn more about it

here: smsna.org/patients/did-you-know/what-is-sensate-focus
-and-how-does-it-work.) One of the things this exercise does
is improve body awareness, which has been found to enhance
sexual well-being for women.[16]

- Do some self-stimulation. Masturbate or use a vibrator to
reignite sexual sensations and/or rediscover areas that may
be especially responsive to stimulation. Vibrators are a particularly effective treatment for orgasm difficulties, and you
can use them on your own or with your partner.[17]

- Expand your views of sexual pleasure. Try outercourse, including extended caressing, mutual masturbation, and sensual
massage instead of intercourse.[18]

- Talk to your partner. Kick around ideas for different ways you
might enhance your level of arousal. Consider making changes
to your sexual routine. Try sharing a bath, experimenting with
different sexual activities, or having sex in the middle of the
day or in a different room in your home. Adding a dose of nov-
elty and freshness often enhances sexual response.

- Exercise for sexual arousal. While any form of exercise can improve your sexual responsiveness partly by enhancing blood
flow, certain forms—like Spinning, doing Kegels or squats, or
using the captain's chair—can prime your G-spot. Research[19]
has found that many women report exercise-induced sexual
pleasure and even orgasms while working out. *Really!*

DEPRESSED MOODS/MOOD SWINGS: If you had PMS
or postpartum depression, or you have been susceptible to mood
swings throughout your life, the menopausal transition may prove
to be challenging in the mood-regulation department. Some
women's brains are particularly sensitive and reactive to hormonal
changes, and mood swings can occur when female reproductive
hormones go on a roller-coaster ride or drop dramatically during
the menopausal transition. Here are some strategies that can help:

- Get moving. Moderate to vigorous exercise can relieve depressive symptoms, boost your mood (thanks to the release of endorphins), and enhance your self-esteem. Whether you walk briskly, cycle, jog, swim, or do another form of aerobic exercise, make an effort to do at least twenty minutes every day for the sake of your mood and mind-set.

- Put your feelings into writing. Whether you do it with pen and paper or on your computer, writing about distressing experiences or emotionally fraught issues in your life can relieve depressive symptoms and enhance your ability to regulate your emotions.[20] Called expressive writing, this activity can be done in just fifteen minutes a day: Simply write your heart out without worrying about spelling, punctuation, or grammar. (It won't be graded; no one else will see this.)

- Expose yourself to bright light. Taking a walk in the sunshine or sitting next to a sun-drenched window can boost your spirits and invigorate you. If that's not possible, consider buying a commercial light box or lamp that emits 10,000 lux—and spend at least thirty minutes in front of it each day. Research has found that light therapy,[21] which is what this essentially is, has a significant effect in reducing depressive symptoms.

- Cultivate an attitude of gratitude. When you focus on what you really appreciate in your life, rather than focusing on your stresses and frustrations, it's like switching on a positivity channel in your brain. Your mood will take an upturn and you're likely to feel more satisfied with your life.[22] To make this happen, spend a few minutes at the end of every day, listing three to five specific things, large or small, that you were grateful for that day.

- Practice mindfulness. Research[23] has found that participating in a mindfulness-based stress reduction (MBSR) intervention involving meditation and yoga reduces depressive symptoms, anxiety, and perceived stress in perimenopausal women. You can find MBSR programs online or at local health and wellness centers.

- Consider therapy. If these measures don't sufficiently ease your depressive symptoms or mood instability, consider going for therapy. These days, there's an array of approaches to choose from, including cognitive behavioral therapy (CBT), which focuses on helping people identify and modify dysfunctional thoughts, feelings, and patterns of behavior; and acceptance and commitment therapy (ACT), which incorporates acceptance, a clarification of your personal values, and a commitment to changing behavior in ways that are in sync with these elements; and others. Do some research and find an approach that appeals to you.

DIFFICULTY CONCENTRATING: Whether it's due to declining estrogen levels, stress overload, or sleep disturbances, many women have trouble focusing or concentrating during the menopausal experience. These bouts can be intermittent or ongoing—and they're often intensely frustrating. Here's what can help:

- Consume caffeine strategically. If you need to jumpstart your focus in the morning or recharge it before giving a presentation in the afternoon, a well-timed cup of coffee or tea can help. But don't drink caffeinated beverages all day long or you could get edgy and anxious.
- Eat foods that are rich in omega-3 fatty acids. Diets rich in omega-3s—from salmon, sardines, anchovies, walnuts, flaxseed, and fortified foods—are associated with improved overall brain function. You may even want to consider taking omega-3 fatty acid supplements (a combination of docosahexaenoic acid, or DHA, and eicosapentaenoic acid, or EPA) if you're frequently struggling with focus; they've been

shown to help kids and teens with attention deficit hyperactivity disorder (ADHD).[24]

- See the advice under "brain fog" for more strategies.

DIZZINESS: Dizziness is a common symptom during the menopausal transition—affecting 36 percent of women ages forty to sixty-five at least once a week, according to a study in a 2018 issue of the journal *BioPsychoSocial Medicine*.[25] The underlying mechanisms aren't entirely clear but it is known that hormonal changes can affect how your body uses insulin, which can lead to blood sugar instability and dizziness.[26] Also, the presence of anxiety, hot flashes, fatigue, high blood pressure, heart palpitations, and inner ear disorders can predispose a menopausal woman to intermittent dizziness. Here's how to deal with it:

- Stay well hydrated. Drink fluids, especially water, throughout the day and consume lots of fruits and veggies, which are high in water.
- Eat small meals frequently. Instead of going for three square meals per day, downsize your meals and have a couple of snacks to help your blood sugar stay on an even keel.
- Try to reduce stress. Exercise, meditate, engage in deep breathing, do yoga or progressive muscle relaxation exercises—just do something every day to calm your physiological response to stress.
- Stand up slowly. Whether you're lying down or sitting down, make a deliberate point to stand up slowly in order to avoid[27] having your blood pressure drop suddenly (a condition called orthostatic hypotension[28]), which can lead to dizziness or feeling faint.
- See your doctor if dizziness persists or worsens. Only a doctor can determine if there's an underlying cause of persistent dizziness that warrants treatment with medication

or vestibular rehabilitation[29] (an exercise program that aims to improve balance, stability, and other factors related to dizziness).

DRY EYES: At first blush, the relationship between menopause and dry eyes may seem to be coincidental. But it turns out that changes in hormone levels—namely, decreases in androgen and estrogen—may play a role because these hormones influence production of all the components of the tear film.[30] Symptoms of dry eye syndrome include dryness (of course), as well as burning, blurred vision, increased tearing, light sensitivity, and sometimes grittiness in the eyes. Here are some measures that can provide relief:

- Lubricate your eyes. Using artificial tears, gels, or ointments several times per day can moisturize the eyes and help them maintain moisture. Placing warm compresses on your eyes (when they're closed) can help, too.
- Give your eyes regular breaks. When you're looking at a computer, you blink about half as frequently as normal, which can exacerbate dry eyes. A good guideline to use: Every twenty minutes, look at a spot twenty feet away for twenty seconds to give your eyes a break. It can also help to occasionally close your eyes for a few minutes or blink repeatedly for a few seconds to spread tears over your eyes.[31]
- Consume omega-3 fatty acids. Including foods—such as salmon, sardines, tuna, trout, anchovies, and flaxseeds—that are rich in omega-3 fatty acids in your diet may help with dry eyes. Alternatively, you could take omega-3 fatty acid supplements.
- Use a humidifier. Especially during the winter when indoor heat is on, add moisture to the air (at least in your bedroom) with a humidifier. Or, put a pan of water on or near your heating vent or radiator.[32]

- Wear wraparound sunglasses. Besides shielding your eyes from sunlight, wraparound glasses will protect your eyes from wind, which can have a drying effect.

DRY SKIN: As estrogen levels drop during the menopausal transition, your skin, which is the largest organ in the body, may pay a price. With menopause, the skin loses some of its ability to generate its own natural moisturizers and hold on to water, which can make it become dry and thin.[33] Besides looking parched or flaky, your skin can become itchy and easily irritated when it's dry. What to do:

- Use a mild cleanser, not soap. Some dermatologists recommend washing your face just once a day, in the evening—to remove dirt and makeup from the day—and simply rinsing it with water in the morning. After washing or rinsing your face, pat it dry then immediately apply a moisturizer that contains hyaluronic acid, lanolin, shea butter, glycerin, or ceramides.
- Steer clear of irritating ingredients. The last thing you want to do is aggravate your already thirsty skin—so avoid skin-care products with alcohol, fragrance, salicylic acid, benzoyl peroxide, or sulfates.
- Choose the right formulation. Different types of moisturizers offer varying degrees of moisture-infusing properties. In a nutshell, lotions are lighter than creams, which tend to be lighter than ointments. If your skin is very dry, you may need to use a cream or an ointment to rehydrate it and help it retain moisture. Reapply moisturizer throughout the day whenever your skin feels dry.
- Make sure you consume enough healthy fats. To keep your skin properly hydrated, consume a balanced diet that includes all the major food groups—but also be sure to get enough fat, preferably from plant-based sources such as olive oil, nuts, seeds, and avocados.

- Use warm, not steaming, hot water. Whether you're taking a shower or doing the dishes (in which case it's a good idea to wear rubber gloves), go with warm H_2O, not hot. Truly hot water will strip your skin of its natural oils,[34] leaving it sapped for moisture.

FATIGUE/LOW ENERGY: If you're feeling more tired than usual, it may be an indirect effect of the loss of estrogen. If you've been experiencing hot flashes, night sweats, sleep problems, anxiety, and/or joint aches, those symptoms can lead to fatigue, too. A study involving more than one thousand women in the Mediterranean region found that 73 percent of the menopausal women reported feelings of tiredness or exhaustion, which was a higher percentage than those reporting hot flashes, anxiety, memory problems, muscle or joint aches, or changes in sexual desire.[35] And if you're caring for children or aging parents and continuing to work during this significant life change, that juggling act can leave you feeling depleted. Here are some ways to boost your energy:

- Get some exercise. It may be the last thing you feel like doing when you're tired but it can actually help recharge your energy. Research published in the journal *Menopause* found that postmenopausal women who engage in regular moderate to vigorous physical activity have greater energy and vitality.[36]
- Downsize your meals. Eating smaller meals more frequently can help you keep your blood sugar steadier, which will help boost your energy. By contrast, having big meals can sap your energy.
- Increase your intake of key nutrients. These include foods that are rich in low-fat protein and high in potassium and magnesium. (Think: nuts, yogurt, beans, lentils, or fish.)
- Drink water throughout the day. Dehydration is a common cause of fatigue, as well as irritability and foggy thinking.

Even before you feel thirsty, your body's hydration will have dropped and you're likely to feel lethargic. While your personal need for water depends on your overall health, your level of physical activity, and your climate, it's a good idea to aim for approximately nine cups per day.

- Breathe right to refresh yourself. Just as engaging in certain breathing patterns can help you relax, the converse is true as well. Here's a yoga-inspired breathing exercise that can boost your energy and alertness[37]: Inhale for a count of two, then exhale for a count of two; inhale for a count of two, then exhale slowly for a count of three; inhale for a count of two, then exhale even more slowly for a count of four; inhale for a count of two, then exhale for a count of five. Repeat the pattern a few times then return to your normal breathing pattern. The flow of oxygen in your blood will have improved and you'll likely feel invigorated.

- Pace yourself. You might be unintentionally adding to your fatigue if you're overbooking yourself or taking on too many (nonessential) projects or responsibilities. If you can delegate or say no to new tasks or obligations, you'll be able to safeguard your energy.

- Consult your doctor. If you feel consistently wiped out and these measures don't help sufficiently, see your health-care provider to determine if an underlying health condition or medication could be making you feel tired all the time.

FREQUENT URINARY TRACT INFECTIONS: As estrogen levels fall, some women are susceptible to frequent urinary tract infections (UTIs). This may be because estrogen helps "good" bacteria thrive in the vagina, keeps "bad" bacteria in check, and because the pH level in the vagina decreases after menopause, making it more susceptible to infections. In addition to these post-menopausal changes, thinning of the vaginal tissue occurs, the pelvic floor becomes weaker, and sometimes the bladder droops (pelvic organ prolapse), and some women have trouble fully emptying their bladder, which can promote the growth of harmful bacteria. Recurrent UTIs can have a significant impact on a woman's quality of life. Here are some ways to prevent them:

- Always wipe from front to back. After having a bowel movement, wipe your bottom from front to back to reduce the chances of transferring E. coli bacteria from the rectal area to the urethra.

- Empty your bladder properly. When you're on the toilet, relax your pelvic floor muscles (instead of straining to pee) and let the stream of urine flow, allowing enough time for your bladder to empty completely. Make it a point to pee after having sexual intercourse to flush away any bacteria that may have entered the urinary tract during sex.

- Consider cranberry supplements. If you're prone to recurring UTIs, taking a cranberry supplement such as the medical-grade Ellura can prevent UTI-causing bacteria from sticking to the bladder. Drink lots of water throughout the day to continuously flush your bladder.

- Treat your genitals well. Whenever possible, take showers instead of baths to reduce exposing your genitourinary tract to bacteria. And avoid using harsh soaps, douches, and feminine hygiene products that can irritate the sensitive skin down there.

- Try D-mannose supplements. Research[38] has found that taking D-mannose supplements protects against recurrent UTIs in women who are susceptible to them; the theory is that D-mannose—a type of sugar found in many fruits—prevents bacteria from adhering to the bladder wall.

HAIR LOSS/HAIR THINNING: The loss of estrogen and other hormonal changes that accompany the menopausal experience can lead to hair loss or hair thinning. Normally, estrogen facilitates hair growth and makes it stay on the head; when estrogen levels decline, hair growth slows down and hair thinning or shedding becomes more pronounced. Meanwhile, a woman's body may produce more androgens during perimenopause and menopause, which can lead to hair loss and sometimes even bald spots. In fact, a study in the April 2022 issue of the journal *Menopause*[39] found that 52 percent of the 178 participating postmenopausal women had some degree of hair loss. Needless to say, most menopausal women I've treated are upset about losing their precious strands. Here's what you can do:

- Increase your intake of key nutrients. Make sure you're consuming enough protein, biotin, folate, and vitamins A, C, and B12, as well as minerals such as zinc, iron, magnesium, copper, and calcium, all of which influence hair growth.[40] If you can't get enough of these nutrients from food, consider supplements.

- Avoid stressing your hair. Brushing your hair too vigorously or too often, using tight rollers, or wearing tight ponytails can cause strands to fall out faster. In addition, overprocessing hair (with coloring, straightening, or perm treatments) or using curling or straightening irons too frequently can cause breakage of the hair shaft.

- Use a satin pillowcase for sleeping instead of a cotton one to prevent breakage during the night.

- Clean your hair carefully. If you're prone to hair loss, you'll want to keep your hair and scalp clean—but without drying them. So use a gentle shampoo, followed by a nourishing conditioner—and lukewarm, not hot, water. Wet hair is more fragile and prone to breakage than dry hair, so after shampooing and conditioning, don't towel-dry it or pull it up in a towel; use your fingers to gently comb it and let it air-dry as much as possible. When styling your hair, stick with a natural bristle brush or a wide-tooth comb and use a blow-dryer on a low setting.

- Consider using an over-the-counter hair growth product. Originally developed for male pattern balding, minoxidil (Rogaine) is available as an over-the-counter liquid or foam that's applied directly to the scalp. It can help hair grow and prevent hair loss and general thinning of the hair on top of the scalp in women, especially in those who have a family history of hair loss. This doesn't work for everyone and you need to use it for at least six months to know if it's going to help you.

- Talk to your doctor about other interventions. In particular, find out if you might benefit from a drug called spironolactone (Aldactone, a diuretic that has anti-androgen effects and hence helps with hair growth) or finasteride (Propecia, which also has anti-androgenic properties). Certain LED light therapies can also help stimulate hair regrowth.

HEART PALPITATIONS: It's not unusual for a woman's heart to race as she's getting a hot flash or even at odd times during the day, especially during perimenopause. As estrogen levels fluctuate and decline, there can be an increase in heart rate and more frequent palpitations, flutterings, or skipped heartbeats and non-threatening arrhythmias.[41] A study in the journal *Menopause*[42] found that 29 to 47 percent of women ages forty-five to fifty-five in four countries experience heart palpitations at midlife. Naturally, heart palpitations can be anxiety provoking, which can make palpitations worse. Here's how to cope:

- Engage in deep breathing. This can cause your parasympathetic nervous system to kick in and calm your body and mind. Doing yoga or meditation can have similarly calming effects.

- Decrease your intake of stimulants. These include caffeine, nicotine, sugar, and weight-loss supplements.

- Pay attention to your hydration status. If your body gets dehydrated, your heart will have to work harder, which can lead to heart palpitations. Also, when levels of certain electrolytes (such as potassium and magnesium) in the body are low, this can result in extra heartbeats or irregular rhythms. Drink water throughout the day and consume plenty of potassium-rich foods (such as potatoes, bananas, legumes, and yogurt) and magnesium-rich foods (such as nuts, seeds, beans, and yogurt).

- Try to identify other triggers. Pay attention to what else may be triggering your racing heart—common culprits include insufficient sleep, stress, spicy foods, and red wine—and try to avoid them.

- Know when to see your doctor. If palpitations are accompanied by trouble breathing, weakness, a squeezing sensation in your chest, or other worrisome symptoms, see a doctor ASAP. Sometimes heart palpitations may be linked to a thyroid problem or a heart condition (such as an arrhythmia), either of which can be treated with medications or procedures.

HOT FLASHES: The drop in estrogen levels that occurs during the menopausal transition causes what's called vasomotor instability—it's as if the thermostat in a woman's brain is being cranked up then down, then up and down again. As a result, you may become more sensitive to slight changes in body temperature,[43] which can trigger hot flashes. Research suggests that more than 80 percent of menopausal women experience hot flashes, often followed by chills, lasting for one to five minutes during the menopausal transition.[44] Here are some strategies that can help you cope with these body-temperature disturbances:

- Avoid common triggers. Spicy foods, alcohol, and hot beverages are known to trigger hot flashes in some women. For others, triggers can be idiosyncratic; try to identify yours and steer clear of them as best you can.
- Dress in layers. That way you can peel them off as necessary and put them back on when you're feeling cool or cold.
- Keep ways to cool yourself handy. Carry cold water and a handheld fan with you, and consider toting around a cooling mist you can spritz on your face as needed.
- Practice paced breathing. When a hot flash starts to come on, engage in deep, diaphragmatic breathing, which will dial down your physiological arousal and reactivity. This may help shorten or decrease the intensity of the hot flash.
- Consider acupuncture. Research has found that acupuncture and electroacupuncture (where a small electric current is passed into pairs of acupuncture needles to enhance the benefits) are effective at relieving hot flashes in menopausal women; the use of electroacupuncture was found to be as effective for relieving hot flashes as the use of non-hormonal drugs.[45]
- Try an over-the-counter remedy. Some women obtain hot-flash relief from taking black cohosh supplements, Equelle (which contains isoflavones), or Estroven (which contains black cohosh, isoflavones, and rhapontic rhubarb extract). The only way to find out if one of these can help you is by giving it a try.

INSOMNIA/TROUBLE STAYING ASLEEP: The hormonal havoc of the menopausal transition can interfere with the quality of your sleep. In particular, the drop in progesterone, which normally makes you sleepy, may be a factor. Insomnia can include having trouble falling asleep, having difficulty staying asleep, or waking up too early and not being able to get back to sleep. Many women experience sleep difficulties during the menopausal transition, with 26 percent of menopausal women experiencing severe symptoms that impact their daytime functioning.[46] Poor or insufficient sleep can also have metabolic consequences such as reduced insulin sensitivity and dysregulation of the hormones that regulate appetite and satiety,[47] among other ill effects. Here's what you can do to regain snooze control:

- Put yourself on a regular sleep schedule. Go to bed and get up at the same time each day, even on weekends, and carve out enough time to get the amount of sleep you need (most adults require seven to nine hours) every night to feel and function optimally.

- Get your sweat on. Do moderate to vigorous exercise at similar times each day but not within three or four hours of bedtime. Research has found that exercise keeps your body's internal clock running smoothly, relieves symptoms of anxiety and depression, and changes your core body temperature in ways that make it easier to fall asleep and stay asleep.

- Remove electronic devices from your bedroom. This includes the TV, computers, tablets, cell phones, and the like. Give yourself a digital curfew an hour or two before you turn in for the night.

- Cultivate a relaxing bedtime routine. Take a warm bath, listen to soothing music, read a book, meditate or do some gentle stretches, have a cup of non-caffeinated tea (such as chamomile or valerian root), or do something else to put yourself in the mood to snooze. Think of this step as a way of downshifting toward sleep.

- Keep your bedroom cool. Some sleep experts say the ideal temperature for sleep is between sixty-five and sixty-seven degrees. If you're prone to night sweats, you may want to go even colder. (In case your partner gets cold, keep an extra blanket at the foot of the bed.)

- Take supplements to help you sleep. Taking 250 to 500 milligrams of magnesium oxide or 5 milligrams of melatonin an hour before bedtime can set the stage for sounder sleep. (Melatonin, a hormone made by the pineal gland in the brain, helps regulate sleep-wake cycles.)

- Consider cognitive behavioral therapy for insomnia (CBT-I). If your sleep-related troubles persist, you may benefit from CBT-I, which is aimed at changing sleep-related habits and misconceptions about snooze control that can perpetuate insomnia.

JOINT ACHES AND PAINS: During the menopausal transition, more than 50 percent of women experience joint pain (a.k.a. arthralgia).[48] It's believed to stem from the loss of estrogen, which keeps the joints healthy and lubricated. These aches and pains can affect a woman's quality of life, including her mood and her willingness to participate in various activities. Here are some measures that can help:

- Take an anti-inflammatory pain reliever. For flare-ups of pain, consider taking a non-steroidal anti-inflammatory drug (NSAID) such as ibuprofen, naproxen, or ketoprofen. But these shouldn't be used day after day, week after week, unless it's under your doctor's direction.

- Apply some relief. Topical preparations such as capsaicin cream or NSAID gels (like Voltaren) or salicylate creams (like Icy Hot and Aspercreme) can provide short-term but effective relief from joint pain.

- Engage in low-impact movement. Physical activity strengthens joints, bathes them in synovial fluid, and promotes greater range of motion. I often say that "motion is lotion"— because movement keeps your musculoskeletal system lubricated by bringing blood to your joints and muscles. If you're already hurting, you may want to avoid high-impact activities and engage in yoga, tai chi, cycling, swimming, or using the elliptical machine.

- Look for supplemental relief. A variety of nutritional supplements—such as glucosamine and chondroitin, fish oil capsules, and collagen supplements[49]—may help relieve joint pain over time. Before taking a new supplement, check with your health-care provider to make sure it won't interact with any medications you're taking.

- Consume anti-inflammatory foods. These include plant-based foods (such as berries, bell peppers, nuts, and seeds), as well as fatty fish like salmon, tuna, and sardines. Various herbs and spices—including turmeric, rosemary, ginger, cardamom, cinnamon, and black pepper—have powerful anti-inflammatory properties as well. If you want to go the extra mile on this, you can take turmeric supplements or put a few drops of turmeric and black pepper extract in a smoothie or cup of tea. These won't help joint pain right away but they can set the stage for easing discomfort in the long term.

The Truth About Menopausal Weight Issues

For some women, gaining weight or the dreaded menopot is one of the most frustrating aspects of the menopausal transition. But what's really going on may surprise you. By themselves, the hormonal changes of menopause don't necessarily cause weight gain.[50,51] What they do cause is a shift in fat distribution and storage from around the hips (the pear shape of fat distribution) to around the waist (more of an apple shape). This means that the number on the scale may not change, but your jeans may suddenly be tight around the waist. That's the menopausal shift of body fat in action.

Meanwhile, some women *do* gain weight during the menopausal transition but this is usually due to genetic factors, age-related loss of muscle mass (which slows the rate at which your body burns calories), lack of exercise, insufficient or poor sleep, and/or changes in eating habits. Beyond the effects weight gain can have on a woman's self-esteem and body image, the concern is that excessive weight, especially around the midsection, is associated with an increased risk of cardiovascular disease, hypertension, type 2 diabetes, sleep apnea, and other chronic diseases, which is why it's important to take steps to control your weight during and after the menopausal transition. Here are strategies that can help:

- **Choose a healthy eating plan.** Don't play the how-low-can-you-go game with severe calorie restriction: While it may produce quick weight loss, it's easy to regain the pounds when you return to your regular eating habits. Instead, aim to shed pounds safely with an enjoyable, balanced eating plan—with 1,500 to 1,800 calories per day, depending on your level of physical activity—one that you can live with in the long run. Following a primarily plant-based plan, such as the Mediterranean diet, is helpful for weight control, as well as heart, brain, gut, and bone

health. Plant-based eating plans can include
dairy, meats, and seafood—but fruits, vegetables,
legumes, whole grains, nuts, and seeds provide
the bulk of the foods and nutrients.

- **Power up with protein.** A higher protein intake
  may provide a calorie-burning edge because your
  body uses more energy (a.k.a. calories) to digest
  protein than carbohydrates and fats. Include at
  least twenty to twenty-five grams of protein at
  every meal and consume high-protein snacks,
  such as Greek or Icelandic yogurt, edamame
  (young, green soybeans), and low-sodium cottage
  cheese. Having adequate amounts of protein
  distributed throughout the day also will help
  you feel fuller for longer—because protein takes
  longer to digest—which means you'll be less
  tempted to snack on high-calorie foods.

- **Focus on fiber.** The basic recommendation[52]
  is for women to consume at least twenty-one
  to twenty-five grams of fiber per day—but
  this is an instance where more may be better.
  Research[53] has found that people who consume
  an extra fourteen grams of fiber daily naturally
  consume about 10 percent fewer calories per
  day, which can lead to weight loss. To get to that
  goal, include at least five servings of fruits and
  vegetables and a minimum of three servings of
  whole grains daily, as well as nuts and seeds.

- **Set yourself up for success.** Plan delicious meals
  and snacks and keep your kitchen stocked with
  the healthy ingredients you'll need to assemble

them. Avoid keeping foods in your home that may cause you to overeat, such as ice cream, chips, cookies, and candy. If you want a treat, turn it into an activity with a goal such as walking to an ice cream shop when you're craving ice cream and getting a single cone rather than keeping a half gallon in the freezer.

- **Use an inverted pyramid to structure your meals.** Have your largest meal in the morning, followed by a smaller meal at lunchtime, and make dinner the lightest meal of the day—and stop eating after dinner. This way, you'll be consuming more of your calories when you're most active during the day and fewer when you're winding down. This is important because when it comes to weight control, when you eat may be as important as what you eat.

- **Account for liquid calories.** Coffee drinks, energy drinks, sweetened teas, beer, wine, and cocktails all have considerable amounts of calories and very few nutrients that promote good health. Also, your body doesn't naturally account for the calories you consume in beverages by leading you to consume fewer calories from food. What's more, drinking alcohol may reduce your eating inhibitions, especially for higher-calorie foods, making it harder to lose weight and keep it off.

- **Practice mindful eating.** Deriving satisfaction from what you eat plays a key role in weight loss and weight maintenance. If you dine at a table without being distracted by your phone or any other screen, it'll help you slow down your eating, which in turn will help increase feelings of fullness and satiety. Whether you're eating at home or at restaurants, make a concerted effort to eat slowly, perhaps putting down your fork or spoon between mouthfuls, and chew your food thoroughly, focusing on the flavors and textures of each bite. Doing this will help you get more enjoyment from your food—and give your brain ample time to register that you've had plenty to eat, before you end up eating too much.

- **Move more.** If you haven't been exercising, it's time to take up aerobic exercise (even brisk walking counts) and strength training (building muscle mass will boost your metabolic rate). If you're already exercising, increase the duration of your workouts by no more than 10 percent per week (to prevent injury) and do more strength training, including core exercises to tone and strengthen the muscles in the midsection. Taking these steps will help offset your body's age-related metabolic slowdown.

- **Be patient.** Losing weight and improving your diet is a long-term process, and it's important to figure out and use strategies that help you stay focused. For example, keeping a food and exercise journal and measuring or weighing food may be helpful for some women, but may generate anxiety or obsessive thoughts for others. Instead, you may find it useful to simply focus on healthy foods to include, such as lean protein choices, fruits, and vegetables, which can foster weight control without calorie counting. Having an exercise buddy (or two or three) will provide healthy support that can help you stay on track.

LEAKING URINE: Weakening of the pelvic floor muscles due to the aging process and the menopausal loss of estrogen can increase your risk of leaking urine when you jump, cough, or sneeze. If you gave birth vaginally or gained considerable weight in the midsection, these factors can take a toll on your pelvic floor as well. Some women accept leaking as a fact of life as they get older and may avoid certain activities or even sex for fear of leakage. But it doesn't have to be that way. Here's what can help:

- Do pelvic floor exercises. To strengthen the muscles around your bladder, do Kegel exercises. You can find the right muscles to contract and relax by stopping the flow of urine while you're peeing; if you can do that, you've identified the right muscles. (Don't make a habit of this, though, because it can lead to incomplete emptying of the bladder.) Once you know which muscles to use, do Kegel exercises when your bladder is empty—by focusing on tightening only your pelvic floor muscles (not the muscles in your abdomen, thighs, or butt): Hold the contractions for two to three seconds then release; work up to doing at least three sets of ten to fifteen repetitions per day. If you have trouble isolating the right muscles, ask your health-care provider for guidance; in some instances, vaginal cones, biofeedback, or pelvic floor physical therapy can help.
- Don't rely on pantyliners or pads. You may think you're doing yourself a favor by keeping your panties dry but liners

and pads can irritate the labia and trap bacteria that can lead to vaginal infections.

- Cut down on caffeine and alcohol. These can irritate the bladder, which can worsen leaking. Drink plenty of water to keep urine flowing and relatively dilute.
- Treat constipation. Having to strain to have a bowel movement can weaken the pelvic floor muscles, and carrying around excess stool can put unnecessary pressure on the bladder.
- Lose weight. Especially if the extra weight is in your midsection, it can weaken the pelvic floor muscles and increase the risk of urinary leakage.
- See a doctor. If these measures don't help sufficiently, see your health-care provider before leakage turns into a chronic problem. A urogynecologist, in particular, may be able to fit you with a device (such as a pessary), give you a medication, or tell if you you're a candidate for surgery.

LOSS OF SEXUAL DESIRE: Sometimes a woman's libido can become diminished during menopause as her estrogen and testosterone levels decline. And women may not feel very sexy when they're besieged by hot flashes or night sweats, which can turn them off to even the prospect of sex. Meanwhile, sex drive often decreases gradually with age in both men and women as they get older.[54] To rekindle your sexual desire, try the following measures:

- Consider what's going on in your relationship.[55] Are unresolved issues or resentments with your partner taking a toll on your libido? Do you feel loved and supported by your partner? When was the last time you felt spontaneously affectionate toward your partner? Try to address these issues on your own or with the help of couples' counseling.

- Examine possible health contributors. Could a medication you're taking be sabotaging your libido? Some diabetes drugs, antidepressants, anti-seizure drugs, and anti-hypertension drugs can quash a woman's sexual interest. Could a medical condition be to blame? Thyroid disorders, depression, diabetes, hypertension, autoimmune disorders, heart disease, and some neurological conditions can KO your sex drive. If any of these are happening to you, talk to your doctor about treatments that might help.

- Talk about what excites you. Spend some time with your partner sharing what pleases each of you sexually, what you fantasize about, and new things (or positions) you'd like to try. Discussing what might help you feel sexy again and what kinds of sexual or sensual activities appeal to you can put you both in the mood again.

- Stimulate your libido. There are many ways to do this—by doing some erotic reading or watching a steamy movie; by thinking or fantasizing about sex; by giving each other sensual massages. Or by shopping for sex toys together; even if you just browse, it may stimulate interest for both of you.

- Get a checkup. See your health-care practitioner for a full examination and blood tests to figure out if an underlying medical condition or low testosterone could be part of the issue.

NAUSEA: Though it's not as common as it is during pregnancy, nausea can occur during the menopausal transition due to the drop in estrogen and progesterone. Nausea also can stem from other menopause-related symptoms, including super-strong hot flashes, dizziness, anxiety, and heart palpitations. Feeling nauseous can throw you off-kilter, ramping up your sensitivity to certain smells or even tactile sensations. Here are some strategies for managing it:

- Alter your eating habits. Avoid spicy, fatty, and sugary foods and stick with bland foods—such as toast and tea—until the digestive distress passes. Don't skip meals; eat small ones throughout the day to prevent blood sugar from plummeting.
- Stay hydrated. Being even mildly dehydrated can worsen nausea so be sure to take small, frequent sips of water throughout the day.
- Put spices on your side. Eating ginger[56]—in tea, candy, or lozenges—can ease nausea from pregnancy, chemotherapy, and other scenarios including menopause. Drinking a cup of chamomile tea can also quell nausea.
- Apply the right pressure. Acupressure has been shown to be effective for reducing nausea and motion sickness—and the same is true of wearing Sea-Bands (acupressure wrist bands).[57] You can find these online or in many drugstores.
- Consider a B6 supplement. Pyridoxine (a.k.a. vitamin B6) has been found to be as effective as ginger in relieving nausea and vomiting during pregnancy.[58] You can take up to two 50 milligram tablets per day.[59]

NIGHT SWEATS: Night sweats are basically hot flashes that occur while you're sleeping. They can disrupt your sleep and make it difficult to get back to sleep, and they can leave you feeling tired the next day. Here are strategies that may help ease them:

- Dress for the occasion. Take a cool shower then wear loose-fitting, lightweight or moisture-wicking sleepwear to bed.
- Cool your bedroom. Turn down your home's thermostat or put on a fan. Keep light, loosely woven blankets handy for when you're chilly.
- Invest in cooling bedding. These days you can buy cooling bedsheets, pillowcases, and mattress pads that can help prevent you from becoming a sweaty sleeper.

- Calm your mind before turning in. Engage in a relaxing bedtime routine that includes practicing mindfulness meditation, progressive muscle relaxation, or deep breathing before you go to sleep.
- Consider a wearable device. Worn on the wrist, Embr Wave (EmbrLabs.com) lets you cool yourself off when you press a button, causing the device to emit cooling pulses that may improve your body's ability to regulate its temperature. You can wear it during the day, too, and there's a sleep mode.

PAIN WITH URINATION: Even if you didn't know there's a word for this—dysuria—you may be familiar with the burning, stinging, and irritation that occurs while you pee. Once again, you can blame the decline in estrogen for this symptom, which is part of the genitourinary syndrome of menopause (GSM).[60] For some women, the pain with urination leads them to believe they have a urinary tract infection and they end up taking unnecessary antibiotics or they rush to their doctor for a urine culture that turns out to be negative. Here are steps that can prevent or ease pain with urination:

- Go to the bathroom when you need to. Don't hold it; urinate when you feel the need to and empty your bladder fully. But don't overdo it by trying to empty your bladder too often, which could worsen or trigger a condition called overactive bladder.
- Avoid bladder irritants. Certain foods and beverages—such as spicy foods, carbonated or caffeinated beverages, acidic foods (like citrus or tomatoes), alcohol, and artificial sweeteners—are known to irritate the bladder. Nicotine does, too. Steer clear of all of these.
- Drink lots of H_2O. Sip water throughout the day and consume lots of water-rich foods such as fruits, vegetables, and

water- or broth-based soups. Consuming plenty of water will help flush out unwanted bacteria in the urinary tract.

- Take ibuprofen. When pain with urination is especially bad, a well-timed dose of ibuprofen can help. But this shouldn't be used as a regular treatment—unless your doctor recommends it.

- See your doctor if it persists. It could be that a bladder, vaginal, or sexually transmitted infection is causing pain during urination, in which case medication is in order. Your healthcare provider can determine the right one.

VAGINAL DRYNESS/PAIN DURING SEXUAL INTERCOURSE: The loss of estrogen due to menopause changes the pH level of the tissues in the genitourinary tract, including the vagina and vulva. This significantly decreases production of natural moisturizers and lubricants, causing the vaginal and vulvar tissues to become thin, dry, and less elastic after menopause. This can lead to substantial discomfort in the genital area, as well as pain, tearing, and bleeding during sex. Here's how to address these issues:

- Use a vaginal moisturizer. I recommend those from SweetSpot Labs or FemmePharma for daily use to keep the skin hydrated. Coconut oil and olive oil also work well and won't cause skin irritation.

- Lube up before sex. To prevent or ease pain with intercourse, over-the-counter lubricants (such as überlube or Slippery Stuff) are essential.

- Avoid harsh cleansers. Don't use soap or body wash on the vulva during a bath or shower; simply use clean water. And don't douche or use powders or fragrances down there because all of these can have a drying or irritating effect on these sensitive tissues.

- Get stimulated. Believe it or not, regular sexual stimulation—with a partner, by yourself, or using a device such as a vibrator—promotes vaginal blood flow and secretions.
- Talk to your doctor. If uncomfortable vaginal dryness persists, consult your health-care provider to see if you're a candidate for a low-dose estrogen product (available by prescription)—such as tablets, creams, gels, or an estrogen ring—which can be applied directly to the vagina without raising blood levels of estrogen.

By now you should have plenty of tools and tips to establish a long-term, evolving menopause treatment plan for yourself. It's up to you to prioritize the introduction of new strategies that make sense for your symptoms and your life. Give some thought to how and when you want to try new symptom-control measures. Some of these you may want to use once in a while, others more regularly. The beauty is that you can mix and match or add or subtract them as your symptoms ebb and flow. The power to improve your well-being is in your own good hands—trust them and your judgment to guide you in the right direction.

The Good, the Bogus, and the Unproven Remedies

When it comes to alternative treatments for menopausal symptoms, there's an underlying assumption that if it's on the shelf or on the market, it must be safe and effective. But that's not always the case. For one thing, dietary supplements, including herbal supplements, are not regulated by the Food and Drug Administration (FDA), and the same is true of many devices. Which means that this is an instance of "buyer beware"! In some instances, the worst that might happen is you waste your money; in others, you could end up with unpleasant side effects but not relief for the menopausal symptoms that are bothering you. Here's a closer look at which so-called remedies may be worth a try and which aren't:

Chaste Tree Berry Extract

The claim: A shrub native to countries in the Mediterranean region and Asia, chaste tree (a.k.a. *Vitex*) produces berries that are often used, as an extract or in powdered form, to treat PMS, menopause symptoms, and infertility issues.

The upshot: In a small 2019 study[61] researchers found that menopausal women who took *Vitex agnus-castus* extracts had diminished anxiety and vasomotor symptoms. Still, more research needs to be done to clarify the degree of effectiveness and its mechanisms of actions. In other words, the jury's out on this one.

Dong Quai Supplements

The claim: An herb used in traditional Chinese medicine, dong quai is purported to relieve hot flashes associated with menopause.

The upshot: Take a hard pass. There's no scientific evidence that dong quai helps with hot flashes—and it can be harmful if you take too much; it can also have dangerous interactions with blood thinners.

Evening Primrose Oil

The claim: Evening primrose oil is a phytoestrogen
(a plant with estrogenic properties) that produces
prostaglandins, a group of compounds that help regulate
blood flow; the extract is believed to relieve hot flashes,
night sweats, and other menopausal symptoms.

The upshot: It may be worth a try. Some studies
have found that taking capsules of evening primrose oil
decreases the severity and frequency of night sweats[62]
and may reduce the intensity of hot flashes.[63]

Maca Supplements

The claim: A medicinal plant that grows in Peru, maca is
sometimes made into capsules that supposedly relieve
hot flashes and improve sexual function in menopausal
women.

The upshot: There have been few rigorous studies
regarding the use of maca for menopausal symptoms
but there is some evidence that it may be helpful for
hot flashes and night sweats. More studies need to be
done to suss out safety and side effect issues. Which
means: The jury's out on this one.

Magnet Therapy

The claim: Magnets can be used to rebalance your
autonomic nervous system, which can relieve stress and
symptoms like hot flashes and insomnia.

The upshot: Save your money. There's absolutely

no evidence that magnets have an effect on any menopausal symptoms.

Wild Yam Extract

The claim: Wild yam (*Dioscorea villosa*) extract, which is applied topically as a cream, is often touted as a natural source of estrogen that can ease menopausal symptoms such as hot flashes.

The upshot: Preliminary research[64] suggests that when women use topical wild yam extract on a short-term basis, they don't experience side effects—but they don't get any relief from menopausal symptoms. Bottom line: Skip this treatment.

13

Self-Care Going Forward

Once you start to get a grip on your menopausal symptoms, it's time to shift your attention to protecting your health for the future. As one chapter of your life—your reproductive years—comes to an end, another beautiful one begins, which is why it's important to adopt lifestyle practices that can help you stay healthy well into the future. In particular, it's important to take steps to lower your risk of developing chronic diseases and conditions that tend to become more common as women become postmenopausal and get into their sixties, seventies, and beyond. This includes heart disease, osteoporosis, type 2 diabetes, pelvic floor dysfunction (including urinary incontinence), and cognitive impairment, the risks of which increase partly from the postmenopausal loss of estrogen and partly from age-related wear and tear on the body.

Fortunately, there's a lot you can do to reduce your risk of developing these diseases and others and improve your ability to age well—without turning your life upside down. I think of this ongoing self-care regimen as building the four pillars of health (diet, exercise, sleep, and mental health). Not only will these measures help you feel good and thrive right now but they also will help protect you from various health conditions that become increasingly common as women get older. Here are the key steps to take:

Adopt a Mediterranean-style diet that's rich in vegetables, fruits, whole grains, legumes, nuts and seeds, lean protein, and healthy fats. Replace saturated fats—found in meats, full-fat dairy products, butter, and tropical oils—in your diet with unsaturated fats such as olive and canola oils, avocados, nuts, seeds, and fatty fish like salmon. Don't engage in excessive dietary restraint or obsess about what you should or shouldn't be eating. Strive to maintain a healthy relationship with food, with even occasional indulgences (such as sweets), because food should be enjoyed and appreciated both for the nutrients and the pleasure it provides.

Also, be sure to stay well hydrated for the sake of your body and mind. Believe it or not, proper hydration contributes to your mental as well as physical performance. So it's important to consume at least sixty-four ounces of fluid daily (more if you are active) to help prevent poor concentration, short-term memory issues, and irritability. Water is the preferred source of fluid, but coffee (yes, even the caffeinated kind), tea (black, green, white, and herbal), milk, juice, and soft drinks count. Produce is also rich in water. Include at least five servings of fruits and vegetables to help meet your fluid needs.

Do thirty to sixty minutes of weight-bearing exercise (including aerobic and strength-training workouts) most days of the week; also engage in exercises that will enhance your balance and flexibility. Human beings were made to move and regular physical activity can improve or protect your health in just about every conceivable way. How? By reducing your risk of heart disease, helping your body manage blood sugar and insulin levels, strengthening your bones and muscles, reducing your risk of falls, improving your sleep and sexual health, and boosting your brain function and mood. It's also one of the best stress-busters around!

Make it a priority to get plenty of good-quality sleep (seven to nine hours *every* night) and stick with healthy habits that set the stage for a sound night's sleep. All too often women skimp on sleep in order to get more done, and they end up paying a price in terms of how they feel and function the next day and in the state of their health. So figure out how much good-quality sleep you need and how much you are currently getting: You can use a tracking device (such as an Apple Watch, Fitbit, or Oura Ring) to see how long you are asleep and how many times you are waking up during the night, perhaps without realizing it. (If you discover something unusual on one of these devices or if your partner tells you that you snore loudly, stop breathing briefly, or move your legs a lot during sleep, you should see a sleep specialist and get checked for sleep apnea and restless legs syndrome; the risks of both increase after menopause.)

Once you've determined how much sleep you need to feel and function at your best, move your bedtime thirty minutes earlier on a weekly basis until you can get the shut-eye you need every night. Maintain a consistent bedtime and awakening time—at least within an hour—even on the weekends. To create an environment that's conducive to good-quality sleep, use your bed only for sleeping and sex. Remove the TV and all electronic devices from your bedroom. Create a relaxing bedtime routine, perhaps with a warm bath, listening to gentle music, reading a not-too-stimulating book, writing in a journal, and the like. If you wake up during the night and struggle to get back to sleep, get out of bed, go to another room, and read a book or listen to soothing music (don't watch TV or use a computer!) until you feel sleepy—then go back to bed.

Take care of your emotional and mental well-being. Carve out private time regularly—whether it's to meditate, write in a journal, take a walk in nature, or do something else you enjoy—and spend time with positive, supportive people you trust. Periodically during the day, pause what you're doing and check your psychological/emotional pulse: Are you constantly worrying about things that are out of your control? Is your mood highly changeable depending on whom you're with or what you're doing?

Are you so focused on what's wrong in your life that you're not enjoying what's going well?

If you answered yes to any of these questions, make an effort to correct course—by focusing on what's within your control and accepting what's not; by making an effort to protect yourself from contagious emotions and steadying your mood as much as you can; and by appreciating the good things in your life even as you make an effort to improve other aspects of your life. In other words, make a concerted effort to support your emotional well-being as much as you can because if it's regularly off-kilter, you're likely to have trouble making complex decisions, working well with challenging people, and managing well in your work and personal relationships. If you find yourself struggling emotionally, consider seeking help from a therapist. You owe it to yourself to take good care of your mental health as well as your physical health.

Supplement Smarts

As far as dietary supplements go, there are some that may be worth taking—but you need to check with your physician first to make sure there aren't concerns about problematic interactions with drugs you may be taking. For menopausal women, I suggest taking vitamin D (800 to 1,000 IU) daily because it's difficult to get enough from food alone. And if your calcium intake from food is falling short of 1,200 milligrams per day, consider taking a calcium supplement (no more than 500 milligrams at a time). If you're a vegan or vegetarian, it can be hard to get enough B12 from your diet; in that case, a B12 supplement may be in order.

If you're concerned about heart disease, cognitive

function, or mood stability, you may want to take omega-3 fatty acid supplements, a combination of docosahexaenoic acid (DHA) and eicosapentaenoic acid (EPA). Meanwhile, a B-complex supplement can help boost energy and protect brain function if those are concerns. Also, if you're taking a statin for cholesterol abnormalities, I advise taking coenzyme Q10 supplements, which help reduce the muscle and joint pains that are common side effects of some statin medications. If you want to enhance your immune function and/or digestion, a probiotic supplement— the most common ones include various strains of Lactobacillus and Bifidobacterium[1]—may make a difference.

Also, if you suffer from insomnia, taking 250 to 500 milligrams of magnesium oxide or 5 milligrams of melatonin an hour before bedtime may help you enter the Land of Nod more easily. Also, it's important to remember that dietary supplements are not regulated by the Food and Drug Administration for safety, purity, or effectiveness. So it's a case of "buyer beware," which means the onus is on you to make good choices. Some independent organizations[2]—including US Pharmacopeia, NSF International, and ConsumerLab .com—offer quality testing and quality assurance that the product was properly manufactured and contains the ingredients it claims to and not harmful ones; their seals of approval may offer you a modicum of comfort or security.

Besides helping with many menopausal symptoms, regardless of your personal menopause type, all of these measures will help set you up for a healthier future. Best of all, these measures have crossover benefits: For example, the Mediterranean diet is widely known for protecting against heart disease and type 2 diabetes; the latest research[3] shows that it is also associated with better cognitive functioning as people get older. Similarly, having sufficient social support has been shown to not only improve people's psychological well-being[4] but also to increase their likelihood of engaging in regular physical activity.[5] And while many people realize that getting consistent aerobic exercise is beneficial for their heart health and bone health, they may not know that studies[6] have shown it to be as effective in treating depression as taking an antidepressant medication. *Movement really is medicine!*

If you need some extra motivation to make these lifestyle changes, think about your why: What do you want to be able to do ten, twenty, or thirty years from now? What do you want your legacy to be? How do you picture your life down the road? What do you want to be able to do? If you want to be able to travel, dance, play tennis or golf, continue working, volunteer in your community, or play with your grandchildren, think about how your health status may help or hinder your ability to do so and what lifestyle modifications might help you get to those gratifying experiences. When you connect something you value to a behavior change you want to make, you increase your chances of succeeding.

I've seen these values-driven results time and time again in my own practice: For example, a patient who connected her compassion for animals to her desire to adopt a vegan diet found it easier to make the switch because it felt personally meaningful to her. Another patient who wanted to clean up the environment took up plogging (picking up trash while jogging), which made building in time for exercise a no-brainer. Research[7] has found, for example, that when people who want to slim down integrate their personal values (a form of persuasion) into changes they want to make in their behavior, their motivation is stimulated and they're more likely to succeed at losing weight and keeping it off.

SET YOURSELF UP FOR SUCCESS

Rather than setting vague goals such as "improving my diet" or "exercising more often," you can help yourself succeed in making health-promoting changes to your lifestyle by drilling down into the details. Otherwise, vague goals tend to lead to vague results, which is probably not what you want to achieve. That's why it's wise to establish SMART goals, which are specific (S), measurable (M), attainable (A), relevant (R), and time-based (T). Let's take a closer look at what this really means:

SPECIFIC: What do you want to accomplish and what exactly will you do?

MEASURABLE: How can you measure your actions and your progress?

ATTAINABLE: Is your goal realistic for you?

RELEVANT: Is the goal meaningful to you personally and relevant to your life?

TIME-BASED: In what kind of timeframe will you complete your goal?

This framework to goal-setting is universally helpful. Whether you want to eat more plant-based foods (and less meat) or you want to increase your physical activity level, you could use the SMART acronym to shape any health-promoting goal, though the steps don't have to be in this exact order. Think of using this template to express what you're aiming for:

"In order to [state your overall goal here], I will [what you will do to achieve it] _____ times per week. This goal matters to me because [mention the relevance here] and I will achieve it by [name your timeframe]."

For example: "I will shift to a more plant-based diet by having meatless meals three days per week. This goal matters to me because I want to reduce my risk of cardiovascular disease. On a monthly basis, I will add an additional meatless meal to my weekly regimen until I get to the point where I am eating meat on an occasional, not regular, basis."

Another example: "I will increase my physical activity level by doing aerobic exercise and strength-training workouts at the gym four times per week for the next two months. This goal is important to me so I can lose weight, get fitter, and have more energy. I will track my progress by keeping a workout diary."

By stating your goals and intentions in clear, simple language, you will essentially create a road map that will help you get to your desired destination. Write down your SMART goals and allow yourself to celebrate reaching certain milestones along the way to your goals. Also, continue to refresh your reasons for wanting to achieve a particular goal so that it feels relevant for the long haul.

WORKING WITH YOUR DOCTOR AFTER MENOPAUSE

Once you segue from treating your menopausal symptoms to focusing on protecting your health into the future, you'll want to work closely with your doctor to make sure that you get the right screening tests at the right times. While various health organizations provide general guidelines about which tests women should have and when, *you* may need to have some sooner or more often than is typically recommended, depending on your personal and family medical histories. Some of these tests can be performed in your doctor's office, while others require a visit to a special radiology or other screening center.

Here's a look at the screening tests you should have, even if you feel fine.

Blood Pressure Screening

High blood pressure (a.k.a. hypertension) significantly increases a woman's risk of developing heart disease, stroke, dementia, kidney problems, and vision problems. Many women don't realize that blood pressure often increases after menopause, whether it's due to the loss of estrogen, weight gain, or an increased sensitivity to salt (which can happen after menopause).[8] In fact, after age forty-five, more women develop hypertension than men do.[9]

It's important to have your blood pressure checked at least every two years. If it's below 120 over 80 mm Hg, which is the upper limit of normal, the American Heart Association recommends having it checked at least every two years, starting at age twenty; for a woman who had gestational hypertension, preeclampsia, or eclampsia, I recommend annually. If your blood pressure is higher or you're being treated for high blood pressure, your doctor may want to check it more frequently.[10]

Cholesterol Screening

Abnormal cholesterol levels increase the risk for heart disease and stroke. Menopause is associated with a progressive increase in total cholesterol, an increase in low-density lipoprotein (LDL, the "bad" cholesterol) and triglycerides, as well as a decrease in high-density lipoprotein (HDL, the "good" cholesterol). Once again, you can blame these changes on the loss of estrogen. In fact, total cholesterol levels peak in women between the ages of fifty-five and sixty-five, about a decade later than in men.[11]

The National Heart, Lung, and Blood Institute recommends that women ages fifty-five to sixty-five have a cholesterol screening every one to two years.[12] You can have this done with a simple blood draw at your doctor's office or a lab. If your cholesterol numbers are not optimal or if you're taking a statin to improve your cholesterol numbers, you may be advised to have yours checked more often.

Diabetes Screening

Diabetes occurs when your blood sugar is too high,[13] and it can affect your health from head to toe, increasing your risks of vision problems and blindness, cardiovascular disease and stroke, high blood pressure, kidney disease, neuropathy (nerve damage), as well as skin and foot problems.[14] Many people are unaware that they have diabetes or prediabetes, a precursor to diabetes[15]—or that the risk of developing diabetes increases after menopause.[16]

To test your blood sugar level, you can have your blood drawn at your doctor's office or a lab. With a fasting blood sugar test, your blood sugar is measured after an overnight fast (not eating or drinking anything since the previous night): If the result is 99 mg/dL or lower, your blood sugar is in the normal range; a level between 100 and 125 mg/dL means you have prediabetes; and 126 mg/dL or higher means you have diabetes.[17] By contrast, the A1C test, which can be used to diagnose type 2 diabetes and prediabetes, provides information about your average blood sugar level over the previous three months[18]; it does not require fasting beforehand. An A1C level below 5.7 percent is considered normal,

5.7 to 6.4 percent indicates prediabetes, and 6.5 percent or higher means you have diabetes.

If you are forty-five or older, have your blood sugar routinely tested; the same is true if you're under forty-four and overweight or obese, or you were diagnosed with polycystic ovary syndrome (PCOS), or you have a family history of diabetes, or you had gestational diabetes.[19] Depending on the results or if you're being treated for diabetes or prediabetes, the frequency of testing is at your doctor's discretion.

These screening tests are especially important because high blood pressure, elevated cholesterol, and diabetes are all risk factors for cardiovascular disease, which is the leading cause of death in women. Many women don't realize this! After menopause women have a notable increase in the risk for cardiovascular disease due to the loss of natural estrogen; this is why women tend to develop heart disease at a later age than men (because women have the protection of estrogen until menopause).[20] But women who experience premature menopause have an elevated risk of cardiovascular disease from a relatively young age.

After Kathryn obtained significant relief from her Full-Throttle menopause symptoms, she began to face the fact that she really wasn't doing as much as she could to improve her high blood pressure—and she definitely wanted to avoid following in her father's footsteps. Not only did her father have high blood pressure and heart disease but he'd had a heart attack a year earlier and he was still recovering slowly. Kathryn had been counting on the anti-hypertension medication she was taking to make her high blood pressure go away completely but between the strain of caring for her father, working as a public relations executive, and managing four kids, that just wasn't happening.

So in addition to continuing her brisk-walking regimen, Kathryn decided to join a running group with other working moms, and she put herself on a more regular sleep-wake schedule with the hope that it would help her gain the energy she needed to train for a 5K race she'd signed up for. By the time she completed the race three months later, her blood pressure had come down considerably, her cholesterol and A1C levels were good—and she had lost weight. By improving her sleep and ramping up her exercise life, she became more aware of making good dietary choices to fuel her goals, which undoubtedly had positive ripple effects on her blood pressure. By setting new priorities for taking charge of her health, she reaped a variety of health improvements and feel-good perks.

Thyroid Screening

Thyroid disorders are common among women, and they become more common as people get older.[21] The latest research[22] suggests that the prevalence of overt and subclinical hypothyroidism (an underactive thyroid) is significantly elevated among women in the late menopausal transition. And while there isn't a consensus among medical groups, I recommend that asymptomatic women ages fifty and older get screened with a simple blood test for thyroid-stimulating hormone (TSH). Depending on the results, treatment and/or follow-up screening recommendations can be made.

Cancer Screening

Breast Cancer

There isn't a true consensus on this but many of the latest guidelines[23] indicate that women ages forty to forty-four should have the choice to start annual breast cancer screening[24] through mammography if they'd like to; women ages forty-five to fifty-four should have mammograms every year, while women fifty-five and older could have mammograms once a year or once every two years, based on shared decision-making with their doctors. These recommendations assume that the findings are normal; if they're not, or if a woman has several risk factors for breast cancer, she may be advised to have mammograms more frequently or additional imaging of the breasts (with ultrasound or a magnetic resonance imaging, or MRI, scan).

A mammogram is basically an X-ray of your breast tissue that's taken when each breast is compressed between two special plates on the machine,[25] usually from two different angles. Mammograms can be performed at a radiology or imaging center or at a hospital.

Breast cancer is the second most common cancer (after skin cancer) among women in the US,[26] and having regular mammograms is the best way for doctors to find breast cancer when it's most treatable and often years before it can be felt as a lump.

Cervical Cancer Screening

While cervical cancer used to be one of the most common causes of cancer-related deaths among women in the US, that's not true anymore. We have the widespread use of the Pap test, which can detect cellular changes on the cervix before they become cancerous,[27] to thank for that. If abnormal cells are found on the cervix during a screening test, they can be removed before they evolve into cancer.

These days, a pair of tests is conducted in a doctor's office or clinic. With the Pap test (a.k.a. Pap smear), a health-care professional lightly scrapes cells from a woman's cervix then sends them to a lab to be evaluated for precancerous changes.[28] With the HPV test, health-care professionals can look for the high-risk types of the human papillomavirus (HPV), the primary cause of cervical cancer, in a sample of cells from the cervix.[29] Best of all, these tests can be performed at the same time.

Between the ages of thirty and sixty-five, women are advised to have a Pap test every three years[30] (assuming the results are normal). Or, you can have a Pap test and an HPV test (what's called co-testing) every five years (if your results are consistently normal). A third option: You can have HPV testing alone every five years. In other words, you have choices! After age sixty-five, there's generally no need for further testing in women who have an average risk of developing cervical cancer and had either three negative Pap test results in a row, two negative HPV tests in a row, or two negative co-test results in a row within the past ten years.

Colorectal Cancer Screening

The third most common form of cancer in the US,[31] colorectal cancer is highly treatable when it's caught early—and even preventable if polyps are removed before they have a chance to turn cancerous. Because the incidence of colorectal cancer has been increasing in adults under age fifty, in 2021 the US Preventive Services Task Force[32] began recommending screening for colorectal cancer beginning at age forty-five, instead of fifty.

There are a variety of screening tests for colorectal cancer.[33] There are stool-based tests—which rely on a chemical to detect blood in the stool, use antibodies to detect blood in the stool, and/or look for altered DNA in the stool. And there are a few direct visualization tests: With a flexible sigmoidoscopy, a short, thin, bendable, illuminated tube is placed into the rectum to check for polyps or cancerous growths inside the rectum and lower part of the colon. With a computed tomography (CT) colonography (a.k.a. a virtual colonoscopy), special X-rays and computers are used to create images of the whole colon for evaluation. And with a colonoscopy, a doctor uses a thin, flexible, lighted tube to look for polyps or cancerous growths inside the rectum and the entire colon; during the procedure, the doctor can remove polyps or other growths that may be found.

The latest recommendations[34] call for adults ages forty-five to seventy-five to be screened for colorectal cancer; after seventy-five, screening decisions should be made selectively, on an individual basis. Depending on the results and the type of test you had, the frequency of follow-up screening will vary. In general, the guidelines advise people to have stool-based tests more often (every one to three years) if they're going that route, a CT colonography or flexible sigmoidoscopy every five years, or a colonoscopy every ten years. This assumes the results are normal. If polyps are found or if colorectal cancer runs in your family or you have inflammatory bowel disease,[35] you may be advised to be screened at a younger age or more frequently.

Bone Density Screening

It's no secret that menopause hastens bone loss in women—significantly!—and increases their risk of osteoporosis. By some estimates, 50 percent of postmenopausal women will have osteoporosis[36] but they may not even realize it until they suffer a fracture. Women aren't routinely advised to be screened for osteoporosis until age sixty-five[37]—unless they are younger women who are at increased risk because they regularly take medications (such as glucocorticoids, aromatase inhibitors, or gonadotropin-releasing hormone agonists)[38] that compromise bone density, have a parent who fractured a hip, or who smokes, consumes excessive alcohol, or has a low body weight. But I don't agree with those guidelines. I recommend having a baseline bone density test two to three years after menopause (the average age is fifty-one) because women lose the most amount of bone when they lose estrogen, which happens during the journey to menopause.

To screen for osteoporosis,[39] which means "porous bone," as well as osteopenia, a condition of low bone density that is often a precursor to osteoporosis, the gold standard is to have a DXA scan. A DXA machine—DXA is short for dual-energy X-ray absorptiometry—is used to measure bone density in the hip or spine,[40] partly because people with osteoporosis have a greater risk of fracturing these bones. In addition, bone density in these areas can predict the risk of future breaks in other bones. You can have this test done at a private radiology group, a hospital radiology department, or at some medical practices.

After Renée, fifty-six, a history professor who had the Mind-Altering Menopause Type, regained a steadier mood and sharper cognitive function, she began feeling a lot more confident. That's when she decided it was time for a full-body tune-up, including catching up with routine screening tests that she had neglected. She scheduled her mammogram (which was two years overdue), a Pap smear, her first colonoscopy, and a bone density test. All the results were in the normal range, except for her bone density: She was diagnosed with osteopenia. By this point, Renée had been engaging in brisk-walking sessions regularly and she decided it was time to up her game—by adding strength training to the equation. So Renée started working with a personal trainer at a gym three times per week and increased her protein intake to help her build muscle; she also began taking vitamin D and calcium supplements with the hope of improving her bone density at least somewhat. When I saw her most recently, she could bench press a lot more weight than I can and she looked lean and strong.

The Postmenopausal Symptom You Should Never Ignore

Sometimes women have a bleeding or spotting event after menopause—and they think, *Hmm, that's weird*, but shrug it off. That's a mistake. If a woman has gone for twelve consecutive months or longer without a menstrual period and suddenly has vaginal bleeding, an investigation is in order. The first step is to have a pelvic ultrasound, which can assess the state of the uterine lining to see if there are signs of polyps or fibroids—and take a look at the ovaries.

If an ultrasound reveals a thickening of the lining of the uterus, the woman should undergo an endometrial biopsy to see if there are signs of uterine cancer. If there are any concerning findings on the biopsy, then she would likely go for a dilation and curettage (D&C), a surgical procedure to remove tissue from inside the uterus. If ovarian cysts are found, they may be able to be followed with routine ultrasounds depending on their size and characteristics; if they're worrisome, a referral is made to a gynecological oncologist.

The most common causes of postmenopausal bleeding or spotting (in order of incidence) are:

1. Atrophy, a natural thinning of the lining of the uterus or vagina after the body no longer makes estrogen
2. Uterine fibroids or polyps
3. Pelvic trauma from infections
4. Postcoital bleeding: When the vaginal tissues get thinner and drier, sexual intercourse can lead to spotting.
5. Excessive growth of the cells that make up the lining of the uterus (endometrial hyperplasia)
6. Bleeding from the rectum or urinary tract
7. Infections
8. Cancer of the uterus, cervix, or vagina

As you can see, cancer—which is unquestionably the scariest possible cause—is the least common cause of postmenopausal bleeding. But it can and does happen. Even the less worrisome causes need to be identified and treated accordingly. The take-home message: Don't ignore postmenopausal bleeding!

What to Know About Pelvic Organ Prolapse

It's not a direct consequence of menopause but pelvic organ prolapse becomes increasingly common with age, particularly *after* menopause. As women get older, the tissues and muscles of the pelvic floor no longer support the pelvic organs the way they should, resulting in one or more of them dropping from their normal position. The phenomenon can involve a woman's bladder, uterus, or rectum descending into the vagina or bulging into the front or back of the vaginal wall. Research[41] suggests that as many as 50 percent of women may experience it, though some don't even recognize the symptoms.

While the most common causes of pelvic organ prolapse are pregnancy and vaginal childbirth (especially with large babies), obesity and long-term constipation also increase the risk because there's more weight or mass pushing on the organs in the pelvis. Jobs that require a lot of heavy lifting can elevate the risk. And having a hysterectomy can compromise support for pelvic organs high up in the vagina, thus increasing the risk of prolapse.

Symptoms of pelvic organ prolapse can vary but can include: a feeling of heaviness in the lower abdomen and genital area, a pulling sensation in the groin area, feeling like something is coming down the vagina, feeling or seeing a bulge or lump in the vagina, discomfort during sex, and difficulty peeing (such as feeling like your bladder isn't emptying fully). Sometimes pelvic organ prolapse doesn't have symptoms; it's found during an internal examination.

It's important for women to stayed attuned to these symptoms or to get checked for pelvic organ prolapse if they have risk factors for it. While it's not life threatening, it can seriously hamper a woman's quality of life and lead to pain, pressure, or other forms of discomfort in the pelvis. Treatment options can include pelvic floor exercises (with a physiotherapist), the use of a vaginal pessary (a small device, usually made of silicone, that's placed in the vagina to support the pelvic organs) or vaginal rings, or surgery.

My hope is that this information helps you formulate a long-term game plan for taking care of your physical and mental health well into the future. Besides helping you make your way onto steady terrain after menopause, I want you to be proactive about protecting your health going forward. Given that women spend a substantial portion of their lives in the postmenopausal zone, thanks to increasing human life expectancy, the goal is to help you arrive at a healthy, feel-good next phase of your life. You've earned it!

Conclusion

Congratulations! You have arrived at the end of this book—but not the end of your feel-good, better-health journey. That will be an ongoing adventure. The good news is, you have identified your menopause type(s) and you now know the optimal ways to handle your personal constellation of symptoms. And you are now armed with the right tools to make this a smoother journey and to troubleshoot any challenges that may crop up along the way. Trust yourself because you have the knowledge and the wherewithal to guide yourself toward feeling and functioning better now and for the foreseeable future. But remember: You don't have to go it alone; don't be afraid to seek additional help from your family, friends, or from medical professionals when you need it.

Menopause is an example of an experience where women don't know what they don't know. Throughout this book, I have filled you in on that crucial 411 and given you the knowledge and power to navigate this tricky terrain along with your clinician. By using the program I have created in these pages, you will be able to not only ease distressing menopausal symptoms and manage your menopause type(s) but also achieve greater physical and emotional well-being. Maybe you'll feel like your old self again or maybe you'll feel even better—it's all good!

Remember to trust your instincts and the plan you've been developing. Don't let yourself be swayed by so-called experts who share super-strong opinions online or on social media about what women should or shouldn't do to treat their menopausal symptoms. You know your body and mind the best and by reading this book, you've learned so much more about healthy measures that are likely to help you, as well as bogus ones you should steer clear of. And if the approaches you've been trying don't help you sufficiently, come back to this book again and try some different strategies. This is your go-to guide for recrafting your approaches to self-care whenever you need to.

After all, there isn't a linear path through the menopausal transition. There are lots of twists and turns that are often challenging to navigate. But now you have a detailed road map to help you get to your desired destination—your feel-good future. And you have the ability to redraw that map whenever you need to. Don't hesitate to do that.

As you obtain relief from your most bothersome symptoms and forge a healthy path into your future, stay open to the possibility that your best self may not be behind you but ahead of you. Some women actually relish settling into the north side of menopause, as they wave a permanent goodbye to monthly cramps and hormonal headaches, worries about unintended pregnancies, premenstrual mood swings, and the like. Many women reach a more peaceful equilibrium in their lives or experience a new sense of self-possession or surges of creativity. If you're lucky you may experience what's referred to as "postmenopausal zest"—a new energy and clarity that stem partly from the absence of unpleasant symptoms but also from deciding to make yourself a priority.

After spending years putting other people first, some of my patients have embarked on new careers, taken up new hobbies or artistic pursuits, enjoyed exciting travel adventures, volunteered for meaningful causes, or discovered the best sex of their lives after menopause. After getting relief from her Full-Throttle menopause symptoms, Joy, fifty-two, a computer science professor and mother of a teenage son, took a sabbatical from work so she could take a yearlong acrobatics course; besides enjoying the adventure to the fullest, she decided to tie her experience and training into her courses on kinesiology and engineering when she returned to work. After getting a grip on her symptoms of the Premature Menopause Type, Erin, thirty-nine, a preschool teacher who enjoyed hiking, began volunteering at a local rock-climbing arena to freshen up her "stale" routine and meet new people. Six months later, she felt physically and emotionally reinvigorated after completing a two-day mountain hike with friends and helping a blind friend win a rock-climbing contest (Erin had coached her the whole way up and down). After menopause, both women's worlds expanded in fantastically gratifying directions. Yours can, too!

What I want most is to help you thrive throughout the menopausal experience and right into the next decades of your life. I'll be cheering you on every step of the way. You deserve to make this your time to shine!

Appendix

HIGH INTENSITY INTERVAL TRAINING (HIIT)

You've probably heard about high-intensity interval training (HIIT for short). A hot concept in the fitness world, this approach alternates short bouts of vigorous exercise with brief periods of exercising at a slightly slower or gentler pace. This cranks up the intensity of your overall workout—more than exercising at a steady pace would—giving you a bigger bang for your efforts.

Besides pushing your heart rate and boosting your overall aerobic capacity, HIIT helps you build muscle strength and endurance and allows you to burn more calories during the workout and afterward (what's called the after-burn effect). As an added bonus: HIIT has been found to improve blood sugar regulation, insulin sensitivity, and blood vessel (endothelial) function. Check with your clinician before starting any exercise plan.

BODY WEIGHT HIIT WORKOUT

SQUATS: **1 minute**
FAST FEET: **30 seconds** Stand with your feet hip-width apart and your knees slightly bent. Jog in place as quickly as you can, keeping your body low; don't bounce up and down.

JUMPING JACKS: **1 minute**

ALTERNATING KNEE-TO-CHEST RAISES: **30 seconds**

BURPEES: **30 seconds** Stand with your feet hip-width apart and assume a squat position, with your knees bent, your back straight, and your feet shoulder-width apart. Place your hands on the floor in front of you, just inside your feet, and with your weight on your hands, kick your feet back into a push-up position. Do one push-up then jump your feet back to their starting position, stand up and reach your arms over your head, jumping quickly into the air and landing back where you started. Repeat.

FORWARD LUNGES: **1 minute, alternating with right and left leg**

180-DEGREE JUMPS: **30 seconds**

SIDE LUNGES: **1 minute, alternating to the right and left side**

MOUNTAIN CLIMBERS: **30 seconds** Get into a plank position, with your hands shoulder-width apart, your back flat, and your head in line with your spine. Lift your right foot and pull your right knee toward your chest. Return it to its start position, and immediately lift your left foot and pull your left knee toward your chest. The goal is to keep your hips down and essentially run your knees in and out as fast as you can.

BIRD DOG: **30 seconds** Get down on all fours, with your hands on the floor directly under both shoulders and your knees directly under your hips. Keep your head in line with your spine and lift your right arm forward and your left leg straight behind you until they are both parallel to the floor. Pause, then return to the starting position. Repeat with the left arm and the right leg. Pause, and return to the starting position. Throughout the exercise, keep your abdominal muscles tight, your back flat, and your hips level throughout the exercise.

PLANK: **hold for 30 seconds**
SUPERMAN: **30 seconds** Lie facedown on the floor with your legs extended straight and your arms extended on the floor above your head. While keeping your neck in line with your body and your eyes focused on the floor, simultaneously raise your arms, legs, and chest a few inches off the floor and hold for two seconds. Slowly return to the starting position. Repeat.
SIDE PLANK: **hold for 30 seconds on each side**
BICYCLE CRUNCHES: **30 seconds**
BRIDGE (A.K.A. HIP RAISES): **30 seconds** Lie on your back with your knees bent at a ninety-degree angle and your feet flat on the floor, your arms at your sides. As you push down through your feet, lift your hips up as high as you can; then, return your hips to the floor in a controlled fashion. Repeat.

Take a thirty-second break then repeat this sequence twice for a twenty-minute workout, three times for a thirty-minute workout. Stretch.

THE DIY HIIT WORKOUT

You can also turn any cardio workout—including walking, jogging, or cycling—into a HIIT session by repeating intense rotations with bouts of active recovery. After warming up for a few minutes, here's how this might look:

Go as hard as you can for thirty seconds.
Walk, jog, or pedal at a comfortable pace for one minute.
Repeat this pattern for the duration of your workout (optimally, twenty or thirty minutes).
Cool down, then stretch.

TRACKING CHART

SYMPTOMS	Mon.	Tues.	Wed.	Thur.	Fri.	Sat.	Sun.
BLEEDING/ SPOTTING							
SLEEP QUALITY/ QUANTITY							
BOTHERSOME SYMPTOMS							
MOOD							
MOVEMENT/ PHYSICAL ACTIVITY							
WHAT YOU'RE DOING FOR SELF-CARE							

Tracking instructions: Spend up to five minutes at the end of the day jotting down notes about your symptoms and experiences for that day. Depending on the item, you can make a check mark (for bleeding, for example), indicate yes or no (for movement), or jot down a quick description of how you're feeling (in the way of mood or bothersome symptoms) or what you did (for self-care). The goal isn't to turn this into a major project—you have enough to do!—but to make this work for you, simply and easily.

Resources

Associations

American Academy of Sleep Medicine (AASM): a professional society dedicated to the specialty of sleep medicine. The site provides patients with information about basic sleep issues and various sleep disorders: AASM.org.

American College of Obstetricians and Gynecologists (ACOG): the professional medical society for obstetricians and gynecologists that's dedicated to providing high-quality, safe medical care for women throughout their reproductive lifespan. The site offers patient information about a variety of topics including contraception, menopause, and more: ACOG.org.

American Council on Exercise (ACE): an organization that certifies exercise professionals and runs programs designed to get people moving. The site offers a healthy living blog and a library of essential exercises: ACEfitness.org.

American Psychological Association (APA): the leading scientific and professional organization representing psychology clinicians, researchers, educators, consultants, and students. The site offers basic information and articles about a variety of timely subjects and links to new research: APA.org.

Endocrine Society: A global community of physicians and scientists who are working at the forefront of hormone science in an effort to improve people's health and well-being. The site is a good source of information and news about various subjects related to hormonal health, from appetite regulation to menopausal issues and thyroid disorders: Endocrine.org.

International Society for the Study of Women's Sexual Health (ISSWSH): a multidisciplinary, scientific, and academic organization focused on women's sexuality, sexual health, experience, and function. The site includes a directory of providers: ISSWSH.org.

The North American Menopause Society (NAMS): a leading nonprofit dedicated to promoting the health and quality of life of women during midlife by providing an understanding of menopause and healthy aging. The site offers an array of helpful information for patients—and it can help you find a menopause practitioner near you: Menopause.org.

Books

The Female Brain (2007) by Dr. Louann Brizendine provides a fascinating look at women's unique brain-body-behavior patterns, including differences in how we think, what we value, how we communicate, and how we love.

Flow: The Psychology of Optimal Experience (2008) by Mihaly Csikszentmihalyi provides insights into the psychology of "optimal experience," or flow, that allows people to experience deep enjoyment, creativity, and full immersion in what they're doing.

The How of Happiness: A New Approach to Getting the Life You Want (2008) by Sonja Lyubomirsky, PhD, offers a comprehensive guide to understanding the elements of happiness and practical strategies for increasing yours.

The XX Brain: The Groundbreaking Science Empowering Women to Maximize Cognitive Health and Prevent Alzheimer's Disease (2020) by Dr. Lisa Mosconi presents groundbreaking research on how women's brains age differently from men's, including evidence-based approaches to protecting the female brain through diet, stress reduction, and sleep.

Body Kindness: Transform Your Health from the Inside Out—and Never Say Diet Again (2016) by Rebecca Scritchfield, RDN, is a practical gem of a book that helps you embrace, love, and honor your body while improving your physical and emotional health.

Women's Moods: What Every Woman Must Know About Hormones, the Brain, and Emotional Health (2000) by Deborah Sichel, MD, and Jeanne Watson Driscoll, MS, RN, CS, takes an intimate look at how and why women's mood issues can change during each stage of their reproductive lives, with advice on steps to take to stabilize the brain and feel better.

The Menopause Diet Plan: A Natural Guide to Managing Hormones, Health, and Happiness (2020) by Hillary Wright, MEd, RDN, and Elizabeth Ward, MS, RDN, provides dietary and lifestyle recommendations for managing your physical and emotional health during perimenopause and menopause; the book also includes lots of tasty recipes.

Websites

Psychology Today: Besides offering a wealth of informative articles about a wide array of psychological subjects, the site offers a free service that allows you to search for a therapist near you: Psychology Today.com/us.

Speaking of Women's Health: a website run by Holly L. Thacker, MD, of the Cleveland Clinic, that provides information about a variety of women's medical conditions and lifestyle recommendations: Speakingof WomensHealth.com.

Glossary

Acceptance and commitment therapy (ACT): a form of psychotherapy that incorporates acceptance, a clarification of one's personal values, and a commitment to changing behavior in ways that are in sync with these elements.

Adaptogens: a class of non-toxic plants, particularly herbs and roots, that are believed to assist the body in better handling physical and mental stress. These include ashwagandha, Asian ginseng, and rhodiola, among others.

Androgens: Often called male hormones, androgens (such as testosterone) contribute to growth and reproductive function; women's bodies produce them, too.

Anovulatory cycles: menstrual cycles in which ovulation doesn't occur for one reason or another.

Anti-mullerian hormone (AMH): a hormone that's produced by cells in the small follicles in the ovaries; levels of AMH are sometimes measured to gauge how well a woman's ovaries are functioning and to determine whether she is nearing menopause.

Bioidentical hormones: The North American Menopause Society uses the term to refer to "compounds that have the same chemical and molecular structure as hormones that are produced in the body." In recent years, "bioidentical" has been used to refer to made-to-order (a.k.a. custom-compounded) hormone treatments that pharmacies create for a particular woman.

Chemopreventive drugs: medications such as tamoxifen, raloxifene, or aromatase inhibitors that are taken to lower a woman's cancer risk or prevent a recurrence of cancer; these can trigger an increased intensity of menopausal symptoms, especially hot flashes.

Cognitive behavioral therapy (CBT): a form of psychotherapy that focuses on helping people identify and modify dysfunctional thoughts, feelings, and patterns of behavior in order to change their responses to challenging situations. There's also a form of CBT that addresses insomnia called CBT-I.

Cognitive distortion: an exaggerated or skewed thought pattern that can affect the way you perceive what's happening around you, often in a negative or unhelpful way; this can increase anxiety, depression, and other unwanted states of mind.

Contraindication: the presence of a medical condition or symptom that serves as a reason for someone not to receive a particular treatment or procedure because it could be harmful.

Dehydroepiandrosterone (DHEA): a hormone naturally produced in the adrenal gland that helps produce other hormones, including estrogen and testosterone.

Diminished ovarian reserve (DOR): a condition in which the ovaries lose their normal reproductive potential, thus compromising fertility.

Early menopause: menopause that occurs between the ages of forty and forty-five (the average age for menopause is fifty-one).

Endocrine-disrupting chemicals (EDCs): Chemicals that can mimic, block, or interfere with hormones in the body, including estrogen and androgens; high levels of EDCs in the body have been linked with an earlier age of menopause.

Endometriosis: an often painful disorder in which tissue that's similar to the tissue that lines the inside of the uterus grows outside of the uterus.

Estrogens: a group of hormones that plays an important role in the reproductive and sexual development of women, among other functions. Men have estrogen, too, and it helps with their sex drive and erectile function.

Fibroids: noncancerous growths made of smooth muscle cells and fibrous connective tissue that develop in the uterus; they can cause pelvic pain and heavy menstrual bleeding.

Follicle-stimulating hormone (FSH): It tells the ovaries to release an egg (a.k.a. ovulate) each month during a woman's reproductive years.

Genitourinary syndrome of menopause (GSM): a variety of changes and symptoms that can occur in the vaginal and vulvar tissue, as well as in the urinary tract, due to the loss of estrogen and changes in the pH level of the tissues that come with menopause.

Hormone therapy (HT): the use of hormones at low doses to treat menopausal symptoms or otherwise help a woman who is experiencing natural menopause; it's also referred to as menopausal hormone therapy (MHT). By contrast, hormone replacement therapy (HRT), which is used for women with premature menopause, early menopause, or premature ovarian insufficiency, contains higher doses of hormones because it's essentially providing or replacing the hormones that the woman's body should be making at her age.

Hypoactive sexual desire disorder (HSDD): a clinical condition that occurs for unknown reasons and produces an ongoing or prolonged lack of interest in sex that causes significant emotional distress.

Hypothalamic pituitary adrenal (HPA) axis: the body's central stress response system that leads to the release of the stress hormone cortisol when something threatening or stressful happens.

Hypothalamic-pituitary-ovarian (HPO) axis: a tightly regulated system that secretes hormones involved in female reproduction.

Hypothalamus: a small region of the brain that plays a significant role in controlling many bodily functions such as releasing hormones and regulating body temperature and sleep cycles, among others.

Hysterectomy: a surgical procedure to remove the uterus.

Kegel exercises: Also known as pelvic floor exercises, Kegel exercises are performed to strengthen the pelvic floor muscles, prevent urine leakage and other pelvic floor problems, and improve sexual response (including orgasms).

Libido: sexual desire.

Medication-induced menopause: a medically induced cessation of ovarian function, often from chemotherapy or other cancer treatments.

Melatonin: a hormone released by the pineal gland that helps regulate the sleep-wake cycle.

Menopause: the milestone when a woman has gone a full year without getting a menstrual period. It's a retrospective event, given that a woman won't know when her final period occurred until she has gone twelve months without another one.

Menopause transition: the time span from perimenopause to your last menstrual period, which can take up to a decade for some women.

Micronized: when a substance is broken into fine particles.

Mindfulness: the ability to be fully present in the here and now and maintain a moment-to-moment awareness of your thoughts, bodily sensations (such as your breath), and surrounding environment.

Natural menopause: menopause that occurs spontaneously or without any intervention after age forty-six.

Neurotransmitters: chemical messengers—such as dopamine and serotonin—that transmit messages from neurons (nerve cells) to target cells throughout the body; they play significant roles in mood, mental health, sleep, and behavior.

Obstructive sleep apnea (OSA): a disorder characterized by repetitive pauses in breathing while you're asleep; this can lead to loud snoring and frequent arousals from sleep, as well as a host of long-term health risks (including heart failure).

Osteopenia: low bone mineral density that's considered a precursor to osteoporosis. The World Health Organization (WHO) defines bones with a T-score—which compares your bone mass to that of a healthy, young adult—between –1 and –2.5 as osteopenic.

Osteoporosis: a progressive condition in which bones become structurally weak and susceptible to fracture. The WHO defines bones with a T-score—which compares your bone mass to that of a healthy, young adult—below –2.5 as osteoporotic.

Oxytocin: a hormone that's produced in the brain's hypothalamus and secreted by the pituitary gland. It's often called the "cuddle hormone" because it's released during hugging or snuggling. It fosters bonding and trust and reduces symptoms of anxiety and depression.

Paced breathing: slow, deliberate, diaphragmatic breathing that can reduce activity in the sympathetic nervous system, decrease hot flashes, and induce the relaxation response.

Parasympathetic nervous system: the part of the autonomic nervous system that controls largely automatic processes such as digestion, respiration, and heart rate—and the relaxation response.

Pelvic floor: a group of muscles and other tissues in the base of the pelvis, between the tailbone and the pubic bone, that supports the pelvic organs.

Pelvic organ prolapse: a condition in which one or more pelvic organs—such as the uterus, bladder, or rectum—drop from their normal position due to weakening of the muscles and tissues that support those organs.

Perimenopause: the long, and sometimes winding, transition to menopause; symptoms can start as early as ten years before your final menstrual period.

Polycystic ovarian syndrome (PCOS): a common reproductive health problem in women that stems from an imbalance in reproductive hormones (namely, excessive male hormones); PCOS can cause irregular periods, weight gain, acne, excessive hair growth, and infertility.

Postmenopause: the time span that follows your official one-year anniversary without menstrual periods and continues into the future; in other words, every day after menopause. It's important to note: Women can still have symptoms related to menopause in postmenopause.

Premature menopause: menopause that occurs before age forty for one reason or another, including genetic disorders.

Premenstrual dysphoric disorder (PMDD): a more severe and sometimes disabling form of PMS (see below).

Premenstrual syndrome (PMS): a combination of physical, emotional, and behavioral symptoms (such as bloating, breast tenderness, mood swings, and cravings) that many women get a week or two before their menstrual period.

Premature ovarian insufficiency (POI): a disorder in which a woman's ovaries stop producing eggs before age forty, which also means they no longer produce sufficient estrogen.

Probiotics: beneficial bacteria found in certain foods—including yogurt, kefir, kimchi, sauerkraut, and miso—and supplements that contribute to increasing the population of "good" or health-promoting bacteria in your gut.

Progesterone: a female sex hormone that's involved in the menstrual cycle, preparing the body for pregnancy, and maintaining pregnancy.

Progressive muscle relaxation: a relaxation technique that involves slowly tensing then relaxing your muscles from head to toe, or vice versa, in order to relieve stress.

Restless legs syndrome (RLS): a condition that causes an intense, often irresistible, urge to move your legs during sleep.

Rumination: the tendency to dwell on or overthink upsetting situations, which can lead to an increase in anxiety, depression, sleep disturbances, and unhealthy behaviors.

Surgical menopause: menopause that's caused by the surgical removal of *both* ovaries; if only one is removed, the other ovary may keep working.

Sympathetic nervous system: the part of the autonomic nervous system that orchestrates the body's fight-or-flight response, including release of the stress hormone cortisol.

Testosterone: the primary male sex hormone (androgen) that plays a critical role in the development of the penis and testes, muscle and bone growth and strength, sex drive, and sperm production. Women have testosterone, too: It's produced in the ovaries and the adrenal gland and assists with ovarian function and sexual behavior (including libido).

Transdermal delivery: the application of a drug (or hormone) through the skin, typically by using an adhesive patch, so that it's absorbed slowly into the body.

Urinary incontinence: loss of bladder control. The primary types are stress incontinence, which occurs when there's increased abdominal pressure from coughing, sneezing, and the like, and urge incontinence, which involves an involuntary loss of urine when a woman suddenly feels the urge to go and can't get to the bathroom fast enough.

Uterine hyperplasia: a buildup of the uterine lining that increases the risk of precancerous or cancerous cells developing. The risk of this happening increases if a woman who has a uterus takes estrogen without progesterone to treat her menopausal symptoms.

Vaginal atrophy: a truly unfortunate term (IMO) that's sometimes used to describe the vaginal tissue becoming thinner and drier due to the loss of estrogen that comes with menopause. This term has largely been replaced by GSM.

Vaginismus: a condition involving the involuntary tensing or contracting of muscles around the vagina, which often makes sexual intercourse painful.

Vaginitis: inflammation of the vagina that can result in discharge, itching, and pain; it can be due to infection or loss of estrogen after menopause.

Vasomotor symptoms: those that occur due to the constriction or dilation of blood vessels resulting in temperature dysfunction; the most common vasomotor symptoms are hot flashes and night sweats.

Selected Bibliography

Introduction

Kling, J. M., K. L. MacLaughlin, P. F. Schnatz, C. J. Crandall, L. J. Skinner, C. A. Stuenkel, A. M. Kaunitz, D. L. Bitner, K. Mara, K. S. Fodmader Hilsaca, and S. S. Faubion. "Menopause Management Knowledge in Postgraduate Family Medicine, Internal Medicine, and Obstetrics and Gynecology Residents: A Cross-Sectional Survey." *Mayo Clinic Proceedings* 94, no. 2 (February 1, 2019): 242–253. https://www.mayoclinicproceedings.org/article/S0025–6196(18)30701–8/fulltext.

Marlatt, K. L, R. A. Beyl, and L. M. Redman. "A Qualitative Assessment of Health Behaviors and Experiences During Menopause: A Cross-sectional, Observational Study." *Maturitas* 116 (October 2018): 36–42. https://www.ncbi.nlm.nih.gov/pmc/articles/PMC6223619/.

Trudeau, K. J., J. L. Ainscough, M. Trant, J. Starker, and T. Cousineau. "Identifying the Educational Needs of Menopausal Women: A Feasibility Study." *Women's Health* 21, no. 2 (March–April 2011). https://www.ncbi.nlm.nih.gov/pmc/articles/PMC3856775/.

1. The Wild, Wild West of Health Experiences

Börü, U. T., C. K. Toksoy, C. Bölük, A. Bilgiç, and M. Taşdemir. "Effects of Multiple Sclerosis and Medications on Menopausal Age." *Journal of International Medical Research* 46, no. 3 (March 2018): 1249–1253. https://www.ncbi.nlm.nih.gov/pmc/articles/PMC5972265/.

Garrard, C. "Coping With Hot Flashes and Other Menopausal Symptoms: What 10 Celebrities Said." EverydayHealth.com (February 22, 2021), https://www.everydayhealth.com/menopause/coping-hot-flashes-menopausal-symptoms-celebrities-said/.

Harlow, S. D., M. Gass, J. E. Hall, R. Lobo, P. Maki, R. W. Rebar, S. Sherman, P. M. Sluss, and T. J. de Villiers. "Executive Summary of STRAW+10: Addressing the Unfinished Agenda of Staging Reproductive Aging." *Climacteric* 15, no. 2 (April 2012): 105–114. https://www.ncbi.nlm.nih.gov/pmc/articles/PMC3580996/.

Katz, E. T. "Kim Cattrall's First Brush With Menopause Was As Samantha on 'Sex And The City.'" HuffPost (September 26, 2014), https://www.huffpost.com/entry/kim-cattrall-menopause_n_5887962.

Mansfield P. K., M. Carey, A. Anderson, S. H. Barsom, and P. B. Koch. "Staging the Menopausal Transition: Data from the TREMIN Research Program on Women's Health." *Women's Health* 14, no. 6 (November–December 2004): 220–226. https://pubmed.ncbi.nlm.nih.gov/15589772/.

Miller, S. R., L. M. Gallicchio, L. M. Lewis, J. K. Babus, P. Langenberg, H. A. Zacur, and J.A. Flaws. "Association Between Race and Hot Flashes in Midlife Women." *Maturitas* 54, no. 3 (June 20, 2006): 260–269. https://pubmed.ncbi.nlm.nih.gov/16423474/.

National Child Development Study. "Childless Women More Likely to Begin Menopause Early, Study Finds" (January 25, 2017). https://ncds.info/childless-women-more-likely-to-begin-menopause-early-study-finds/.

The North American Menopause Society. "Menopause 101: A Primer for the Perimenopausal." https://www.menopause.org/for-women/menopauseflashes/menopause-symptoms-and-treatments/menopause-101-a-primer-for-the-perimenopausal.

Okeke, T. C., U. B. Anyaehie, and C. C. Ezenyeaku. "Premature Menopause." *Annals of Medical & Health Sciences Research* 3, no. 1 (January–March 2013): 90–95. https://www.ncbi.nlm.nih.gov/pmc/articles/PMC3634232/.

Sammaritano, L. R. "Menopause in Patients with Autoimmune Diseases." *Autoimmunity Reviews* 11, no. 6 (May 2012): A430–A436. https://www.sciencedirect.com/science/article/abs/pii/S1568997211002680.

Schmidt, C. W. "Age at Menopause: Do Chemical Exposures Play a Role?" *Environmental Health Perspectives* 125, no. 6 (June 2017): 062001. https://www.ncbi.nlm.nih.gov/pmc/articles/PMC5743449/.

Schnatz, P. F., J. Serra, D. M. O'Sullivan, and J. I. Sorosky. "Menopausal Symptoms in Hispanic Women and the Role of Socioeconomic Factors." *Obstetrical & Gynecological Survey* 61, no. 3 (March 2006): 187–193. https://pubmed.ncbi .nlm.nih.gov/16490118/.

Zhu, D., et al. "Relationships Between Intensity, Duration, Cumulative Dose, and Timing of Smoking with Age at Menopause: A Pooled Analysis of Individual Data from 17 Observational Studies." *PLoS Medicine* 15, no. 11 (November 2018): https://www.ncbi.nlm.nih.gov/pmc/articles/PMC6258514/.

2. Myths and Misconceptions About Menopause

Ayers, B., M. Forshaw, and M. S. Hunter. "The Impact of Attitudes Towards the Menopause on Women's Symptom Experience: A Systematic Review." *Maturitas* 65, no. 1 (January 2010): 28–36. https://www.sciencedirect.com/science/article /abs/pii/S0378512209003971.

Bjelland, E. K., S. Hofvind, L. Byberg, and A. Eskild. "The Relation of Age at Menarche with Age at Natural Menopause: A Population Study of 336,788 Women in Norway." *Human Reproduction* 33, no. 6 (June 2018): 1149–1157. https://www.ncbi.nlm.nih.gov/pmc/articles/PMC5972645/.

Breastcancer.org. "Breast Cancer Risk Seems More Affected by Total Body Fat Than Abdominal Fat" (June 27, 2017). https://www.breastcancer.org/research -news/total-body-fat-affects-risk-more-than-belly-fat.

Centers for Disease Control and Prevention. "Percentage of Adults Aged 65 and Over With Osteoporosis or Low Bone Mass at the Femur Neck or Lumbar Spine: United States, 2005–2010." https://www.cdc.gov/nchs/data/hestat/osteoporsis /osteoporosis2005_2010.htm.

Cohen, L. S. C. N. Soares, A. F. Vitonis, M. W. Otto, and B. L. Harlow. "Risk for New Onset of Depression During the Menopausal Transition: The Harvard Study of Moods and Cycles." *JAMA Psychiatry* 63, no. 4 (April 2006): 385–390. https://jamanetwork.com/journals/jamapsychiatry/fullarticle /209471.

Endocrine Society. "Menopause and Bone Loss." (January 23, 2022): https: //www.endocrine.org/patient-engagement/endocrine-library/menopause-and -bone-loss.

Gould, D. C. and R. Petty. "The Male Menopause: Does it Exist?" *Western Journal of Medicine* 173, no. 2 (August 2000): 76–78. https://www.ncbi.nlm.nih.gov/pmc/articles/PMC1070997/.

Kameda, T., H. Mano, T. Yuasa, Y. Mori, K. Miyazawa, M. Shiokawa, Y. Nakamaru, E. Hiroi, K. Hiura, A. Kameda, N. N. Yang, Y. Hakeda, and M. Kumegawa. "Estrogen Inhibits Bone Resorption by Directly Inducing Apoptosis of the Bone-resorbing Osteoclasts." *Journal of Experimental Medicine* 186, no. 4 (August 1997): 489–495. https://www.ncbi.nlm.nih.gov/pmc/articles/PMC2199029/.

Kravitz, H. M., R. Kazlauskaite, and H. Joffe. "Sleep, Health, and Metabolism in Midlife Women and Menopause: Food for Thought." *Obstetrics and Gynecology Clinics of North America* 45, no. 4 (December 2018): 679–694. https://www.ncbi.nlm.nih.gov/pmc/articles/PMC6338227/.

Mair, K. M., R. Gaw, and M. R. MacLean. "Obesity, Estrogens, and Adipose Tissue Dysfunction—Implications for Pulmonary Arterial Hypertension." *Pulmonary Circulation* 10, no. 3 (September 18, 2020): https://journals.sagepub.com/doi/full/10.1177/2045894020952023.

Mayo Clinic. "Male Menopause: Myth or Reality?" https://www.mayoclinic.org/healthy-lifestyle/mens-health/in-depth/male-menopause/art-20048056.

Moilanen, A., J. Kopra, H. Kroger, R. Sund, R. Rikkonen, and J. Sirola. "Characteristics of Long-Term Femoral Neck Bone Loss in Postmenopausal Women: A 25-Year Follow-Up." *Journal of Bone and Mineral Research* 37, no. 2 (February 2022): 173–178. https://asbmr.onlinelibrary.wiley.com/doi/10.1002/jbmr.4444.

Muka, T., C. Oliver-Williams, V. Colpani, S. Kunutsor, S. Chowdhury, R. Chowdhury, M. Kavousi, and O. H. Franco. "Association of Vasomotor and Other Menopausal Symptoms with Risk of Cardiovascular Disease: A Systematic Review and Meta-Analysis." *PLoS One* 11, no. 6 (2016): e0157417. https://www.ncbi.nlm.nih.gov/pmc/articles/PMC4912069/.

Romani, W. A., L. Gallicchio, and J. A. Flaws. "The Association Between Physical Activity and Hot Flash Severity, Frequency, and Duration in Mid-Life Women." *American Journal of Human Biology* 21, no. 1 (January–February 2009): 127–129. https://www.ncbi.nlm.nih.gov/pmc/articles/PMC2753173/.

Rush University Medical Center. "How the Body Regulates Heat." https://www.rush.edu/news/how-body-regulates-heat.

Ryu, K. J., H. Park, J. S. Park, Y. W. Lee, S. Y. Kim, H. Kim, Y. Jeong, Y. J. Kim, K. W. Yi, J. H. Shin, J. Y. Hur, and T. Kim. "Vasomotor Symptoms:

More Than Temporary Menopausal Symptoms." *Journal of Menopausal Medicine* 26, no. 3 (December 2020): 147–153. https://e-jmm.org/DOIx.php?id=10.6118/jmm.20030.

Ryu, K. J., H. K. Kim, Y. J. Lee, H. Park, and T. Kim. "Association Between Vasomotor Symptoms and Sarcopenia Assessed by L3 Skeletal Muscle Index Among Korean Menopausal Women." *Menopause* 29, no. 1 (January 2022): 48–53. https://journals.lww.com/menopausejournal/Fulltext/2022/01000/Association_between_vasomotor_symptoms_and.10.aspx.

Smith, M. "Doctor, just what is a hot flash?" *Contemporary OB/GYN* (October 7, 2011): https://www.contemporaryobgyn.net/view/doctor-just-what-hot-flash.

Sood, R., C. L. Kuhle, E. Kapoor, J. M. Thielen, K. S. Frohmader, K. C. Mara, and S. S. Faubion. "Association of Mindfulness and Stress with Menopausal Symptoms in Midlife Women." *Climacteric* 22, no. 4 (August 2019): 377–382. https://pubmed.ncbi.nlm.nih.gov/30652511/.

The North American Menopause Society. "Management of Osteoporosis in Postmenopausal Women: The 2021 Position Statement of the North American Menopause Society." *Menopause* 28, no. 9 (September 2021): 973–997. https://journals.lww.com/menopausejournal/Abstract/2021/09000/Management_of_osteoporosis_in_postmenopausal.3.aspx.

Thomas, A., and A. J. Daley. "Women's Views About Physical Activity as a Treatment for Vasomotor Menopausal Symptoms: A Qualitative Study." *BMC Women's Health* 20, no. 203 (2020): https://bmcwomenshealth.biomedcentral.com/articles/10.1186/s12905-020-01063-w.

3. The Hormone Conundrum

Al-Imari, L., and W. L. Wolfman. "The Safety of Testosterone Therapy in Women." *Journal of Obstetrics and Gynaecology Canada* 34, no. 9 (September 2012): 859–865. https://www.jogc.com/article/S1701-2163(16)35385-3/pdf.

Canonico, M., E. Oger, G. Plu-Bureau, J. Conard, G. Meyer, H. Lévesque, N. Trillot, M. T. Barrellier, D. Wahl, J. Emmerich, P. Y. "Hormone Therapy and Venous Thromboembolism Among Postmenopausal Women: Impact of the Route of Estrogen Administration and Progestogens: The ESTHER Study." *Circulation* 115, no. 7 (February 20, 2007): 840–845. https://pubmed.ncbi.nlm.nih.gov/17309934/.

Chlebowski, R. T., G. L. Anderson, A. K. Aragaki, J. E. Manson, M. L. Stefanick, K. Pan, W. Barrington, L. H. Kuller, M. S. Simon, D. Lane, K. C. Johnson, T. E. Rohan, M. L. S. Gass, J. A. Cauley, E. D. Paskett, M. Sattari, R. L. Prentice. "Association of Menopausal Hormone Therapy With Breast Cancer Incidence and Mortality During Long-term Follow-up of the Women's Health Initiative Randomized Clinical Trials." *JAMA* 324, no. 4 (July 28, 2020): 369–380. https://www.ncbi.nlm.nih.gov/pmc/articles/PMC7388026/.

Davis, S. R., R. Baber, N. Panay, J. Bitzer, S. C. Perez, R. M. Islam, A. M. Kaunitz, S. A. Kingsberg, I. Lambrinoudaki, J. Liu, S. J. Parish, J. Pinkerton, J. Rymer, J. A. Simon, L. Vignozzi, and M. E. Wierman. "Global Consensus Position Statement on the Use of Testosterone Therapy for Women." *The Journal of Clinical Endocrinology & Metabolism* 104, no. 10. (October 2019): 4660–4666. https://academic.oup.com/jcem/article/104/10/4660/5556103#165873304.

Delamater, L., and N. Santoro. "Management of the Perimenopause." *Clinical Obstetrics and Gynecology* 61, no. 3 (September 2018): 419–432. https://www.ncbi.nlm.nih.gov/pmc/articles/PMC6082400/.

"Design of the Women's Health Initiative Clinical Trial and Observational Study. The Women's Health Initiative Study Group." *Controlled Clinical Trials* 19, no. 1 (February 1998): 61–109. https://pubmed.ncbi.nlm.nih.gov/9492970/.

Kim, H. K., S. Y. Kang, Y. J. Chung, J. H. Kim, and M. R. Kim. "The Recent Review of the Genitourinary Syndrome of Menopause." *Journal of Menopausal Medicine* 21, no. 2 (August 2015): 65–71. https://www.ncbi.nlm.nih.gov/pmc/articles/PMC4561742/.

Manson, J. E., A. K. Aragaki, J. E. Rossouw, G. L. Anderson, R. L. Prentice, A. Z. LaCroix, R. T. Chlebowski, B. V. Howard, C. A. Thomson, K. L. Margolis, C. E. Lewis, M. L. Stefanick, R. D. Jackson, K. C. Johnson, L. W. Martin, S. A. Shumaker, M. A. Espeland, and J. Wactawski-Wende. "Menopausal Hormone Therapy and Long-term All-Cause and Cause-Specific Mortality: The Women's Health Initiative Randomized Trials." *JAMA* 318, no. 10 (September 12, 2017): 927–938. https://jamanetwork.com/journals/jama/fullarticle/2653735.

Manson, J. E., et al. "The Women's Health Initiative Hormone Therapy Trials: Update and Overview of Health Outcomes During the Intervention and Post-Stopping Phases." *JAMA* 310, no. 13 (October 2, 2013): 1353–1368. https://www.ncbi.nlm.nih.gov/pmc/articles/PMC3963523/.

The North American Menopause Society. "Changes in Hormone Levels." http://www.menopause.org/for-women/sexual-health-menopause-online/changes-at-midlife/changes-in-hormone-levels.

The North American Menopause Society. "Hormone Help Desk: ET, EPT, and More." http://www.menopause.org/for-women/menopauseflashes/menopause-symptoms-and-treatments/hormone-help-desk-et-ept-and-more.

The North American Menopause Society. "Menopause FAQs: Hormone Therapy for Menopause Symptoms." http://www.menopause.org/for-women/menopause-faqs-hormone-therapy-for-menopause-symptoms.

The North American Menopause Society. "News You Can Use About Hormone Therapy." http://www.menopause.org/for-women/menopauseflashes/menopause-symptoms-and-treatments/news-you-can-use-about-hormone-therapy.

The North American Menopause Society. "The North American Menopause Society Statement on Continuing Use of Systemic Hormone Therapy After Age 65." http://www.menopause.org/docs/default-source/2015/2015-nams-hormone-therapy-after-age-65.pdf.

The North American Menopause Society. "The 2017 Hormone Therapy Position Statement of the North American Menopause Society." *Menopause* 24, no. 7 (2017): 728–753. https://www.menopause.org/docs/default-source/2017/nams-2017-hormone-therapy-position-statement.pdf.

U.S. Department of Health & Human Services, Office on Women's Health. "Largest Women's Health Prevention Study Ever—Women's Health Initiative." https://www.womenshealth.gov/30-achievements/25.

U.S. Food and Drug Administration. "Menopause & Hormones: Common Questions." https://www.fda.gov/media/130242/download.

5. The Premature Menopause Type

Boughton, M. A. "Premature Menopause: Multiple Disruptions Between the Woman's Biological Body Experience and Her Lived Body." *Journal of Advanced Nursing* 37, no. 5 (March 2002): 423–430. https://pubmed.ncbi.nlm.nih.gov/11843980/.

Choe, S. A., and J. Sung. "Trends of Premature and Early Menopause: A Comparative Study of the US National Health and Nutrition Examination Survey and the Korea National Health and Nutrition Examination Survey." *Journal of Korean Medical Science* 35, no. 14 (April 13, 2020): e97. https://www.ncbi.nlm .nih.gov/pmc/articles/PMC7152531/.

Dobashi, S., S. Kawaguchi, D. Ando, and K. Koyama. "Alternating Work Posture Improves Postprandial Glucose Response Without Reducing Computer Task Performance in the Early Afternoon." *Physiology & Behavior* (August 1, 2021): 237. https://pubmed.ncbi.nlm.nih.gov/33887321/.

Franco, L. S., D. F. Shanahan, and R. A. Fuller. "A Review of the Benefits of Nature Experiences: More Than Meets the Eye." *International Journal of Environmental Research and Public Health* 14, no. 8 (August 2017): 864. https://www .ncbi.nlm.nih.gov/pmc/articles/PMC5580568/.

Gaiam. "1-Minute Breathing Exercise For Energy and Productivity." https:// www.gaiam.com/blogs/discover/1-minute-breathing-exercise-for-energy-and -productivity.

Gao, Y., M. Silvennoinen, A. J. Pesola, H. Kainulainen, N. J. Cronin, and T. Finni. "Acute Metabolic Response, Energy Expenditure, and EMG Activity in Sitting and Standing." *Medicine and Science in Sports and Exercise* 49, no. 9 (September 2017): 1927–1934. https://pubmed.ncbi.nlm.nih.gov/28463899/.

Gibbs, B. B., R. J. Kowalsky, S. J. Perdomo, M. Grier, and J. M. Jakicic. "Energy Expenditure of Deskwork when Sitting, Standing, or Alternating Positions." *Occupational Medicine* 67, no. 2 (March 1, 2017): 121–127. https://pubmed.ncbi .nlm.nih.gov/27515973/.

Kovar, E. "Music and Exercise: How Music Affects Exercise Motivation." ACE Fitness. (December 7, 2015): https://www.acefitness.org/education-and -resources/lifestyle/blog/5763/music-and-exercise-how-music-affects-exercise -motivation/.

Liao, K. L., N. Wood, and G. S. Conway. "Premature Menopause and Psychological Well-being." *Journal of Psychosomatic Obstetrics and Gynaecology* 21, no. 3 (September 2000): 167–174. https://pubmed.ncbi.nlm.nih.gov/11076338/.

Luborsky, J. L., P. Meyer, M. F. Sowers, E. B. Gold, and N. Santoro. "Premature Menopause in a Multi-ethnic Population Study of the Menopause Transition." *Human Reproduction* 18, no. 1 (January 2003): 199–206. https://academic.oup .com/humrep/article/18/1/199/880307.

Mishra, G. D., H. F. Chung, A. Cano, P. Chedraui, D. G. Goulis, P. Lopes, A. Mueck, M. Rees, L. M. Senturk, T. Simoncini, J. C. Stevenson, P. Stute,

P. Tuomikoski, and I. Lambrinoudaki. "EMAS Position Statement: Predictors of Premature and Early Natural Menopause." *Maturitas* 123 (May 2019): 82–88. https://pubmed.ncbi.nlm.nih.gov/31027683/.

Okele, T. C., U. B. Anyaehie, and C. C. Ezenyeaku. "Premature Menopause." *Annals of Medical and Health Sciences Research* 3, no. 1 (January–March 2013): 90–95. https://www.ncbi.nlm.nih.gov/pmc/articles/PMC3634232/.

Schroder, H. S., T. P. Moran, and J. S. Moser. "The Effect of Expressive Writing on the Error-related Negativity Among Individuals with Chronic Worry." *Psychophysiology* 55, no. 2 (February 2018): 10.1111/psyp.12990. https://www.ncbi.nlm.nih.gov/pmc/articles/PMC8543488/.

Shuster, L. T., D. J. Rhodes, B. S. Gostout, B. R. Grossardt, and W. A. Rocca. "Premature Menopause or Early Menopause: Long-term Health Consequences." *Maturitas* 65, no. 2 (February 2010): 161. https://www.ncbi.nlm.nih.gov/pmc/articles/PMC2815011/.

Sullivan, S. D., P. M. Sarrel, and L. M. Nelson. "Hormone Replacement Therapy in Young Women with Primary Ovarian Insufficiency and Early Menopause." *Fertility and Sterility* 106, no. 7 (December 1, 2016): 1588–1599. https://www.fertstert.org/article/S0015–0282(16)62877–7/fulltext.

The North American Menopause Society. "Effective Treatments for Sexual Problems." http://www.menopause.org/for-women/sexual-health-menopause-online/effective-treatments-for-sexual-problems.

Zhu, D., et al. "Age at Natural Menopause and Risk of Incident Cardiovascular Disease: A Pooled Analysis of Individual Patient Data." *The Lancet Public Health* 4, no. 11 (November 1, 2019): E553–E564. https://www.thelancet.com/journals/lanpub/article/PIIS2468–2667(19)30155–0/fulltext.

6. The Sudden Menopause Type

Costantino, D. and C. Guaraldi. "Effectiveness and Safety of Vaginal Suppositories for the Treatment of the Vaginal Atrophy in Postmenopausal Women: An Open, Non-controlled Clinical Trial." *European Review for Medical and Pharmacological Sciences* 12, no. 6 (November–December 2008): 411–416. https://pubmed.ncbi.nlm.nih.gov/19146203/.

Elkjaer, E., M. B. Mikkelsen, J. Michalak, D. S. Mennin, and M. S. O'Toole. "Expansive and Contractive Postures and Movement: A Systematic Review and

Meta-Analysis of the Effect of Motor Displays on Affective and Behavioral Responses." *Perspectives on Psychological Science* 17, no. 1 (January 1, 2022): 276–304. https://journals.sagepub.com/doi/abs/10.1177/1745691620919358.

Fischer, J., P. Fischer, B. Englich, N. Aydin, and D. Frey. "Empower My Decisions: The Effects of Power Gestures on Confirmatory Information Processing." *Journal of Experimental Social Psychology* 47, no. 6 (November 2011): 1146–1154. https://www.sciencedirect.com/science/article/abs/pii/S0022 103111001697.

Garg, A. and L. Robinson. "Surgical Menopause: A Toolkit for Healthcare Professionals." *Post Reproductive Health* 27, no. 4 (December 2021): 222–225. https://pubmed.ncbi.nlm.nih.gov/34761721/.

Miragall, M., A. Borrego, A. Cebolla, E. Etchemendy, J. Navarro-Siurana, R. Llorens, S. E. Blackwell, and R. M. Baños. "Effect of an Upright (vs. Stooped) Posture on Interpretation Bias, Imagery, and Emotions." *Journal of Behavior Therapy and Experimental Psychiatry* 68 (September 2020): 101560. https://www .sciencedirect.com/science/article/abs/pii/S0005791619301594.

National Institutes of Health, Office of Dietary Supplements. "Omega-3 Fatty Acids." https://ods.od.nih.gov/factsheets/Omega3FattyAcids-Consumer/.

National Institutes of Health, Office of Dietary Supplements. "Probiotics." https://ods.od.nih.gov/factsheets/Probiotics-HealthProfessional/.

Nelson, J. B. "Mindful Eating: The Art of Presence While You Eat." *Diabetes Spectrum* 30, no. 3 (August 2017): 171–174. https://www.ncbi.nlm.nih.gov /pmc/articles/PMC5556586/.

The North American Menopause Society. "MenoNote: Vaginal Dryness." https://www.menopause.org/docs/default-source/for-women/mn-vaginal-dryness .pdf.

The North American Menopause Society. "The 2017 Hormone Therapy Position Statement of the North American Menopause Society." *Menopause* 24, no. 7 (2017): 728–753. https://www.menopause.org/docs/default-source/2017/nams -2017-hormone-therapy-position-statement.pdf.

Robinson, J. G., N. Ijioma, and W. Harris. "Omega-3 Fatty Acids and Cognitive Function in Women." *Women's Health* 6, no. 1 (January 2010): 119–134. https://www.ncbi.nlm.nih.gov/pmc/articles/PMC2826215/.

Schaffer, R. "Nonhormonal Therapy Reduces Moderate to Severe Menopausal Hot Flashes." *Healio Endocrinology* (September 28, 2021): https://www.healio

.com/news/endocrinology/20210927/nonhormonal-therapy-reduces-moderate -to-severe-menopausal-hot-flashes.

Shuster, L. T., D. J. Rhodes, B. S. Gostout, B. R. Grossardt, and W. A. Rocca. "Premature Menopause or Early Menopause: Long-term Health Consequences." *Maturitas* 65, no. 2 (February 2010): 161. https://www.ncbi.nlm.nih .gov/pmc/articles/PMC2815011/.

7. The Full-Throttle Menopause Type

Barton, D. L., K. C. F. Schroeder, T. Banerjee, S. Wolf, T. Z. Keith, and G. Elkins. "Efficacy of a Biobehavioral Intervention for Hot Flashes: A Randomized Controlled Pilot Study." *Menopause* 24, no. 7 (July 2017): 774–782. https://www .ncbi.nlm.nih.gov/pmc/articles/PMC5747247/.

Be Well at Work. University of California, Berkeley. "Breathing Exercises." https://uhs.berkeley.edu/sites/default/files/breathing_exercises_0.pdf.

Garcia, M. C., E. J. Kozasa, S. Tufik, L. E. A. M. Mello, and H. Hachul. "The Effects of Mindfulness and Relaxation Training for Insomnia (MRTI) on Postmenopausal Women: A Pilot Study." *Menopause* 25, no. 9 (September 2018): 992–1003. https://pubmed.ncbi.nlm.nih.gov/29787483/.

Jalambadani, Z., Z. Rezapour, and S. M. Zadeh. "Investigating the Relationship between Menopause Specific Quality of Life and Perceived Social Support among Postmenopausal Women in Iran." *Experimental Aging Research* 46, 4 (July–September 2020): 359–366. https://pubmed.ncbi.nlm.nih.gov /32496973/.

Joffe, H., K. A. Guthrie, A. Z. LaCroix, S. D. Reed, K. E. Ensrud, J. E. Manson, K. M. Newton, E. W. Freeman, G. L. Anderson, J. C. Larson, J. Hunt, J. Shifren, K. M. Rexrode, B. Caan, B. Sternfeld, J. S. Carpenter, and L. Cohen. "Randomized Controlled Trial of Low-Dose Estradiol and the SNRI Venlafaxine for Vasomotor Symptoms." *JAMA Internal Medicine* 174, no. 7 (July 2014): 1058–1066. https://www.ncbi.nlm.nih.gov/pmc/articles/PMC4179877/.

Li, L., Y. Lv, L. Xu, and Q. Zheng. "Quantitative Efficacy of Soy Isoflavones on Menopausal Hot Flashes." *Pharmacodynamics* (October 15, 2014): https: //bpspubs.onlinelibrary.wiley.com/doi/full/10.1111/bcp.12533.

Lisa Health. "Manage Your Menopause Mood Swings with the CTFO Technique." https://blog.lisahealth.com/blog/2020/1/24/ctfo.

Meyers, H. "Why Is My Dog Shaking? Causes & Solutions." American Kennel Club. (April 18, 2022): https://www.akc.org/expert-advice/health/why-do-dogs -shake/.

Mirabi, P. and F. Mojab. "The Effects of Valerian Root on Hot Flashes in Menopausal Women." *Iranian Journal of Pharmaceutical Research* 12, no. 1 (Winter 2013): 217–222. https://www.ncbi.nlm.nih.gov/pmc/articles/PMC3813196/.

National Institutes of Health, Office of Dietary Supplements. "Black Cohosh." https://ods.od.nih.gov/factsheets/BlackCohosh-HealthProfessional/.

National Institutes of Health, Office of Dietary Supplements. "Vitamin B6." https://ods.od.nih.gov/factsheets/VitaminB6-HealthProfessional/.

Otte, J. L., J. S. Carpenter, L. Roberts, and G. R. Elkins. "Self-Hypnosis for Sleep Disturbances in Menopausal Women." *Journal of Women's Health* 29, no. 3 (March 2020): 461–463. https://www.ncbi.nlm.nih.gov/pmc/articles /PMC7097677/.

Payne, P., and M. A. Crane-Godreau. "Meditative Movement for Depression and Anxiety." *Frontiers in Psychiatry* (July 24,2013): https://www.frontiersin.org /articles/10.3389/fpsyt.2013.00071/full#h5.

Pereira, N., M. F. Naufel, E. B. Ribeiro, S. Tufik, and H. Hachul. "Influence of Dietary Sources of Melatonin on Sleep Quality: A Review." *Journal of Food Science* (December 19, 2019): https://ift.onlinelibrary.wiley.com/doi/full/10.1111 /1750–3841.14952

Polat, F., I. Orhan, and D. Ş. Küçükkelepçe. "Does Social Support Affect Menopausal Symptoms in Menopausal Women?" *Perspectives in Psychiatric Care* (July 2, 2021): https://pubmed.ncbi.nlm.nih.gov/34212380/.

Roberts, R. L., J. R. Rhodes, and G. R. Elkins. "Effect of Hypnosis on Anxiety: Results from a Randomized Controlled Trial with Women in Postmenopause." *Journal of Clinical Psychology in Medical Settings* 28, no. 4 (December 2021): 868–881. https://pubmed.ncbi.nlm.nih.gov/34403019/.

Sahni, S., A. Lobo-Romero, and T. Smith. "Contemporary Non-hormonal Therapies for the Management of Vasomotor Symptoms Associated with Menopause: A Literature Review." *touchREVIEWS in Endocrinology* 17, no. 2 (October 13, 2021): 133–137. https://www.touchendocrinology.com/reproductive -endocrinology/journal-articles/contemporary-non-hormonal-therapies-for-the -management-of-vasomotor-symptoms-associated-with-menopause-a-literature -review/.

Sarrel, P., D. Portman, P. Lefebvre, M. H. Lafeuille, A. M. Grittner, J. Fortier, J. Gravel, M. S. Duh, and P. M. Aupperle. "Incremental Direct and Indirect Costs of Untreated Vasomotor Symptoms." *Menopause* 22, no. 3 (March 2015): 260–266. https://pubmed.ncbi.nlm.nih.gov/25714236/.

SleepScoreLabs. "Alcohol & Insomnia: How Alcohol Affects Sleep Quality." (July 15, 2017): https://www.sleepscore.com/blog/how-a-nightcap-can-ruin -your-sleep/.

Shepherd-Banigan, M. K., M. Goldstein, R. R. Coeytaux, J. R. McDuffie, A. P. Goode, A. S. Kosinski, M. G. Van Noord, D. Befus, S. Adam, V. Masila-mani, A. Nagi, and J. W. Williams Jr. "Improving Vasomotor Symptoms; Psychological Symptoms; and Health-related Quality of Life in Peri-or Post-menopausal Women Through Yoga: An Umbrella Systematic Review and Meta-analysis." *Complementary Therapies in Medicine* 34 (October 2017): 156–164. https://www .sciencedirect.com/science/article/abs/pii/S0965229917300596.

Sood, R., A. Sood, S. L. Wolf, B. M. Linquist, H. Liu, J. A. Sloan, D. V. Satele, C. L. Loprinzi, and D. L. Barton. "Paced Breathing Compared with Usual Breathing for Hot Flashes." *Menopause* 20, no. 2 (February 2013): 179–184. https://pubmed.ncbi.nlm.nih.gov/22990758/.

The North American Menopause Society. "Chapter 8: Prescription Therapies." http://www.menopause.org/publications/clinical-care-recommendations /chapter-8-prescription-therapies.

The North American Menopause Society. "Menopause FAQs: Hot Flashes." https://www.menopause.org/for-women/menopause-faqs-hot-flashes.

U.S. Food and Drug Administration. "FDA Approves New Treatment for Hypoactive Sexual Desire Disorder in Premenopausal Women." (June 21, 2019): https://www.fda.gov/news-events/press-announcements/fda-approves-new -treatment-hypoactive-sexual-desire-disorder-premenopausal-women.

U.S. Pain Foundation. "How Flow State and The Nervous System Interact." (July 28, 2021): https://uspainfoundation.org/news/how-flow-state-and-the -nervous-system-interact/.

Yeung, A., J. S. M. Chan, J. C. Cheung, and L. Zou. "Qigong and Tai-Chi for Mood Regulation." *Focus: The Journal of Lifelong Learning in Psychiatry* 16, no. 1 (Winter 2018): 40–47. https://www.ncbi.nlm.nih.gov/pmc/articles /PMC6519567/.

8. The Mind-Altering Menopause Type

Abedi, P., P. Nikkhah, and S. Najar. "Effect of Pedometer-based Walking on Depression, Anxiety and Insomnia Among Postmenopausal Women." *Climacteric* 18, no. 6 (2015): 841–845. https://pubmed.ncbi.nlm.nih.gov/26100101/.

Aibar-Almazán, A., F. Hita-Contreras, D. Cruz-Díaz, M. de la Torre-Cruz, J. D. Jiménez-García, and A. Martínez-Amat. "Effects of Pilates Training on Sleep Quality, Anxiety, Depression and Fatigue in Postmenopausal Women: A Randomized Controlled Trial." *Maturitas* 124 (June 2019): 62–67. https://pubmed.ncbi.nlm.nih.gov/31097181/.

Anderson, D., C. Seib, and L. Rasmussen. "Can Physical Activity Prevent Physical and Cognitive Decline in Postmenopausal Women? A Systematic Review of the Literature." *Maturitas* 79, no. 1 (September 2014): 14–33. https://pubmed.ncbi.nlm.nih.gov/25008420/.

Bach, D., G. Groesbeck, P. Stapleton, R. Sims, K. Blickheuser, and D. Church. "Clinical EFT (Emotional Freedom Techniques) Improves Multiple Physiological Markers of Health." *Journal of Evidence-Based Integrative Medicine* 24 (2019): https://www.ncbi.nlm.nih.gov/pmc/articles/PMC6381429/.

Bromberger, J. T., Y. Chang, A. B. Colvin, H. M. Kravitz, and K. A. Matthews. "Does Childhood Maltreatment or Current Stress Contribute to Increased Risk for Major Depression During the Menopause Transition?" *Psychological Medicine* (December 10, 2020): 1–8. https://pubmed.ncbi.nlm.nih.gov/33298219/.

Chae, M., and K. Park. "Association Between Dietary Omega-3 Fatty Acid Intake and Depression in Postmenopausal Women." *Nutrition Research and Practice* 15, no. 4 (August 2021): 468–478. https://www.ncbi.nlm.nih.gov/pmc/articles/PMC8313386/.

Colvin, A., G. A. Richardson, J. M. Cyranowski, A. Youk, and J. T. Bromberger. "The Role of Family History of Depression and the Menopausal Transition in the Development of Major Depression in Midlife Women: Study of Women's Health Across the Nation Mental Health Study (SWAN MHS)." *Depression & Anxiety* 34, no. 9 (September 2017): 826–835. https://www.ncbi.nlm.nih.gov/pmc/articles/PMC5585035/.

Craig, M. C., P. M. Maki, and D. G. M. Murphy. "The Women's Health Initiative Memory Study: Findings and Implications for Treatment." *The Lancet Neurology* 493 (March 2005): 190–194. https://pubmed.ncbi.nlm.nih.gov/15721829/.

Dąbrowska-Galas, M., and J. Dąbrowska. "Physical Activity Level and Self-Esteem in Middle-Aged Women." *International Journal of Environmental Research and Public Health* 18, no. 14 (July 2021): 7293. https://www.ncbi.nlm.nih.gov/pmc/articles/PMC8305857/.

Drake, C. L., D. A. Kalmbach, J. T. Arnedt, P. Cheng, C. V. Tonnu, A. Cuamatzi-Castelan, and C. Fellman-Couture. "Treating Chronic Insomnia in Postmenopausal Women: A Randomized Clinical Trial Comparing Cognitive-Behavioral Therapy for Insomnia, Sleep Restriction Therapy, and Sleep Hygiene Education." *Sleep* 42, no. 2 (February 2019): https://academic.oup.com/sleep/article/42/2/zsy217/5179856.

Epperson, C. N., B. Pittman, K. A. Czarkowski, J. Bradley, D. M. Quinlan, and T. E. Brown. "Impact of Atomoxetine on Subjective Attention and Memory Difficulties in Perimenopausal and Postmenopausal Women." *Menopause* 18, no. 5 (May 2011): 542–548. https://www.ncbi.nlm.nih.gov/pmc/articles/PMC4076798/.

Freeman, E. W. "Depression in the Menopause Transition: Risks in the Changing Hormone Milieu as Observed in the General Population." *Women's Midlife Health* (August 11, 2015): https://www.ncbi.nlm.nih.gov/pmc/articles/PMC6214217/.

Greendale, G. A., M. H. Huang, R. G. Wight, T. Seeman, C. Luetters, N. E. Avis, J. Johnston, and A. S. Karlamangla. "Effects of the Menopause Transition and Hormone Use on Cognitive Performance in Midlife Women." *Neurology* 72, no. 21 (May 26, 2009): 1850–1857. https://www.ncbi.nlm.nih.gov/pmc/articles/PMC2690984/.

Gujral, S., H. Aizenstein, C. F. Reynolds, III, M. A. Butters, and K. I. Erickson. "Exercise Effects on Depression: Possible Neural Mechanisms." *General Hospital Psychiatry* 49 (November 2017): 2–10. https://www.ncbi.nlm.nih.gov/pmc/articles/PMC6437683/.

Hoffman, B. M., M. A. Babyak, W. E. Craighead, A. Sherwood, P. M. Doraiswamy, M. J. Coons, and J. A. Blumenthal. "Exercise and Pharmacotherapy in Patients With Major Depression: One-Year Follow-Up of the SMILE Study." *Psychosomatic Medicine* 73, no. 2 (February–March 2011): 127–133. https://www.ncbi.nlm.nih.gov/pmc/articles/PMC3671874/.

Jaff, N. G., and P. M. Maki. "Scientific Insights into Brain Fog During the Menopausal Transition." *Climacteric* 24, no. 4 (2021): 317–318. https://www.tandfonline.com/doi/full/10.1080/13697137.2021.1942700.

Jones, H. J., P. A. Minarik, C. L. Gilliss, and K. A. Lee. "Depressive Symptoms Associated with Physical Health Problems in Midlife Women: A Longitudinal Study." *Journal of Affective Disorders* 263 (February 15, 2020): 301–309. https://www.ncbi.nlm.nih.gov/pmc/articles/PMC6989369/.

Jorge, M. P., D. F. Santaella, I. M. O. Pontes, V. K. M. Shiramizu, E. B. Nascimento, A. Cabral, T. M. A. M. Lemos, R. H. Silva, and A. M. Ribeiro. "Hatha Yoga Practice Decreases Menopause Symptoms and Improves Quality of Life: A Randomized Controlled Trial." *Complementary Therapies in Medicine* 26 (June 2016): 128–135. https://pubmed.ncbi.nlm.nih.gov/27261993/.

Jung, S. J., A. Shin, and D. Kang. "Hormone-Related Factors and Post-Menopausal Onset Depression: Results from KNHANES (2010–2012)." *Journal of Affective Disorders* 175 (April 1, 2015): 176–183. https://www.sciencedirect.com/science/article/pii/S0165032715000038.

Kalmbach, D. A., P. Cheng, J. T. Arnedt, J. R. Anderson, T. Roth, C. Fellman-Couture, R. A. Williams, and C. L. Drake. "Treating Insomnia Improves Depression, Maladaptive Thinking, and Hyperarousal in Postmenopausal Women: Comparing Cognitive-Behavioral Therapy for Insomnia (CBTI), Sleep Restriction Therapy, and Sleep Hygiene Education." *Sleep Medicine* 55 (March 2019): 124–134. https://www.ncbi.nlm.nih.gov/pmc/articles/PMC6503531/.

Koçak, D. Y., and Y. Varişoğlu. "The Effect of Music Therapy on Menopausal Symptoms and Depression: A Randomized-Controlled Study." *Menopause* 29, no. 5 (May 2022): 545–552. https://journals.lww.com/menopausejournal/Abstract/9000/The_effect_of_music_therapy_on_menopausal_symptoms.96827.aspx.

Konishi, M., B. Berberian, V. de Gardelle, and J. Sackur. "Multitasking Costs on Metacognition in a Triple-task Paradigm." *Psychonomic Bulletin & Review* 28, no. 6 (December 2021): 2075–2084. https://pubmed.ncbi.nlm.nih.gov/34173189/.

Maki, P. M., G. Springer, K. Anastos, D. R. Gustafson, K. Weber, D. Vance, D. Dykxhoorn, J. Milam, A. A. Adimora, S. G. Kassaye, D. Waldrop, and L. H. Rubin. "Cognitive Changes During the Menopausal Transition: A Longitudinal Study in Women with and without HIV." *Menopause* 28, no. 4 (April 2021): 360–368. https://journals.lww.com/menopausejournal/Citation/2021/04000/Cognitive_changes_during_the_menopausal.5.aspx.

Maki, P. M. and V. W. Henderson. "Cognition and the Menopause Transition." *Menopause* 23, no. 7 (July 2016): 803–805. https://pubmed.ncbi.nlm.nih.gov/27272226/.

Mandolesi, L., A. Polverino, S. Montuori, F. Foti, G. Ferraioli, P. Sorrentino, and G. Sorrentino. "Effects of Physical Exercise on Cognitive Functioning and Wellbeing: Biological and Psychological Benefits." *Frontiers in Psychology* 9 (2018): 509. https://www.ncbi.nlm.nih.gov/pmc/articles/PMC5934999/.

Mangweth-Matzek, B., H. W. Hoek, C. I. Rupp, G. Kemmler, H. G. Pope, and J. Kinzl. "The Menopausal Transition—A Possible Window of Vulnerability for Eating Pathology." *International Journal of Eating Disorders* 46, no. 6 (September 2013): 609–616. https://pubmed.ncbi.nlm.nih.gov/23847142/.

Mangweth-Matzek, B., C. I. Rupp, S. Vedova, V. Dunst, P. Hennecke, M. Daniaux, and H. G. Pope. "Disorders of Eating and Body Image During the Menopausal Transition: Associations with Menopausal Stage and with Menopausal Symptomatology." *Eating and Weight Disorders* 26, no. 8 (December 2021): 2763–2769. https://pubmed.ncbi.nlm.nih.gov/33595812/.

Marcus, M. D., J. T. Bromberger, H. L. Wei, C. Brown, and H. M. Kravitz. "Prevalence and Selected Correlates of Eating Disorder Symptoms Among a Multiethnic Community Sample of Midlife Women." *Annals of Behavioral Medicine* 33, no. 3 (June 2007): 269–277. https://pubmed.ncbi.nlm.nih.gov/17600454/.

Morgan, M. L., I. A. Cook, A. J. Rapkin, and A. F. Leuchter. "Estrogen Augmentation of Antidepressants in Perimenopausal Depression: A Pilot Study." *Journal of Clinical Psychiatry* 66, no. 6 (June 2005): 774–780. https://pubmed.ncbi.nlm.nih.gov/15960574/.

Morita, E., S. Fukuda, J. Nagano, N. Hamajima, H. Yamamoto, Y. Iwai, T. Nakashima, H. Ohira, and T. Shirakawa. "Psychological Effects of Forest Environments on Healthy Adults: Shinrin-yoku (Forest-air Bathing, Walking) as a Possible Method of Stress Reduction." *Public Health* 121, 1 (January 2007): 54–63. https://pubmed.ncbi.nlm.nih.gov/17055544/.

Mosconi, L., V. Berti, J. Dyke, E. Schelbaum, S. Jett, L. Loughlin, G. Jang, A. Rahman, H. Hristov, S. Pahlajani, R. Andrews, D. Matthews, O. Etingin, C. Ganzer, M. de Leon, R. Isaacson, and R. D. Brinton. "Menopause Impacts Human Brain Structure, Connectivity, Energy Metabolism, and Amyloid-beta

Deposition." *Scientific Reports* 11 (2021): Article number 10867. https://www.nature.com/articles/s41598-021-90084-y.

Mulhall, S., R. Andel, and K. J. Anstey. "Variation in Symptoms of Depression and Anxiety in Midlife Women by Menopausal Status." *Maturitas* 108 (February 2018): 7–12. https://pubmed.ncbi.nlm.nih.gov/29290217/.

National Institutes of Health, Office of Dietary Supplements. "Choline." https://ods.od.nih.gov/factsheets/Choline-HealthProfessional/.

Paolucci, E. M., D. Loukov, D. W. E. Bowdish, and J. J. Heisz. "Exercise Reduces Depression and Inflammation but Intensity Matters." *Biological Psychology* 133 (March 2018): 79–84. https://pubmed.ncbi.nlm.nih.gov/29408464/.

Robinson, J. G., N. Ijioma, and W. Harris. "Omega-3 Fatty Acids and Cognitive Function in Women." *Women's Health* 6, no. 1 (January 2010): 119–134. https://www.ncbi.nlm.nih.gov/pmc/articles/PMC2826215/.

Samuels, K. L., M. M. Maine, and M. Tantillo. "Disordered Eating, Eating Disorders, and Body Image in Midlife and Older Women." *Current Psychiatry Reports* 21, no. 8 (July 1, 2019): 70. https://pubmed.ncbi.nlm.nih.gov/31264039/.

Schuch, F. B., S. S. Pinto, N. C. Bagatine, P. Zaffari, C. L. Alberton, E. L. Cadore, R. F. Silva, and L. F. M. Kruel. "Water-based Exercise and Quality of Life in Women: The Role of Depressive Symptoms." *Women & Health* 54, no. 2 (2014): 161–175. https://pubmed.ncbi.nlm.nih.gov/24329155/.

Schwert, C., S. Aschenbrenner, M. Weisbrod, and A. Schröder. "Cognitive Impairments in Unipolar Depression: The Impact of Rumination." *Psychopathology* 50, no. 5 (2017): 347–354. https://pubmed.ncbi.nlm.nih.gov/28850956/.

Shea, A. K., N. Sohel, A. Gilsing, A. J. Mayhew, L. E. Griffith, and P. Raina. "Depression, Hormone Therapy, and the Menopausal Transition Among Women Aged 45 to 64 Years Using Canadian Longitudinal Study on Aging Baseline Data." *Menopause* 27, no. 7 (July 2020): 763–770. https://pubmed.ncbi.nlm.nih.gov/32217892/.

Thompson, K. A., and A. M. Bardone-Cone. "Evaluating Attitudes about Aging and Body Comparison as Moderators of the Relationship Between Menopausal Status and Disordered Eating and Body Image Concerns Among Middle-aged Women." *Maturitas* 124 (June 2019): 25–31. https://pubmed.ncbi.nlm.nih.gov/31097174/.

Wariso, B. A., G. M. Guerrieri, K. Thompson, D. E. Koziol, N. Haq, P. E. Martinez, D. R. Rubinow, and P. J. Schmidt. "Depression During the

Menopause Transition: Impact on Quality of Life, Social Adjustment, and Disability." *Archives of Women's Mental Health* 20, no. 2 (April 2017): 273–282. https://www.ncbi.nlm.nih.gov/pmc/articles/PMC6309889/.

Wong, C. B., H. K. Yip, T. Gao, K. Y. U. Lam, D. M. S. Woo, A. L. K. Yip, C. Y. Chin, W. P. Y. Tang, M. M. T. Choy, K. W. K. Tsang, S. C. Ho, H. S. W. Ma, and S. Y. S. Wong. "Mindfulness-Based Stress Reduction (MBSR) or Psychoeducation for the Reduction of Menopausal Symptoms: A Randomized, Controlled Clinical Trial." *Scientific Reports* 8 (2018): 6609. https://www.ncbi.nlm.nih.gov/pmc/articles/PMC5919973/.

Yagi, A., R. Nouchi, L. Butler, and R. Kawashima. "Lutein Has a Positive Impact on Brain Health in Healthy Older Adults: A Systematic Review of Randomized Controlled Trials and Cohort Studies." *Nutrients* 13 (2021): 1746. https://mdpi-res.com/d_attachment/nutrients/nutrients-13-01746/article_deploy/nutrients-13-01746.pdf.

Yu, Q., C. X. Yin, Y. Hui, J. Yu, F. F. He, J. Wei, and Y. Y. Wu. "[Comparison of the Effect of Fluoxetine Combined with Hormone Replacement Therapy (HRT) and Single HRT in Treating Menopausal Depression]." *Zhonghua Fu Chan Ke Za Zhi* 39, no. 7 (July 2004): 461–464. https://pubmed.ncbi.nlm.nih.gov/15347469/.

9. The Seemingly Never-Ending Menopause Type

Avis, N. E., S. L. Crawford, G. Greendale, J. T. Bromberger, S. A. Everson-Rose, E. B. Gold, R. Hess, H. Joffe, H. M. Kravitz, P. G. Tepper, R. C. Thurston. "Duration of Menopausal Vasomotor Symptoms Over the Menopause Transition." *JAMA Internal Medicine* 175, no. 4 (April 1, 2015): 531–539. https://www.ncbi.nlm.nih.gov/pmc/articles/PMC4433164/.

Berg, J. "The Stress of Caregiving in Midlife Women." The North American Menopause Society 36 (July 2011): 33–36. http://www.menopause.org/docs/default-document-library/careberg.pdf?sfvrsn=2.

Brown, L., C. Bryant, V. Brown, B. Bei, and F. Judd. "Investigating how Menopausal Factors and Self-Compassion Shape Well-being: An Exploratory Path Analysis." *Maturitas* 81, no. 2 (June 2015): 293–299. https://pubmed.ncbi.nlm.nih.gov/25818770/.

DiBonaventura, M., X. Luo, M. Moffatt, A. G. Bushmakin, M. Kumar, and J. Bobula. "The Association Between Vulvovaginal Atrophy Symptoms and Quality of Life Among Postmenopausal Women in the United States and Western Europe." *Journal of Women's Health* 24, no. 9 (September 2015): 713–722. https://pubmed.ncbi.nlm.nih.gov/26199981/.

Grandner, M. A., S. Nowakowski, J. D. Kloss, and M. L. Perlis. "Insomnia Symptoms Predict Physical and Mental Impairments Among Postmenopausal Women." *Sleep Medicine* 16, no. 3 (March 2015): 317–318. https://www.ncbi.nlm.nih.gov/pmc/articles/PMC4375439/.

Greenstein, A., L. Abramov, H. Matzkin, and J. Chen. "Sexual Dysfunction in Women Partners of Men with Erectile Dysfunction." *International Journal of Impotence Research* 18 (2006): 44–46. https://www.nature.com/articles/3901367.

Halis, F., P. Yildirim, R. Kocaaslan, K. Cecen, and A. Gokce. "Pilates for Better Sex: Changes in Sexual Functioning in Healthy Turkish Women After Pilates Exercise." *Journal of Sex & Marital Therapy* 42, no. 4 (May 18, 2016): 302–308. https://pubmed.ncbi.nlm.nih.gov/25826474/.

Kline, C. E., Colvin, A. B., K. P. Gabriel, C. A. Karvonen-Gutierrez, J. A. Cauley, M. H. Hall, K. A. Matthews, K. M. Ruppert, G. S. Neal-Perry, E. S. Strotmeyer, and B. Sternfeld. "Associations Between Longitudinal Trajectories of Insomnia Symptoms and Sleep Duration with Objective Physical Function in Postmenopausal Women: The Study of Women's Health Across the Nation." *Sleep* 44, no. 8 (August 2021): https://www.ncbi.nlm.nih.gov/pmc/articles/PMC8361301/.

Kołodyńska, G., M. Zalewski, and K. Rożek-Piechura. "Urinary Incontinence in Postmenopausal Women—Causes, Symptoms, Treatment." *Przegląd Menopauzalny* 18, no. 1 (April 2019): 46–50. https://www.ncbi.nlm.nih.gov/pmc/articles/PMC6528037/.

Mayo Clinic. "Kegel Exercises: A How-to Guide for Women." https://www.mayoclinic.org/healthy-lifestyle/womens-health/in-depth/kegel-exercises/art-20045283.

Mili, N., S. A. Paschou, A. Armeni, N. Georgopoulos, D. G. Goulis, and I. Lambrinoudaki. "Genitourinary Syndrome of Menopause: A Systematic Review on Prevalence and Treatment." *Menopause* 28, no. 6 (March 15, 2021): 706–716. https://pubmed.ncbi.nlm.nih.gov/33739315/.

Motzer, A. A., and V. Hertig. "Stress, Stress Response, and Health." *The Nursing Clinics of North America* 39, no. 1 (March 2004): 1–17. https://pubmed.ncbi.nlm.nih.gov/15062724/.

Moyneur, E., K. Dea, L. R. Derogati, F. Vekeman, A. Y. Dury, and F. Labrie. "Prevalence of Depression and Anxiety in Women Newly Diagnosed with Vulvovaginal Atrophy and Dyspareunia." *Menopause* 27, no. 2 (February 2020): 134–142. https://pubmed.ncbi.nlm.nih.gov/31688416/.

National Institutes of Health, Office of Dietary Supplements. "Black Cohosh." https://ods.od.nih.gov/factsheets/BlackCohosh-HealthProfessional/.

National Institutes of Health, Office of Dietary Supplements. "Vitamin B6." https://ods.od.nih.gov/factsheets/VitaminB6-HealthProfessional/.

Parish, S. J., and S. R. Hahn. "Hypoactive Sexual Desire Disorder: A Review of Epidemiology, Biopsychology, Diagnosis, and Treatment." *Sexual Medicine Reviews* 4, no. 2 (April 2016): 103–120. https://pubmed.ncbi.nlm.nih.gov /27872021/.

Pereira, N., M. F. Naufel, E. B. Ribeiro, S. Tufik, and H. Hachul. "Influence of Dietary Sources of Melatonin on Sleep Quality: A Review." *Journal of Food Science* 85, no. 1 (January 2020): 5–13. https://ift.onlinelibrary.wiley.com/doi /full/10.1111/1750–3841.14952.

Pérez-Herrezuelo, I., A. Aibar-Almazán, A. Martínez-Amat, R. Fábrega-Cuadros, E. Díaz-Mohedo, R. Wangensteen, and F. Hita-Contreras. "Female Sexual Function and Its Association with the Severity of Menopause-Related Symptoms." *International Journal of Environmental Research and Public Health* 17, no. 19 (October 2020): 7235. https://www.ncbi.nlm.nih.gov/pmc/articles /PMC7579461/.

Pingarrón Santofimia, M. C., S. P. González Rodríguez, M. Lilue, and S. Palacios. "Experience with Ospemifene in Patients with Vulvar and Vaginal Atrophy: Case Studies with Bone Marker Profiles." *Drugs in Context* 9 (2020). https:// www.ncbi.nlm.nih.gov/pmc/articles/PMC7337603/.

Sahni, S., A. Lobo-Romero, and T. Smith. "Contemporary Non-hormonal Therapies for the Management of Vasomotor Symptoms Associated with Menopause: A Literature Review." *touchREVIEWS in Endocrinology* 17, no. 2: 133–137. https: //www.touchendocrinology.com/reproductive-endocrinology/journal-articles /contemporary-non-hormonal-therapies-for-the-management-of-vasomotor -symptoms-associated-with-menopause-a-literature-review/.

Science Daily. "Anticipating A Laugh Reduces Our Stress Hormones, Study Shows." April 10, 2008. https://www.sciencedaily.com/releases/2008/04 /080407114617.htm.

Shih, E., H. Hirsch, and H. L. Thacker. "Medical Management of Urinary Incontinence in Women." *Cleveland Clinic Journal of Medicine* 84, no. 2 (February 2017): 151–158. https://www.ccjm.org/content/84/2/151.long.

The North American Menopause Society. "The North American Menopause Society Statement on Continuing Use of Systemic Hormone Therapy After Age 65." http://www.menopause.org/docs/default-source/2015/2015-nams-hormone-therapy-after-age-65.pdf.

The North American Menopause Society. "Urinary Incontinence." https://www.menopause.org/for-women/sexual-health-menopause-online/causes-of-sexual-problems/urinary-incontinence.

The North American Menopause Society. "Vaginal Dryness." https://www.menopause.org/docs/default-source/for-women/mn-vaginal-dryness.pdf.

Woods, N. F., E. S. Mitchell, D. B. Percival, and K. Smith-DiJulio. "Is the Menopausal Transition Stressful? Observations of Perceived Stress from the Seattle Midlife Women's Health Study." *Menopause* 16, no. 1 (January–February 2009). https://www.ncbi.nlm.nih.gov/pmc/articles/PMC3842691/.

10. The Silent Menopause Type

Centers for Disease Control and Prevention. "Diabetes Tests." https://www.cdc.gov/diabetes/basics/getting-tested.html.

Centers for Disease Control and Prevention. "Prediabetes—Your Chance to Prevent Type 2 Diabetes." https://www.cdc.gov/diabetes/basics/prediabetes.html.

Cleveland Clinic. "Postmenopause." https://my.clevelandclinic.org/health/diseases/21837-postmenopause.

Cleveland Clinic. "Restless Legs Syndrome." https://my.clevelandclinic.org/health/diseases/9497-restless-legs-syndrome.

Cleveland Clinic Health Essentials. "Statins Giving You Achy Muscles? Ask Your Doctor About These 4 Potential Fixes." https://health.clevelandclinic.org/statins-giving-you-achy-muscles-ask-your-doctor-about-these-4-potential-fixes/.

Currie, H. and C. Williams. "Menopause, Cholesterol and Cardiovascular Disease." *US Cardiology* 5, no. 1 (2008): 12–14. https://www.uscjournal.com/articles/menopause-cholesterol-and-cardiovascular-disease-0.

Edwards, B. A., D. M. O'Driscoll, A. Ali, A. S. Jordan, J. Trinder, and A. Malhotra. "Aging and Sleep: Physiology and Pathophysiology." *Seminars in Respiratory and Critical Care Medicine* 31, no. 5 (October 2010): 618–633. https://www.ncbi.nlm.nih.gov/pmc/articles/PMC3500384/.

Greater Good in Action. "Body Scan Meditation." https://ggia.berkeley.edu/practice/body_scan_meditation.

Hord, N. G., Y. Tang, and N. S. Bryan. "Food Sources of Nitrates and Nitrites: The Physiologic Context for Potential Health Benefits." *The American Journal of Clinical Nutrition* 90, no. 1 (July 2009): 1–10. https://academic.oup.com/ajcn/article/90/1/1/4596750.

Huo, M., L. M. S. Miller, K. Kim, and S. Liu. "Volunteering, Self-Perceptions of Aging, and Mental Health in Later Life." *Gerontologist* 61, no. 7 (September 13, 2021): 1131–1140. https://pubmed.ncbi.nlm.nih.gov/33103726/.

Mayo Clinic. "Metabolic Syndrome." https://www.mayoclinic.org/diseases-conditions/metabolic-syndrome/diagnosis-treatment/drc-20351921.

Mayo Clinic. "Nutrition and Healthy Eating: 3 Diet Changes Women over 50 Should Make Right Now." https://www.mayoclinic.org/healthy-lifestyle/nutrition-and-healthy-eating/in-depth/3-diet-changes-women-over-50-should-make-right-now/art-20457589.

Mayo Clinic Health System. "5, 4, 3, 2, 1: Countdown to Make Anxiety Blast Off." (June 6, 2020): https://www.mayoclinichealthsystem.org/hometown-health/speaking-of-health/5-4-3-2-1-countdown-to-make-anxiety-blast-off.

Miner, B., and M. H. Kryger. "Sleep in the Aging Population." *Sleep Medicine Clinics* 15, no. 2 (June 2020): 311–318. https://pubmed.ncbi.nlm.nih.gov/32386704/.

Morrow-Howell, N., J. Hinterlong, P. A. Rozario, and F. Tang. "Effects of Volunteering on the Well-being of Older Adults." *The Journals of Gerontology. Series B, Psychological Sciences and Social Sciences* 58, no. 3 (May 2003): S137–145. https://pubmed.ncbi.nlm.nih.gov/12730314/.

Musich, S., S. S. Wang, S. Kraemer, K. Hawkins, and E. Wicker. "Purpose in Life and Positive Health Outcomes Among Older Adults." *Population Health Management* 21, no. 2 (April 1, 2018): 139–147. https://www.ncbi.nlm.nih.gov/pmc/articles/PMC5906725/.

National Institutes of Health, Office of Dietary Supplements. "Calcium." https://ods.od.nih.gov/factsheets/Calcium-HealthProfessional/.

National Institutes of Health, Office of Dietary Supplements. "Vitamin C." https://ods.od.nih.gov/factsheets/VitaminC-HealthProfessional/.

National Institutes of Health, Office of Dietary Supplements. "Vitamin D." https://ods.od.nih.gov/factsheets/VitaminD-HealthProfessional/.

National Institutes of Health, Office of Dietary Supplements. "Vitamin K." https://ods.od.nih.gov/factsheets/vitaminK-HealthProfessional/.

National Library of Medicine. MedlinePlus. "Obstructive Sleep Apnea." https://medlineplus.gov/genetics/condition/obstructive-sleep-apnea/.

Nelson, J. B. "Mindful Eating: The Art of Prescence While You Eat." *Diabetes Spectrum* 30, no. 3 (August 2017): 171–174. https://www.ncbi.nlm.nih.gov/pmc/articles/PMC5556586/.

Ockermann, P., L. Headley, R. Lizio, and J. Hansmann. "A Review of the Properties of Anthocyanins and Their Influence on Factors Affecting Cardiometabolic and Cognitive Health." *Nutrients* 13, no. 8 (August 2021): 2831. https://www.ncbi.nlm.nih.gov/pmc/articles/PMC8399873/.

Qu, H., M. Guo, H. Chai, W. T. Wang, Z. Y. Gao, and D. Z. Shi. "Effects of Coenzyme Q10 on Statin-Induced Myopathy: An Updated Meta-Analysis of Randomized Controlled Trials." *Journal of the American Heart Association* 7, no. 19 (September 25, 2018). https://www.ahajournals.org/doi/10.1161/JAHA.118.009835.

Romero-Peralta, S., I. Cano-Pumarega, C. Garcia-Malo, L. A. Ramos, and D. García-Borreguero. "Treating Restless Legs Syndrome in the Context of Sleep Disordered Breathing Comorbidity." *European Respiratory Review* 28 (2019): 190061. https://err.ersjournals.com/content/28/153/190061.

Seeman, M. V. "Why Are Women Prone to Restless Legs Syndrome?" *International Journal of Environmental Research and Public Health* 17, no. 1 (January 2020): 368. https://www.ncbi.nlm.nih.gov/pmc/articles/PMC6981604/.

Swarup, S., A. Goyal, Y. Grigorova, and R. Zeltser. "Metabolic Syndrome." *StatPearls.* https://www.ncbi.nlm.nih.gov/books/NBK459248/.

Varacallo, M., T. J. Seaman, J. S. Jandu, and P. Pizzutillo. "Osteopenia." *StatPearls.* https://www.ncbi.nlm.nih.gov/books/NBK499878/.

Zolfaghari, S., C. Yao, C. Thompson, N. Gosselin, A. Desautels, T. T. Dang-Vu, R. B. Postuma, and J. Carrier. "Effects of Menopause on Sleep Quality and Sleep Disorders: Canadian Longitudinal Study on Aging." *Menopause* 27, no. 3 (March 2020): 295–304. https://pubmed.ncbi.nlm.nih.gov/31851117/.

11. Prioritizing Relief and Your Safety

Leproult, R., and E. Van Cauter. "Role of Sleep and Sleep Loss in Hormonal Release and Metabolism." *Endocrine Development* 17 (2010): 11–21. https://www.ncbi.nlm.nih.gov/pmc/articles/PMC3065172/.

Women's Health Network. "Talking to Your Doctor About Hormone Therapy." https://www.womenshealthnetwork.com/hrt/hormone-therapy-talking-to-your -doctor/.

12. Personalizing Your Treatment Plan

Aibar-Almazán, A., F. Hita-Contreras, D. Cruz-Díaz, M. de la Torre-Cruz, J. D. Jiménez-García, and A. Martínez-Amat. "Effects of Pilates Training on Sleep Quality, Anxiety, Depression and Fatigue in Postmenopausal Women: A Randomized Controlled Trial." *Maturitas* 124 (June 2019): 62–67. https://pubmed.ncbi.nlm.nih.gov/31097181/.

American Academy of Dermatology Association. "Caring For Your Skin in Menopause." https://www.aad.org/public/everyday-care/skin-care-secrets/anti -aging/skin-care-during-menopause.

Aylett, E., N. Small, and P. Bower. "Exercise in the Treatment of Clinical Anxiety in General Practice—A Systematic Review and Meta-analysis." *BMC Health Services Research* 18 (2018): 559. https://www.ncbi.nlm.nih.gov/pmc /articles/PMC6048763/.

Baker, F. C., M. de Zambott, I. M. Colrain, and B. Bei. "Sleep Problems During the Menopausal Transition: Prevalence, Impact, and Management Challenges." *Nature and Science of Sleep* 10 (2018): 73–95. https://www.ncbi.nlm.nih.gov /pmc/articles/PMC5810528/.

Balci, F. L., C. Uras, and S. Feldman. "Clinical Factors Affecting the Therapeutic Efficacy of Evening Primrose Oil on Mastalgia." *Annals of Surgical Oncology*

27, no. 12 (November 2020): 4844–4852. https://pubmed.ncbi.nlm.nih.gov /32748152/.

Bansal, R. and N. Aggarwal. "Menopausal Hot Flashes: A Concise Review." *Journal of Mid-Life Health* 10, no. 1 (January–March 2019): 6–13. https://www .ncbi.nlm.nih.gov/pmc/articles/PMC6459071/.

Barati, F., A. Nasiri, N. Akbari, and G. Sharifzadeh. "The Effect of Aroma-therapy on Anxiety in Patients." *Nephro-Urology Monthly* 8, no. 5 (September 2016): e38347. https://www.ncbi.nlm.nih.gov/pmc/articles/PMC5111093/.

Boyd, K. "What Is Dry Eye? Symptoms, Causes and Treatment." American Academy of Ophthalmology (September 15, 2021): https://www.aao.org/eye -health/diseases/what-is-dry-eye#treatment.

Chaikittisilpa, S., N. Rattanasirisin, R. Panchaprateep, N. Orprayoon, P. Phutrakul, A. Suwan, and U. Jaisamrarn. "Prevalence of Female Pattern Hair Loss in Postmenopausal Women: A Cross-sectional Study." *Menopause* 29, no. 4 (April 2022): 415–420. https://journals.lww.com/menopausejournal/Abstract /2022/04000/Prevalence_of_female_pattern_hair_loss_in.7.aspx.

Chang, J. P. C., K. P. Su, V. Mondelli, and C. M. Pariante. "Omega-3 Poly-unsaturated Fatty Acids in Youths with Attention Deficit Hyperactivity Disor-der: A Systematic Review and Meta-Analysis of Clinical Trials and Biological Studies." *Neuropsychopharmacology* 43, no. 3 (February 2018): 534–545. https: //www.ncbi.nlm.nih.gov/pmc/articles/PMC5669464/.

Clark, K. L., W. Sebastianelli, K. R. Flechsenhar, D. F. Aukermann, F. Meza, R. L. Millard, J. R. Deitch, P. S. Sherbondy, and A. Albert. "24-Week Study on the Use of Collagen Hydrolysate as a Dietary Supple-ment in Athletes with Activity-Related Joint Pain." *Current Medical Re-search and Opinion* 24, no. 5 (May 2008): 1485–1496. https://pubmed.ncbi .nlm.nih.gov/18416885/.

Cleveland Clinic. "Here's How Menopause Affects Your Skin and Hair." https://health.clevelandclinic.org/heres-how-menopause-affects-your-skin -and-hair/.

Cleveland Clinic. "Low Blood Pressure (Orthostatic Hypotension)." https: //my.clevelandclinic.org/health/diseases/9385-low-blood-pressure-orthostatic -hypotension.

Cleveland Clinic. "Vestibular Rehabilitation." https://my.clevelandclinic.org /health/treatments/15298-vestibular-rehabilitation.

Cleveland Clinic. "Women and Heart Rate." https://my.clevelandclinic.org /health/diseases/17644-women—abnormal-heart-beats.

Cunha, L. F., L. C. Pellanda, and C. T. Reppold. "Positive Psychology and Gratitude Interventions: A Randomized Clinical Trial." *Frontiers in Psychology* 10 (March 21, 2019): 584. https://pubmed.ncbi.nlm.nih.gov/30949102/.

Dahiya, P., R. Kamal, M. Kumar, Niti, R. Gupta, and K. Chaudhary. "Burning Mouth Syndrome and Menopause." *International Journal of Preventive Medicine* 4, no. 1 (January 2013): 15–20. https://www.ncbi.nlm.nih.gov/pmc/articles /PMC3570906/.

Davis, S. R., C. Castelo-Branco, P. Chedraui, M. A. Lumsden, R. E. Nappi, D. Shah, P. Villaseca. "Understanding Weight Gain at Menopause." *Climacteric* 15, no. 5 (September 2012): 419–429. https://www.tandfonline.com/doi /full/10.3109/13697137.2012.707385.

El Hajj, A., N. Wardy, S. Haidar, D. Bourgi, M. El Haddad, D. El Chammas, N. El Osta, L. R. Khabbaz, and T. Papazian. "Menopausal Symptoms, Physical Activity Level and Quality of Life of Women Living in the Mediterranean Region." *PLoS ONE* 15, no. 3: e0230515. https://journals.plos.org/plosone/article ?id=10.1371/journal.pone.0230515.

Farzaneh, F., S. Fatehi, M. R. Sohrabi, and K. Alizadeh. "The Effect of Oral Evening Primrose Oil on Menopausal Hot Flashes: A Randomized Clinical Trial." *Archives of Gynecology and Obstetrics* 288, no. 5 (November 2013): 1075–1079. https://pubmed.ncbi.nlm.nih.gov/23625331/.

Gaiam. "1-Minute Breathing Exercise for Energy and Productivity." https:// www.gaiam.com/blogs/discover/1-minute-breathing-exercise-for-energy-and -productivity.

Goluch-Koniuszy, Z. S. "Nutrition of Women with Hair Loss Problem During the Period of Menopause." *Menopause Review* 15, no. 1 (March 2016): 56–61. https://www.ncbi.nlm.nih.gov/pmc/articles/PMC4828511/.

Gong, M., H. Dong, Y. Tang, W. Huang, and F. Lu. "Effects of Aromatherapy on Anxiety: A Meta-analysis of Randomized Controlled Trials." *Journal of Affective Disorders* 274 (September 1, 2020): 1028–1040. https://www.sciencedirect .com/science/article/abs/pii/S016503271933160X.

Gordon, J. L., M. Halleran, S. Beshai, T. A. Eisenlohr-Moul, J. Frederick, and T. S. Campbell. "Endocrine and Psychosocial Moderators of Mindfulness-Based Stress Reduction for the Prevention of Perimenopausal Depressive Symptoms: A

Randomized Controlled Trial." *Psychoneuroendocrinology* 130 (August 2021): 105277. https://pubmed.ncbi.nlm.nih.gov/34058560/.

Gortner, E. M., S. S. Rude, and J. W. Pennebaker. "Benefits of Expressive Writing in Lowering Rumination and Depressive Symptoms." *Behavior Therapy* 37, no. 3 (September 2006): 292–303. https://pubmed.ncbi.nlm.nih.gov/16942980/.

Gurvich, C., C. Zhu, and S. Arunogiri. "'Brain Fog' During Menopause Is Real—It Can Disrupt Women's Work and Spark Dementia Fears." *The Conversation* (December 13, 2021): https://theconversation.com/brain-fog-during -menopause-is-real-it-can-disrupt-womens-work-and-spark-dementia-fears -173150.

Herbenick, D. and J. D. Fortenberry. "Exercise-Induced Orgasm and Pleasure Among Women." *Sexual and Relationship Therapy* 26, no. 4 (2011): 378–388. https://www.tandfonline.com/doi/abs/10.1080/14681994.2011.647902.

Howarth, N. C., E. Saltzman, and S. B. Roberts. "Dietary Fiber and Weight Regulation." *Nutrition Reviews* 59, no. 5 (May 2001): 129–139. https://pubmed .ncbi.nlm.nih.gov/11396693/.

Kapoor, E., M. L. Collazo-Clavell, and S. S. Faubion. "Weight Gain in Women at Midlife: A Concise Review of the Pathophysiology and Strategies for Management." *Mayo Clinic Proceedings* 92, no. 10 (October 2017): 1552–1558. https: //pubmed.ncbi.nlm.nih.gov/28982486/.

Katz, V. L., L. Rozas, R. Ryder, and R. C. Cefalo. "Effect of Daily Immersion on the Edema of Pregnancy." *American Journal of Perinatalogy* 9, no. 4 (July 1992): 225–227. https://pubmed.ncbi.nlm.nih.gov/1627208/.

Kazemi, F., A. Z. Masoumi, A. Shayan, and K. Oshvandi. "The Effect of Evening Primrose Oil Capsule on Hot Flashes and Night Sweats in Postmenopausal Women: A Single-Blind Randomized Controlled Trial." *Journal of Menopausal Medicine* 27, no. 1 (April 2021): 8–14. https://www.ncbi.nlm.nih .gov/pmc/articles/PMC8102809/.

Khan, J., M. Anwer, N. Noboru, D. Thomas, and M. Kalladka. "Topical Application in Burning Mouth Syndrome." *Journal of Dental Sciences* 14, no. 4 (December 2019): 352–357. https://www.sciencedirect.com/science/article/pii /S1991790219301692.

Khunger, N. and K. Mehrotra. "Menopausal Acne—Challenges And Solutions." *International Journal of Women's Health* 11 (2019): 555–567. https://www .ncbi.nlm.nih.gov/pmc/articles/PMC6825478/.

Kim, H. K., S. Y. Kang, Y. J. Chung, J. H. Kim, and M. R. Kim. "The Recent Review of the Genitourinary Syndrome of Menopause." *Journal of Menopausal Medicine* 21, no. 2 (August 2015): 65–71. https://www.ncbi.nlm.nih.gov/pmc /articles/PMC4561742/.

Komesaroff, P. A., C. V. Black, V. Cable, and K. Sudhir. "Effects of Wild Yam Extract on Menopausal Symptoms, Lipids and Sex Hormones in Healthy Menopausal Women." *Climacteric* 4, no. 2 (June 2001): 144–150. https://pubmed.ncbi .nlm.nih.gov/11428178/.

Lenger, S. M., M. S. Bradley, D. A. Thomas, M. H. Bertolet, J. L. Lowder, and S. Sutcliffe. "D-mannose vs Other Agents for Recurrent Urinary Tract Infection Prevention in Adult Women: A Systematic Review and Meta-analysis." *American Journal of Obstetrics and Gynecology* 223, no. 2 (August 2020): 265 .e1–265.e.13. https://www.ncbi.nlm.nih.gov/pmc/articles/PMC7395894/.

Li, T., Y. Zhang, Q. Cheng, M. Hou, X. Zheng, Q. Zheng, and L. Li. "Quantitative Study on the Efficacy of Acupuncture in the Treatment of Menopausal Hot Flashes and its Comparison with Nonhormonal Drugs." *Menopause* 28, no. 5 (March 15, 2021): 564–572. https://pubmed.ncbi.nlm.nih.gov /33739313/.

Magliano, M. "Menopausal Arthralgia: Fact or Fiction." *Maturitas* 67, no. 1 (September 2010): 29–33. https://pubmed.ncbi.nlm.nih.gov/20537472/.

Mahdood, B., B. Imani, and S. Khazaei. "Effects of Inhalation Aromatherapy With Rosa damascena (Damask Rose) on the State Anxiety and Sleep Quality of Operating Room Personnel During the COVID-19 Pandemic: A Randomized Controlled Trial." *Journal of PeriAnesthesia Nursing.* (October 29, 2021): https://www.ncbi.nlm.nih.gov/pmc/articles/PMC8554138/.

Mayo Clinic. "Chart of High-Fiber Foods." https://www.mayoclinic.org /healthy-lifestyle/nutrition-and-healthy-eating/in-depth/high-fiber-foods/art -20050948.

Mayo Clinic. "Dry Eyes." https://www.mayoclinic.org/diseases-conditions/dry -eyes/symptoms-causes/syc-20371863.

Mayo Clinic. "Orthostatic Hypotension (Postural Hypotension)." https://www .mayoclinic.org/diseases-conditions/orthostatic-hypotension/diagnosis -treatment/drc-20352553.

Medical News Today. "Does Menopause Cause Dizziness?" https://www .medicalnewstoday.com/articles/319860.

Naseri, R., V. Farnia, K. Yazdchi, M. Alikhani, B. Basanj, and S. Salemi. "Comparison of Vitex Agnus-castus Extracts with Placebo in Reducing Menopausal Symptoms: A Randomized Double-Blind Study." *Korean Journal of Family Medicine* 40, no. 6 (November 2019): 362–367. https://www.ncbi.nlm.nih.gov/pmc/articles/PMC6887765/.

National Institute of Dental and Craniofacial Research. "Burning Mouth Syndrome." https://www.nidcr.nih.gov/health-info/burning-mouth.

National Institutes of Health, Office of Dietary Supplements. "Vitamin B6." https://ods.od.nih.gov/factsheets/VitaminB6-Consumer/.

Peck, T., L. Olsakovsky, and S. Aggarwal. "Dry Eye Syndrome in Menopause and Perimenopausal Age Group." *Journal of Mid-Life Health* 8, no. 2 (April–June 2017): 51–54. https://www.ncbi.nlm.nih.gov/pmc/articles/PMC5496280/.

Sanaati, F., S. Najafi, Z. Kashaninia, and M. Sadeghi. "Effect of Ginger and Chamomile on Nausea and Vomiting Caused by Chemotherapy in Iranian Women with Breast Cancer." *Asian Pacific Journal of Cancer Prevention* 17, no. 8 (2016): 4125–4129. https://pubmed.ncbi.nlm.nih.gov/27644672/.

Seal, B. N., and C. M. Meston. "The Impact of Body Awareness on Women's Sexual Health: A Comprehensive Review." *Sexual Medicine Reviews* 8, no. 2 (April 2020): 242–255. https://pubmed.ncbi.nlm.nih.gov/29678474/.

Sexual Medicine Society of North America (SMSNA). "What Is Sensate Focus and How Does It Work?" https://www.smsna.org/patients/did-you-know/what-is-sensate-focus-and-how-does-it-work.

Sharifzadeh, F., M. Kashanian, J. Koohpayehzadeh, F. Rezaian, N. Sheikhansari, and N. Eshraghi. "A Comparison Between the Effects of Ginger, Pyridoxine (Vitamin B6) and Placebo for the Treatment of the First Trimester Nausea and Vomiting of Pregnancy (NVP)." *Journal of Maternal-Fetal and Neonatal Medicine* 31, no. 19 (October 2018): 2509–2514. https://pubmed.ncbi.nlm.nih.gov/28629250/.

Sharma, S. and M. Kavuru. "Sleep and Metabolism: An Overview." *International Journal of Endocrinology* (2010): 270832. https://www.ncbi.nlm.nih.gov/pmc/articles/PMC2929498/.

Shifren, J. L. "Patient Education: Sexual Problems in Women (Beyond the Basics)." UpToDate. https://www.uptodate.com/contents/sexual-problems-in-women-beyond-the-basics.

Sievert, L. L., and C. M. Obermeyer. "Symptom Clusters at Midlife: A Four-Country Comparison of Checklist and Qualitative Responses." *Menopause* 19, no. 2 (February 2012): 133–144. https://www.ncbi.nlm.nih.gov/pmc/articles/PMC3267011/.

Simon, N. M., S. G. Hofmann, D. Rosenfield, S. S. Hoeppner, E. A. Hoge, E. Bui, and S. B. S. Khalsa. "Efficacy of Yoga vs Cognitive Behavioral Therapy vs Stress Education for the Treatment of Generalized Anxiety Disorder: A Randomized Clinical Trial." *JAMA Psychiatry* 78, no. 1 (January 1, 2021): 13–20. https://pubmed.ncbi.nlm.nih.gov/32805013/.

Steele, N. M., J. French, J. Gatherer-Boyles, S. Newman, and S. Leclaire. "Effect of Acupressure by Sea-Bands on Nausea and Vomiting of Pregnancy." *Journal of Obstetric, Gynecologic, and Neonatal Nursing* 30, no. 1 (January–February 2001): 61–70. https://pubmed.ncbi.nlm.nih.gov/11277163/.

Tao, L., R. Jiang, K. Zhang, Z. Qian, P. Chen, Y. Lv, and Y. Yao. "Light Therapy in Non-seasonal Depression: An Update Meta-analysis." *Psychiatry Research* 291 (September 2020): 113247. https://pubmed.ncbi.nlm.nih.gov/32622169/.

Terauchi, M., T. Odai, A. Hirose, K. Kato, M. Akiyoshi, M. Masuda, R. Tsunoda, H. Fushiki, and N. Miyasaka. "Dizziness in Peri-and Postmenopausal Women is Associated with Anxiety: A Cross-sectional Study." *BioPsychoSocial Medicine* 12 (2018): 21. https://www.ncbi.nlm.nih.gov/pmc/articles/PMC6291970/.

Teruel, A. and S. Patel. "Burning Mouth Syndrome: A Review of Etiology, Diagnosis, and Management." *General Dentistry* (March/April 2019): 25–29. https://www.agd.org/docs/default-source/self-instruction-(gendent)/gendent_ma19_patel.pdf?sfvrsn=266273b1_0.

The North American Menopause Society. "Decreased Desire." https://www.menopause.org/for-women/sexual-health-menopause-online/sexual-problems-at-midlife/decreased-desire.

The North American Menopause Society. "Effective Treatments for Sexual Problems." https://www.menopause.org/for-women/sexual-health-menopause-online/effective-treatments-for-sexual-problems.

The North American Menopause Society. "MenoNote: Vaginal Dryness." https://www.menopause.org/docs/default-source/for-women/mn-vaginal-dryness.pdf.

The North American Menopause Society. "Menopause FAQS: Hot Flashes." https://www.menopause.org/for-women/menopause-faqs-hot-flashes.

Ward-Ritacco, C. L., A. L. Adrian, P. J. O'Connor, J. A. Binkowski, L. Q. Rogers, M. A., Johnson, and E. M. Evans. "Feelings of Energy Are Associated with Physical Activity and Sleep Quality, but not Adiposity, in Middle-aged Postmenopausal Women." *Menopause* 22, no. 3 (March 2015): 304–311. https://journals.lww.com/menopausejournal/Abstract/2015/03000/Feelings_of_energy_are_associated_with_physical.11.aspx.

13. Self-Care Going Forward

American Cancer Society. "American Cancer Society Guidelines for the Early Detection of Cancer." https://www.cancer.org/healthy/find-cancer-early/american-cancer-society-guidelines-for-the-early-detection-of-cancer.html.

American Cancer Society. "Key Statistics for Cervical Cancer." https://www.cancer.org/cancer/cervical-cancer/about/key-statistics.html.

American Cancer Society. "Key Statistics for Colorectal Cancer." https://www.cancer.org/cancer/colon-rectal-cancer/about/key-statistics.html.

American Cancer Society. "The Pap (Papanicolaou) Test." https://www.cancer.org/cancer/cervical-cancer/detection-diagnosis-staging/screening-tests/pap-test.html.

American College of Obstetricians and Gynecologists. "Updated Cervical Cancer Screening Guidelines." (April 2021): https://www.acog.org/clinical/clinical-guidance/practice-advisory/articles/2021/04/updated-cervical-cancer-screening-guidelines.

American Diabetes Association. "Diabetes Overview: The Path to Understanding Diabetes Starts Here." https://www.diabetes.org/diabetes.

American Heart Association. "Heart-Health Screenings." https://www.heart.org/en/health-topics/consumer-healthcare/what-is-cardiovascular-disease/heart-health-screenings.

Asbjørnsen, R. A., J. Wentzel, M. L. Smedsrød, J. Hjelmesæth, M. M. Clark, L. S. Nes, and J. E. W. C. Van Gemert-Pijnen. "Identifying Persuasive Design Principles and Behavior Change Techniques Supporting End User Values and Needs in eHealth Interventions for Long-Term Weight Loss Maintenance: Qualitative Study." *Journal of Medical Internet Research* 22, no. 11 (November 2020): e22598. https://www.ncbi.nlm.nih.gov/pmc/articles /PMC7735908/.

Barber, M. D. and C. Maher. "Epidemiology and Outcome Assessment of Pelvic Organ Prolapse." *International Urogynecology Journal* 24, no. 11 (November 2013): 1783–1790. https://pubmed.ncbi.nlm.nih.gov/24142054/.

Bone Health and Osteoporosis Foundation. "What Is Osteoporosis and What Causes It?" https://www.nof.org/patients/what-is-osteoporosis/.

Bone Health and Osteoporosis Foundation. "Evaluation of Bone Health/ Bone Density Testing." https://www.bonehealthandosteoporosis.org/patients /diagnosis-information/bone-density-examtesting/.

Centers for Disease Control and Prevention. "Breast Cancer Screening Guidelines for Women." https://www.cdc.gov/cancer/breast/pdf/breast-cancer-screening -guidelines-508.pdf.

Centers for Disease Control and Prevention. "Breast Cancer Statistics." https: //www.cdc.gov/cancer/breast/statistics/index.htm.

Centers for Disease Control and Prevention. "Breast Cancer: What Is a Mammogram?" https://www.cdc.gov/cancer/breast/basic_info/mammograms.htm.

Centers for Disease Control and Prevention. "Colorectal Cancer Screening Tests." https://www.cdc.gov/cancer/colorectal/basic_info/screening/tests.htm.

Centers for Disease Control and Prevention. "Diabetes Tests." https://www.cdc .gov/diabetes/basics/getting-tested.html.

Corley, J., S. R. Cox, A. M. Taylor, M. V. Hernandez, S. M. Maniega, L. Ballerini, S. Wiseman, R. Meijboom, E. V. Backhouse, M. E. Bastin, J. M. Wardlaw, and I. J. Deary. "Dietary Patterns, Cognitive Function, and Structural Neuroimaging Measures of Brain Aging." *Experimental Gerontology* 142 (December 2020): https://www.sciencedirect.com/science/article/abs/pii/S0531556520304654.

Currie, H. and C. Williams. "Menopause, Cholesterol and Cardiovascular Disease." *US Cardiology* 5, no. 1 (2008): 12–14. https://www.uscjournal.com /articles/menopause-cholesterol-and-cardiovascular-disease-0.

De Brito, T. R. P., D. P. Nunes, L. P. Corona, T. da Silva Alexandre, and Y. A. de Oliveira Duarte. "Low Supply of Social Support as Risk Factor for Mortality in the Older Adults." *Archives of Gerontology and Geriatrics* 73 (November 2017): 77–81. https://pubmed.ncbi.nlm.nih.gov/28783514/.

El Khoudary, S. R., B. Aggarwal, T. M. Beckie, H. N. Hodis, A. E. Johnson, R. D. Langer, M. C. Limacher, J. E. Manson, M. L. Stefanick, M. A. Allison. "Menopause Transition and Cardiovascular Disease Risk: Implications for Timing of Early Prevention: A Scientific Statement From the American Heart Association." *Circulation* 142, no. 25 (November 30, 2020): e506-e532. https://www.ahajournals.org/doi/10.1161/CIR.0000000000000912.

Endocrine Society. "Menopause and Bone Loss." January 23, 2022. https://www.endocrine.org/patient-engagement/endocrine-library/menopause-and-bone-loss.

Gesing, A. "The Thyroid Gland and the Process of Aging." *Thyroid Research* 8 (June 22, 2015): A8. https://www.ncbi.nlm.nih.gov/pmc/articles/PMC4480281/.

Hoffman, B. M., M. A. Babyak, W. E. Craighead, A. Sherwood, P. M. Doraiswamy, M. J. Coons, and J. A. Blumenthal. "Exercise and Pharmacotherapy in Patients With Major Depression: One-Year Follow-Up of the SMILE Study." *Psychosomatic Medicine* 73, no. 2 (February–March 2011): 127–133. https://www.ncbi.nlm.nih.gov/pmc/articles/PMC3671874/.

Kim, Y., Y. Chang, I. Y. Cho, R. Kwon, G. Y. Lim, J. H. Jee, S. Ryu, and M. Kang. "The Prevalence of Thyroid Dysfunction in Korean Women Undergoing Routine Health Screening: A Cross-Sectional Study." *Thyroid* (May 16, 2022): https://pubmed.ncbi.nlm.nih.gov/35293242/.

Mayo Clinic. "Colon Cancer." https://www.mayoclinic.org/diseases-conditions/colon-cancer/symptoms-causes/syc-20353669.

Medical News Today. "What to Know About Menopause and High Blood Pressure." https://www.medicalnewstoday.com/articles/menopause-and-high-blood-pressure-link-and-treatment.

National Heart, Lung, and Blood Institute. "Blood Cholesterol: Diagnosis." https://www.nhlbi.nih.gov/health/blood-cholesterol/diagnosis.

National Institute of Diabetes and Digestive and Kidney Diseases. "Diabetes Tests & Diagnosis." https://www.niddk.nih.gov/health-information/diabetes/overview/tests-diagnosis#who.

National Institute of Diabetes and Digestive and Kidney Diseases. "The A1C Test & Diabetes." https://www.niddk.nih.gov/health-information/diagnostic-tests/a1c-test.

National Institute of Diabetes and Digestive and Kidney Diseases. "What is Diabetes?" https://www.niddk.nih.gov/health-information/diabetes/overview/what-is-diabetes.

National Institutes of Health, Office of Dietary Supplements. "Dietary Supplements: What You Need to Know." https://ods.od.nih.gov/factsheets/WYNTK-Consumer/.

National Institutes of Health, Office of Dietary Supplements. "Probiotics." https://ods.od.nih.gov/factsheets/Probiotics-HealthProfessional/.

National Library of Medicine. Medline. "Health Screenings for Women ages 40 to 64." https://medlineplus.gov/ency/article/007467.htm.

Smith, G. L., L. Banting, R. Eime, G. O'Sullivan, J. G. Z. van Uffelen. "The Association Between Social Support and Physical Activity in Older Adults: A Systematic Review." *International Journal of Behavioral Nutrition and Physical Activity* 14, no. 1 (April 27, 2017): 56. https://www.ncbi.nlm.nih.gov/pmc/articles/PMC5408452/.

U.S. Preventive Services Task Force. "Colorectal Cancer: Screening." (May 18, 2021): https://www.uspreventiveservicestaskforce.org/uspstf/recommendation/colorectal-cancer-screening.

U.S. Preventive Services Task Force. "Osteoporosis to Prevent Fractures: Screening." (June 26, 2018): https://www.uspreventiveservicestaskforce.org/uspstf/recommendation/osteoporosis-screening#bootstrap-panel—6.

U.S. Preventive Services Task Force. "Prediabetes and Type 2 Diabetes: Screening." (August 24, 2021): https://www.uspreventiveservicestaskforce.org/uspstf/recommendation/screening-for-prediabetes-and-type-2-diabetes.

Acknowledgments

The path to achieving a major goal in life is rarely straight, which often makes the journey that much more interesting. While I didn't always know I would become a menopause doctor, helping patients with difficult health-related challenges, dealing with full-frontal mistakes, and trusting my gut brought me to where I am today. And I'm thrilled about that!

Also, my grandfather, an ob-gyn, inspired me with his clarity on the importance of preventive care in the 1950s when that concept seemed irrelevant.

This book would not be in your hands without the fabulous and talented writer Stacey Colino, my partner in crime, who I consider the doula who helped birth this book. Without Stacey, this book would simply not exist. For her incredible intuition, intelligence, and support, I hope every reader can acknowledge her genius.

I would not be the clinician I am without my mentor and fellowship director, Dr. Holly Thacker, professor of obstetrics and gynecology and director of the Center for Specialized Women's Health at the Cleveland Clinic. Dr. Thacker taught me everything I know about menopause, midlife, and hormone therapy. She also taught me that medicine is political, whether we agree with that or not. Not only did she grace me with this knowledge, she armed me with a readiness for social change that ignited a fire under my a$$.

A special thank-you to many other clinician and research

mentors and heroes of mine including Dr. Megan McNamara, Dr. Rebecca Flyct, Dr. Pelin Batur, Dr. Rebecca Jackson, Dr. Sarah Jonaus, Elizabeth Gandee, CNP, Dr. JoAnn Manson, Dr. Philip Sarrel, Dr. Stephanie McClellan, Dr. Jim Simon, Dr. Avrum Bluming, Dr. Kari Braaten, the leaders of both the North American Menopause Society (NAMS) and the International Society for the Study of Women's Sexual Health (ISSWSH), and the incredible Dr. Kathryn Rexrode, chief of the Division of Women's Health at the Brigham and Women's Hospital in Boston, Massachusetts, who saw clear potential in me and advocated for the expansion of women's health to include a specialized center for menopause. There has never been a greater reward than teaching some of the most talented clinicians, researchers, and scientists at Harvard and throughout Boston and New England.

Many thanks to those who helped me with specialized knowledge for this book including Elizabeth Ward, RD, and Dr. Allison Deutch. Also, a huge thank-you to my literary agent, Jane von Mehren, who saw the potential in this book from day one, as well as St. Martin's editors Daniela Rapp and Elizabeth Beier who have been big proponents behind the book. I would also like to thank Melissa Nasson and Veronica Ramirez, Yemi Morrison (web design), and Katheryn Costello (photography).

In truth, there has been no bigger cheerleader for me throughout my life than my mother, who drove me to every medical school interview, residency interview (that she could), and marathon that I ever ran. Heck, she often had to drive me to homeroom to ensure I made it through high school. She has listened to every trial and tribulation in my life, those big and small, and without her this book would absolutely not exist.

I also want to thank my husband, Blaze, for his incredible patience and parenting of three kids under five while I snuck away to write this book. My husband frequently picked up the slack in our household—as well as the proverbial pom-poms to cheer me on whenever I needed it. Blaze, DeMille, Bryson, and Brody, I love you!

Finally, I would like to thank you, dear reader, and all the women who have asked me questions about menopause, advocated for their health, or engaged with any of my social media posts. I see you. I hear you. I've got you. This book is for *you*.

Notes

Introduction

1. K. J. Trudeau, J. L. Ainscough, M. Trant, J. Starker, and T. Cousineau, "Identifying the Educational Needs of Menopausal Women: A Feasibility Study," *Women's Health* 21, no. 2 (March–April 2011), https://www.ncbi.nlm.nih.gov/pmc/articles/PMC3856775/.

2. K. L. Marlatt, R. A. Beyl, and L. M. Redman, "A Qualitative Assessment of Health Behaviors and Experiences During Menopause: A Cross-sectional, Observational Study," *Maturitas* 116 (October 2018), 36–42, https://www.ncbi.nlm.nih.gov/pmc/articles/PMC6223619/.

3. J. M. Kling, K. L. MacLaughlin, P. F. Schnatz, C. J. Crandall, L. J. Skinner, C. A. Stuenkel, A. M. Kaunitz, D. L. Bitner, K. Mara, K. S. Fodmader Hilsaca, and S. S. Faubion, "Menopause Management Knowledge in Postgraduate Family Medicine, Internal Medicine, and Obstetrics and Gynecology Residents: A Cross-Sectional Survey," *Mayo Clinic Proceedings* 94, no. 2 (February 1, 2019), 242–253, https://www.mayoclinicproceedings.org/article/S0025–6196(18)30701–8/fulltext.

Chapter 1: The Wild, Wild West of Health Experiences

1. C. Garrard, "Coping With Hot Flashes and Other Menopausal Symptoms: What 10 Celebrities Said," EverydayHealth.com (February 22, 2021), https://www.everydayhealth.com/menopause/coping-hot-flashes-menopausal-symptoms-celebrities-said/.

2. E. T. Katz, "Kim Cattrall's First Brush With Menopause Was As Samantha on 'Sex And The City,'" HuffPost (September 26, 2014), https://www.huffpost.com/entry/kim-cattrall-menopause_n_5887962.

3. The North American Menopause Society, "Menopause 101: A Primer for the Perimenopausal," https://www.menopause.org/for-women/menopauseflashes /menopause-symptoms-and-treatments/menopause-101-a-primer-for-the -perimenopausal.

4. P. K. Mansfield, M. Carey, A. Anderson, S. H. Barsom, and P. B. Koch, "Staging the Menopausal Transition: Data from the TREMIN Research Program on Women's Health," *Women's Health* 14, no. 6 (November–December 2004), 220–226. https://pubmed.ncbi.nlm.nih.gov/15589772/.

5. S. D. Harlow, M. Gass, J. E. Hall, R. Lobo, P. Maki, R. W. Rebar, S. Sherman, P. M. Sluss, and T. J. de Villiers, "Executive Summary of STRAW+10: Addressing the Unfinished Agenda of Staging Reproductive Aging," *Climacteric* 15, no. 2 (April 2012), 105–114, https://www.ncbi.nlm.nih.gov/pmc /articles/PMC3580996/.

6. T. C. Okeke, U. B. Anyaehie, and C. C. Ezenyeaku, "Premature Menopause," *Annals of Medical & Health Sciences Research* 3, no. 1 (January–March 2013), 90–95, https://www.ncbi.nlm.nih.gov/pmc/articles/PMC3634232/.

7. L. R. Sammaritano, "Menopause in Patients with Autoimmune Diseases," *Autoimmunity Reviews* 11, no. 6 (May 2012), A430–A436, https://www .sciencedirect.com/science/article/abs/pii/S1568997211002680.

8. U. T. Börü, C. K. Toksoy, C. Bölük, A. Bilgiç, and M. Taşdemir, "Effects of Multiple Sclerosis and Medications on Menopausal Age," *Journal of International Medical Research* 46, no. 3 (March 2018), 1249–1253, https://www .ncbi.nlm.nih.gov/pmc/articles/PMC5972265/.

9. D. Zhu et al., "Relationships Between Intensity, Duration, Cumulative Dose, and Timing of Smoking with Age at Menopause: A Pooled Analysis of Individual Data from 17 Observational Studies," *PLoS Medicine* 15, no. 11 (November 2018), https://www.ncbi.nlm.nih.gov/pmc/articles /PMC6258514/.

10. C. W. Schmidt, "Age at Menopause: Do Chemical Exposures Play a Role?" *Environmental Health Perspectives* 125, no. 6 (June 2017), 062001, https: //www.ncbi.nlm.nih.gov/pmc/articles/PMC5743449/.

11. P. F. Schnatz, J. Serra, D. M. O'Sullivan, and J. I. Sorosky, "Menopausal Symptoms in Hispanic Women and the Role of Socioeconomic Factors," *Obstetrical & Gynecological Survey* 61, no. 3 (March 2006), 187–193, https: //pubmed.ncbi.nlm.nih.gov/16490118/.

Chapter 2: Myths and Misconceptions About Menopause

1. E. K. Bjelland, S. Hofvind, L. Byberg, and A. Eskild, "The Relation of Age at Menarche with Age at Natural Menopause: A Population Study of

336,788 Women in Norway," *Human Reproduction* 33, no. 6 (June 2018), 1149–1157, https://www.ncbi.nlm.nih.gov/pmc/articles/PMC5972645/.

2. S. Witkowski, "A Sedentary Lifestyle Can Lead to More Nighttime Hot Flashes," presented during the North American Menopause Society (NAMS) Annual Meeting in Washington, DC, September 22–25, 2021, https://www.eurekalert.org/news-releases/928804, https://www.newswise.com/articles/a-sedentary-lifestyle-can-lead-to-more -nighttime-hot-flashes.

3. W. A. Romani, L. Gallicchio, and J. A. Flaws, "The Association Between Physical Activity and Hot Flash Severity, Frequency, and Duration in Mid-Life Women," *American Journal of Human Biology* 21, no. 1 (January–February 2009), 127–129, https://www.ncbi.nlm.nih.gov/pmc/articles/PMC2753173/.

4. K. J. Ryu, H. K. Kim, Y. J. Lee, H. Park, and T. Kim, "Association Between Vasomotor Symptoms and Sarcopenia Assessed by L3 Skeletal Muscle Index Among Korean Menopausal Women," *Menopause* 29, no. 1 (January 2022), 48–53, https://journals.lww.com/menopausejournal/Fulltext/2022/01000 /Association_between_vasomotor_symptoms_and.10.aspx.

5. A. Thomas and A. J. Daley, "Women's Views About Physical Activity as a Treatment for Vasomotor Menopausal Symptoms: A Qualitative Study," *BMC Women's Health* 20, no. 203 (2020), https://bmcwomenshealth .biomedcentral.com/articles/10.1186/s12905-020-01063-w.

6. B. Ayers, M. Forshaw, and M. S. Hunter, "The Impact of Attitudes Towards the Menopause on Women's Symptom Experience: A Systematic Review," *Maturitas* 65, no. 1 (January 2010), 28–36, https://www.sciencedirect.com /science/article/abs/pii/S0378512209003971.

7. R. Sood, C. L. Kuhle, E. Kapoor, J. M. Thielen, K. S. Frohmader, K. C. Mara, and S. S. Faubion, "Association of Mindfulness and Stress with Menopausal Symptoms in Midlife Women," *Climacteric* 22, no. 4 (August 2019), 377–382, https://pubmed.ncbi.nlm.nih.gov/30652511/.

8. T. Muka, C. Oliver-Williams, V. Colpani, S. Kunutsor, S. Chowdhury, R. Chowdhury, M. Kavousi, and O. H. Franco, "Association of Vasomotor and Other Menopausal Symptoms with Risk of Cardiovascular Disease: A Systematic Review and Meta-Analysis," *PLoS One* 11, no. 6 (2016), https: //www.ncbi.nlm.nih.gov/pmc/articles/PMC4912069/.

9. Rush University Medical Center, "How the Body Regulates Heat," https: //www.rush.edu/news/how-body-regulates-heat.

10. H. M. Kravitz, R. Kazlauskaite, and H. Joffe, "Sleep, Health, and Metabolism in Midlife Women and Menopause: Food for Thought," *Obstetrics and Gynecology Clinics of North America* 45, no. 4 (December 2018), 679–694, https://www.ncbi.nlm.nih.gov/pmc/articles/PMC6338227/.

11. L. S. Cohen, C. N. Soares, A. F. Vitonis, M. W. Otto, and B. L. Harlow, "Risk for New Onset of Depression During the Menopausal Transition: The Harvard Study of Moods and Cycles," *JAMA Psychiatry* 63, no. 4 (April 2006), 385–390, https://jamanetwork.com/journals/jamapsychiatry /fullarticle/209471.

12. A. Moilanen, J. Kopra, H. Kroger, R. Sund, R. Rikkonen, and J. Sirola, "Characteristics of Long-Term Femoral Neck Bone Loss in Postmenopausal Women: A 25-Year Follow-Up," *Journal of Bone and Mineral Research* 37, no. 2 (February 2022), 173–178, https://asbmr.onlinelibrary.wiley.com/doi /10.1002/jbmr.4444.

13. T. Kameda, H. Mano, T. Yuasa, Y. Mori, K. Miyazawa, M. Shiokawa, Y. Nakamaru, E. Hiroi, K. Hiura, A. Kameda, N. N. Yang, Y. Hakeda, and M. Kumegawa, "Estrogen Inhibits Bone Resorption by Directly Inducing Apoptosis of the Bone-resorbing Osteoclasts," *Journal of Experimental Medicine* 186, no. 4 (August 1997), 489–495, https://www.ncbi.nlm.nih.gov /pmc/articles/PMC2199029/.

14. Centers for Disease Control and Prevention, "Percentage of Adults Aged 65 and Over With Osteoporosis or Low Bone Mass at the Femur Neck or Lumbar Spine: United States, 2005–2010," https://www.cdc.gov/nchs/data /hestat/osteoporsis/osteoporosis2005_2010.htm.

15. Mayo Clinic, "Male Menopause: Myth or Reality?" https://www.mayoclinic .org/healthy-lifestyle/mens-health/in-depth/male-menopause/art -20048056.

16. D. C. Gould and R. Petty, "The Male Menopause: Does it Exist?" *Western Journal of Medicine* 173, no. 2 (August 2000), 76–78, https://www.ncbi.nlm .nih.gov/pmc/articles/PMC1070997/.

Chapter 3: The Hormone Conundrum

1. The Women's Health Initiative Study Group, "Design of the Women's Health Initiative Clinical Trial and Observational Study," *Controlled Clinical Trials* 19, no. 1 (February 1998), 61–109, https://pubmed.ncbi.nlm.nih .gov/9492970/.

2. U.S. Department of Health & Human Services, Office on Women's Health, "Largest Women's Health Prevention Study Ever—Women's Health Initiative," https://www.womenshealth.gov/30-achievements/25.

3. J. E. Manson et al., "Menopausal Hormone Therapy and Long-term All-Cause and Cause-Specific Mortality: The Women's Health Initiative Randomized Trials," *JAMA* 318, no. 10 (September 12, 2017), 927–938, https://jamanetwork.com/journals/jama/fullarticle/2653735.

4. The North American Menopause Society, "News You Can Use About Hormone Therapy," http://www.menopause.org/for-women/menopauseflashes /menopause-symptoms-and-treatments/news-you-can-use-about-hormone -therapy.

5. The North American Menopause Society, "The North American Menopause Society Statement on Continuing Use of Systemic Hormone Therapy After Age 65," http://www.menopause.org/docs/default-source/2015/2015 -nams-hormone-therapy-after-age-65.pdf.

6. The North American Menopause Society, "News You Can Use About Hormone Therapy," http://www.menopause.org/for-women/menopauseflashes /menopause-symptoms-and-treatments/news-you-can-use-about-hormone -therapy.

7. The North American Menopause Society, "Menopause FAQs: Hormone Therapy for Menopause Symptoms," http://www.menopause.org/for-women /menopause-faqs-hormone-therapy-for-menopause-symptoms.

8. J. E. Manson et al., "The Women's Health Initiative Hormone Therapy Trials: Update and Overview of Health Outcomes During the Intervention and Post-Stopping Phases," *JAMA* 310, no. 13 (October 2, 2013), 1353–1368, https://www.ncbi.nlm.nih.gov/pmc/articles/PMC3963523/.

9. The North American Menopause Society, "Changes in Hormone Levels," http://www.menopause.org/for-women/sexual-health-menopause-online /changes-at-midlife/changes-in-hormone-levels.

10. The North American Menopause Society, "Hormone Help Desk: ET, EPT, and More," http://www.menopause.org/for-women/menopauseflashes/menopause -symptoms-and-treatments/hormone-help-desk-et-ept-and-more.

11. L. Al-Imari and W. L. Wolfman, "The Safety of Testosterone Therapy in Women," *Journal of Obstetrics and Gynaecology Canada* 34, no. 9 (September 2012), 859–865, https://www.jogc.com/article/S1701–2163(16)35385–3/ pdf.

12. R. T. Chlebowski, et al., "Association of Menopausal Hormone Therapy With Breast Cancer Incidence and Mortality During Long-term Follow-up of the Women's Health Initiative Randomized Clinical Trials," *JAMA* 324, no. 4 (July 28, 2020), 369–380, https://www.ncbi.nlm.nih.gov/pmc /articles/PMC7388026/.

13. The North American Menopause Society, "The 2017 Hormone Therapy Position Statement of the North American Menopause Society," *Menopause* 24, no. 7 (2017), 728–753, https://www.menopause.org/docs/default -source/2017/nams-2017-hormone-therapy-position-statement.pdf.

14. L. Delamater and N. Santoro, "Management of the Perimenopause," *Clinical Obstetrics and Gynecology* 61, no. 3 (September 2018), 419–432, https: //www.ncbi.nlm.nih.gov/pmc/articles/PMC6082400/.

15. H. K. Kim, S. Y. Kang, Y. J. Chung, J. H. Kim, and M. R. Kim, "The Recent Review of the Genitourinary Syndrome of Menopause," *Journal of Menopausal Medicine* 21, no. 2 (August 2015), 65–71, https://www.ncbi.nlm.nih.gov/pmc/articles/PMC4561742/.

16. The North American Menopause Society, "The 2017 Hormone Therapy Position Statement of the North American Menopause Society," *Menopause* 24, no. 7 (2017), 728–753, https://www.menopause.org/docs/default-source/2017/nams-2017-hormone-therapy-position-statement.pdf.

17. The North American Menopause Society, "The North American Menopause Society Statement on Continuing Use of Systemic Hormone Therapy After Age 65," http://www.menopause.org/docs/default-source/2015/2015-nams-hormone-therapy-after-age-65.pdf.

18. M. Canonico, E. Oger, G. Plu-Bureau, J. Conard, G. Meyer, H. Lévesque, N. Trillot, M. T. Barrellier, D. Wahl, J. Emmerich, P. Y. Scarabin, "Hormone Therapy and Venous Thromboembolism Among Postmenopausal Women: Impact of the Route of Estrogen Administration and Progestogens: The ESTHER Study," *Circulation* 115, no. 7 (February 20, 2007), 840–845, https://pubmed.ncbi.nlm.nih.gov/17309934/.

Chapter 5: The Premature Menopause Type

1. S. A. Choe and J. Sung, "Trends of Premature and Early Menopause: A Comparative Study of the US National Health and Nutrition Examination Survey and the Korea National Health and Nutrition Examination Survey," *Journal of Korean Medical Science* 35, no. 14 (April 13, 2020), https://www.ncbi.nlm.nih.gov/pmc/articles/PMC7152531/.

2. J. L. Luborsky, P. Meyer, M. F. Sowers, E. B. Gold, and N. Santoro, "Premature Menopause in a Multi-ethnic Population Study of the Menopause Transition," *Human Reproduction* 18, no. 1 (January 2003), 199–206, https://academic.oup.com/humrep/article/18/1/199/880307.

3. D. Zhu, et al., "Age at Natural Menopause and Risk of Incident Cardiovascular Disease: A Pooled Analysis of Individual Patient Data," *The Lancet Public Health* 4, no. 11 (November 1, 2019), https://www.thelancet.com/journals/lanpub/article/PIIS2468–2667(19)30155–0/fulltext.

4. T. C. Okele, U. B. Anyaehie, and C. C. Ezenyeaku, "Premature Menopause," *Annals of Medical and Health Sciences Research* 3, no. 1 (January–March 2013), 90–95, https://www.ncbi.nlm.nih.gov/pmc/articles/PMC3634232/.

5. G. D. Mishra, H. F. Chung, A. Cano, P. Chedraui, D. G. Goulis, P. Lopes, A. Mueck, M. Rees, L. M. Senturk, T. Simoncini, J. C. Stevenson, P. Stute, P. Tuomikoski, and I. Lambrinoudaki, "EMAS Position Statement: Predictors

of Premature and Early Natural Menopause," *Maturitas* 123 (May 2019), 82–88, https://pubmed.ncbi.nlm.nih.gov/31027683/.

6. M. A Boughton, "Premature Menopause: Multiple Disruptions Between the Woman's Biological Body Experience and Her Lived Body," *Journal of Advanced Nursing* 37, no. 5 (March 2002), 423–430, https://pubmed.ncbi.nlm.nih.gov/11843980/.

7. K. L. Liao, N. Wood, and G. S. Conway, "Premature Menopause and Psychological Well-being," *Journal of Psychosomatic Obstetrics and Gynaecology* 21, no. 3 (September 2000), 167–174, https://pubmed.ncbi.nlm.nih.gov/11076338/.

8. L. T. Shuster, D. J. Rhodes, B. S. Gostout, B. R. Grossardt, and W. A. Rocca, "Premature Menopause or Early Menopause: Long-term Health Consequences," *Maturitas* 65, no. 2 (February 2010), 161, https://www.ncbi.nlm.nih.gov/pmc/articles/PMC2815011/.

9. The North American Menopause Society, "Effective Treatments for Sexual Problems," http://www.menopause.org/for-women/sexual-health-menopause-online/effective-treatments-for-sexual-problems.

10. S. D. Sullivan, P. M. Sarrel, and L. M. Nelson, "Hormone Replacement Therapy in Young Women with Primary Ovarian Insufficiency and Early Menopause," *Fertility and Sterility* 106, no. 7 (December 1, 2016), https://www.fertstert.org/article/S0015-0282(16)62877-7/fulltext.

11. H. S. Schroder, T. P. Moran, and J. S. Moser, "The Effect of Expressive Writing on the Error-related Negativity Among Individuals with Chronic Worry," *Psychophysiology* 55, no. 2 (February 2018), https://www.ncbi.nlm.nih.gov/pmc/articles/PMC8543488/.

12. E. Kovar, "Music and Exercise: How Music Affects Exercise Motivation," ACE Fitness (December 7, 2015), https://www.acefitness.org/education-and-resources/lifestyle/blog/5763/music-and-exercise-how-music-affects-exercise-motivation/.

13. L. S. Franco, D. F. Shanahan, and R. A. Fuller, "A Review of the Benefits of Nature Experiences: More Than Meets the Eye," *International Journal of Environmental Research and Public Health* 14, no. 8 (August 2017) 864, https://www.ncbi.nlm.nih.gov/pmc/articles/PMC5580568/.

14. R. M. Ryan, N. Weinstein, J. Bernstein, K. W. Broan, L. Mistretta, and M. Gagné, "Vitalizing Effects of Being Outdoors and in Nature," *Journal of Environmental Psychology,* 30, no. 2 (June 2010), 159–168, https://www.sciencedirect.com/science/article/abs/pii/S0272494409000838?via%3Dihub.

Chapter 6: The Sudden Menopause Type

1. A. Garg and L. Robinson, "Surgical Menopause: A Toolkit for Healthcare Professionals," *Post Reproductive Health* 27, no. 4 (December 2021), 222–225, https://pubmed.ncbi.nlm.nih.gov/34761721/.

2. The North American Menopause Society, "MenoNote: Vaginal Dryness," https://www.menopause.org/docs/default-source/for-women/mn-vaginal-dryness.pdf.

3. L. T. Shuster, D. J. Rhodes, B. S. Gostout, B. R. Grossardt, and W. A. Rocca, "Premature Menopause or Early Menopause: Long-term Health Consequences," *Maturitas* 65, no. 2 (February 2010), 161, https://www.ncbi.nlm.nih.gov/pmc/articles/PMC2815011/.

4. The North American Menopause Society, "The 2017 Hormone Therapy Position Statement of the North American Menopause Society," *Menopause* 24, no. 7 (2017), 728–753, https://www.menopause.org/docs/default-source/2017/nams-2017-hormone-therapy-position-statement.pdf.

5. D. Costantino and C. Guaraldi, "Effectiveness and Safety of Vaginal Suppositories for the Treatment of the Vaginal Atrophy in Postmenopausal Women: An Open, Non-controlled Clinical Trial," *European Review for Medical and Pharmacological Sciences* 12, no. 6 (November–December 2008), 411–416, https://pubmed.ncbi.nlm.nih.gov/19146203/.

6. R. Schaffer, "Nonhormonal Therapy Reduces Moderate to Severe Menopausal Hot Flashes," *Healio Endocrinology* (September 28, 2021), https://www.healio.com/news/endocrinology/20210927/nonhormonal-therapy-reduces-moderate-to-severe-menopausal-hot-flashes.

7. J. G. Robinson, N. Ijioma, and W. Harris, "Omega-3 Fatty Acids and Cognitive Function in Women," *Women's Health* 6, no. 1 (January 2010), 119–134, https://www.ncbi.nlm.nih.gov/pmc/articles/PMC2826215/.

8. National Institutes of Health, Office of Dietary Supplements, "Omega-3 Fatty Acids," https://ods.od.nih.gov/factsheets/Omega3FattyAcids-Consumer/.

9. J. B. Nelson, "Mindful Eating: The Art of Presence While You Eat," *Diabetes Spectrum* 30, no. 3 (August 2017), 171–174, https://www.ncbi.nlm.nih.gov/pmc/articles/PMC5556586/.

10. National Institutes of Health, Office of Dietary Supplements, "Probiotics," https://ods.od.nih.gov/factsheets/Probiotics-HealthProfessional/.

11. A. Nortje, "10+ Best Grounding Techniques & Exercises For Your Mindfulness Practice," PositivePsychology.com (July 1, 2020), https://positivepsychology.com/grounding-techniques/.

12. E. Elkjaer, M. B. Mikkelsen, J. Michalak, D. S. Mennin, and M. S. O'Toole, "Expansive and Contractive Postures and Movement: A Systematic Review

and Meta-Analysis of the Effect of Motor Displays on Affective and Behavioral Responses," *Perspectives on Psychological Science* 17, no. 1 (January 1, 2022), 276–304, https://journals.sagepub.com/doi/abs/10.1177/1745691 620919358.

13. J. Fischer, P. Fischer, B. Englich, N. Aydin, and D. Frey, "Empower My decisions: The Effects of Power Gestures on Confirmatory Information Processing," *Journal of Experimental Social Psychology* 47, no. 6 (November 2011), 1146–1154, https://www.sciencedirect.com/science/article/abs/pii /S0022103111001697.

14. M. Miragall, A. Borrego, A. Cebolla, E. Etchemendy, J. Navarro-Siurana, R. Llorens, S. E. Blackwell, and R. M. Baños, "Effect of an Upright (vs. Stooped) Posture on Interpretation Bias, Imagery, and Emotions," *Journal of Behavior Therapy and Experimental Psychiatry* 68 (September 2020), 101560, https://www.sciencedirect.com/science/article/abs/pii/S0005791619301594.

Chapter 7: The Full-Throttle Menopause Type

1. The North American Menopause Society, "Menopause FAQS: Hot Flashes," https://www.menopause.org/for-women/menopause-faqs-hot-flashes.

2. P. Sarrel, D. Portman, P. Lefebvre, M. H. Lafeuille, A. M. Grittner, J. Fortier, J. Gravel, M. S. Duh, and P. M. Aupperle, "Incremental Direct and Indirect Costs of Untreated Vasomotor Symptoms," *Menopause* 22, no. 3 (March 2015), 260–266, https://pubmed.ncbi.nlm.nih.gov/25714236/.

3. The North American Menopause Society, "Chapter 8: Prescription Therapies," http://www.menopause.org/publications/clinical-care-recommendations /chapter-8-prescription-therapies.

4. H. Joffe, K. A. Guthrie, A. Z. LaCroix, S. D. Reed, K. E. Ensrud, J. E. Manson, K. M. Newton, E. W. Freeman, G. L. Anderson, J. C. Larson, J. Hunt, J. Shifren, K. M. Rexrode, B. Caan, B. Sternfeld, J. S. Carpenter, and L. Cohen, "Randomized Controlled Trial of Low-Dose Estradiol and the SNRI Venlafaxine for Vasomotor Symptoms," *JAMA Internal Medicine* 174, no. 7 (July 2014), 1058–1066, https://www.ncbi.nlm.nih.gov/pmc/articles/PMC4179877/.

5. S. Sahni, A. Lobo-Romero, and T. Smith "Contemporary Non-hormonal Therapies for the Management of Vasomotor Symptoms Associated with Menopause: A Literature Review," *touchREVIEWS in Endocrinology* 17, no. 2 (October 13, 2021), 133–137 https://www.touchendocrinology.com /reproductive-endocrinology/journal-articles/contemporary-non-hormonal -therapies-for-the-management-of-vasomotor-symptoms-associated-with -menopause-a-literature-review/.

6. U.S. Food and Drug Administration, "FDA Approves New Treatment for Hypoactive Sexual Desire Disorder in Premenopausal Women," (June 21,

2019), https://www.fda.gov/news-events/press-announcements/fda-approves-new-treatment-hypoactive-sexual-desire-disorder-premenopausal-women.

7. SleepScoreLabs, "Alcohol & Insomnia: How Alcohol Affects Sleep Quality," (July 15, 2017), https://www.sleepscore.com/blog/how-a-nightcap-can-ruin-your-sleep/.

8. L. Li, Y. Lv, L. Xu, and Q. Zheng, "Quantitative Efficacy of Soy Isoflavones on Menopausal Hot Flashes," *Pharmacodynamics* (October 15, 2014) https://bpspubs.onlinelibrary.wiley.com/doi/full/10.1111/bcp.12533.

9. N. Pereira, M. F. Naufel, E. B. Ribeiro, S. Tufik, and H. Hachul, "Influence of Dietary Sources of Melatonin on Sleep Quality: A Review," *Journal of Food Science* (December 19, 2019), https://ift.onlinelibrary.wiley.com/doi/full/10.1111/1750–3841.14952.

10. National Institutes of Health, Office of Dietary Supplements, "Vitamin B6," https://ods.od.nih.gov/factsheets/VitaminB6-HealthProfessional/.

11. National Institutes of Health, Office of Dietary Supplements, "Black Cohosh," https://ods.od.nih.gov/factsheets/BlackCohosh-HealthProfessional/.

12. P. Mirabi and F. Mojab, "The Effects of Valerian Root on Hot Flashes in Menopausal Women," *Iranian Journal of Pharmaceutical Research* 12, no. 1 (Winter 2013), 217–222, https://www.ncbi.nlm.nih.gov/pmc/articles/PMC3813196/.

13. M. Shepherd-Banigan, K. M. Goldstein, R. R. Coeytaux, J. R. McDuffie, A. P. Goode, A. S. Kosinski, M. G. Van Noord, D. Befus, S. Adam, V. Masilamani, A. Nagi, and J. W. Williams, Jr., "Improving Vasomotor Symptoms; Psychological Symptoms; and Health-related Quality of Life in Peri-or Post-menopausal Women Through Yoga: An Umbrella Systematic Review and Meta-analysis," *Complementary Therapies in Medicine* 34 (October 2017), 156–164, https://www.sciencedirect.com/science/article/abs/pii/S0965229917300596.

14. A. Yeung, J. S. M. Chan, J. C. Cheung, and L. Zou, "Qigong and Tai-Chi for Mood Regulation," *Focus: The. Journal of Lifelong Learning in Psychiatry* 16, no. 1 (Winter 2018), 40–47, https://www.ncbi.nlm.nih.gov/pmc/articles/PMC6519567/.

15. P. Payne and M. A. Crane-Godreau, "Meditative Movement for Depression and Anxiety," *Frontiers in Psychiatry* (July 24, 2013), https://www.frontiersin.org/articles/10.3389/fpsyt.2013.00071/full#h5.

16. R. Sood, A. Sood, S. L. Wolf, B. M. Linquist, H. Liu, J. A. Sloan, D. V. Satele, C. L. Loprinzi, and D. L. Barton, "Paced Breathing Compared with Usual Breathing for Hot Flashes," *Menopause* 20, no. 2 (February 2013), 179–184, https://pubmed.ncbi.nlm.nih.gov/22990758/.

17. University of California, Berkeley, "Breathing Exercises," https://uhs.berkeley.edu/sites/default/files/breathing_exercises_0.pdf.

18. U.S. Pain Foundation, "How Flow State and the Nervous System Interact," (July 28, 2021), https://uspainfoundation.org/news/how-flow-state-and-the -nervous-system-interact/.

19. M. C. Garcia, E. J. Kozasa, S. Tufik, L. E. A. M. Mello, and H. Hachul, "The Effects of Mindfulness and Relaxation Training for Insomnia (MRTI) on Postmenopausal Women: A Pilot Study," *Menopause* 25, no. 9 (September 2018), 992–1003, https://pubmed.ncbi.nlm.nih.gov/29787483/.

20. F. Polat, I. Orhan, and D. Ş. Küçükkelepçe, "Does Social Support Affect Menopausal Symptoms in Menopausal Women?" *Perspectives in Psychiatric Care* (July 2, 2021), https://pubmed.ncbi.nlm.nih.gov/34212380/.

21. Z. Jalambadani, Z. Rezapour, and S. M. Zadeh, "Investigating the Relationship between Menopause Specific Quality of Life and Perceived Social Support among Postmenopausal Women in Iran," *Experimental Aging Research* 46, no. 4 (July–September 2020), 359–366, https://pubmed.ncbi .nlm.nih.gov/32496973/.

22. J. L. Otte, J. S. Carpenter, L. Roberts, and G. R. Elkins, "Self-Hypnosis for Sleep Disturbances in Menopausal Women," *Journal of Women's Health* 29, no. 3 (March 2020), 461–463, https://www.ncbi.nlm.nih.gov/pmc/articles /PMC7097677/.

23. R. L. Roberts, J. R. Rhodes, and G. R. Elkins, "Effect of Hypnosis on Anxiety: Results from a Randomized Controlled Trial with Women in Postmenopause," *Journal of Clinical Psychology in Medical Settings* 28, no. 4 (December 2021), 868–881, https://pubmed.ncbi.nlm.nih.gov /34403019/.

24. D. L. Barton, K. C. F. Schroeder, T. Banerjee, S. Wolf, T. Z. Keith, and G. Elkins, "Efficacy of a Biobehavioral Intervention for Hot Flashes: A Randomized Controlled Pilot Study," *Menopause* 24, no. 7 (July 2017), 774–782, https://www.ncbi.nlm.nih.gov/pmc/articles/PMC5747247/.

25. Lisa Health, "Manage Your Menopause Mood Swings with the CTFO Technique," https://blog.lisahealth.com/blog/2020/1/24/ctfo.

26. H. Meyers, "Why Is My Dog Shaking? Causes & Solutions," American Kennel Club (April 18, 2022), https://www.akc.org/expert-advice/health /why-do-dogs-shake/.

Chapter 8: The Mind-Altering Menopause Type

1. C. N. Epperson, B. Pittman, K. A. Czarkowski, J. Bradley, D. M. Quinlan, and T. E. Brown, "Impact of Atomoxetine on Subjective Attention and Memory Difficulties in Perimenopausal and Postmenopausal Women," *Menopause* 18, no. 5 (May 2011), 542–548, https://www.ncbi.nlm.nih.gov /pmc/articles/PMC4076798/.

2. P. M. Maki and V. W. Henderson, "Cognition and the Menopause Transition," *Menopause* 23, no. 7 (July 2016), 803–805, https://pubmed.ncbi.nlm.nih.gov/27272226/.

3. P. M. Maki, G. Springer, K. Anastos, D. R. Gustafson, K. Weber, D. Vance, D. Dykxhoorn, J. Milam, A. A. Adimora, S. G. Kassaye, D. Waldrop, and L. H. Rubin, "Cognitive Changes During the Menopausal Transition: A Longitudinal Study in Women with and without HIV," *Menopause* 28, no. 4 (April 2021), 360–368, https://journals.lww.com/menopausejournal/Citation/2021/04000/Cognitive_changes_during_the_menopausal.5.aspx.

4. S. Mulhall, R. Andel, and K. J. Anstey, "Variation in Symptoms of Depression and Anxiety in Midlife Women by Menopausal Status," *Maturitas* 108 (February 2018), 7–12, https://pubmed.ncbi.nlm.nih.gov/29290217/.

5. B. A. Wariso, G. M. Guerrieri, K. Thompson, D. E. Koziol, N. Haq, P. E. Martinez, D. R. Rubinow, and P. J. Schmidt, "Depression During the Menopause Transition: Impact on Quality of Life, Social Adjustment, and Disability," *Archives of Women's Mental Health* 20, no. 2 (April 2017), 273–282, https://www.ncbi.nlm.nih.gov/pmc/articles/PMC6309889/.

6. J. T. Bromberger, Y. Chang, A. B. Colvin, H. M. Kravitz, and K. A. Matthews, "Does Childhood Maltreatment or Current Stress Contribute to Increased Risk for Major Depression During the Menopause Transition?" *Psychological Medicine* (December 10, 2020), 1–8, https://pubmed.ncbi.nlm.nih.gov/33298219/.

7. A. Colvin, G. A. Richardson, J. M. Cyranowski, A. Youk, and J. T. Bromberger, "The Role of Family History of Depression and the Menopausal Transition in the Development of Major Depression in Midlife Women: Study of Women's Health Across the Nation Mental Health Study (SWAN MHS)," *Depression & Anxiety* 34, no. 9 (September 2017), 826–835, https://www.ncbi.nlm.nih.gov/pmc/articles/PMC5585035/.

8. H. J. Jones, P. A. Minarik, C. L. Gilliss, and K. A. Lee, "Depressive Symptoms Associated with Physical Health Problems in Midlife Women: A Longitudinal Study," *Journal of Affective Disorders* 263 (February 15, 2020), 301–309, https://www.ncbi.nlm.nih.gov/pmc/articles/PMC6989369/.

9. S. J. Jung, A. Shin, and D. Kang, "Hormone-related Factors and Postmenopausal Onset Depression: Results from KNHANES (2010–2012)," *Journal of Affective Disorders* 175 (April 1, 2015), 176–183, https://www.sciencedirect.com/science/article/pii/S0165032715000038.

10. A. K. Shea, N. Sohel, A. Gilsing, A. J. Mayhew, L. E. Griffith, and P. Raina, "Depression, Hormone Therapy, and the Menopausal Transition Among Women Aged 45 to 64 Years Using Canadian Longitudinal Study on Aging Baseline Data," *Menopause* 27, no. 7 (July 2020), 763–770, https://pubmed.ncbi.nlm.nih.gov/32217892/.

11. D. A. Kalmbach, P. Cheng, J. T. Arnedt, J. R. Anderson, T. Roth, C. Fellman-Couture, R. A. Williams, and C. L. Drake, "Treating Insomnia Improves Depression, Maladaptive Thinking, and Hyperarousal in Post-menopausal Women: Comparing Cognitive-Behavioral Therapy for Insomnia (CBTI), Sleep Restriction Therapy, and Sleep Hygiene Education," *Sleep Medicine* 55 (March 2019), 124–134, https://www.ncbi.nlm.nih.gov/pmc/articles/PMC6503531/.

12. N. G. Jaff and P. M. Maki, "Scientific Insights into Brain Fog During the Menopausal Transition," *Climacteric* 24, no. 4 (2021), 317–318, https://www.tandfonline.com/doi/full/10.1080/13697137.2021.1942700.

13. M. C. Craig, P. M. Maki, and D. G. M. Murphy, "The Women's Health Initiative Memory Study: Findings and Implications for Treatment," *The Lancet Neurology* 493 (March 2005), 190–194, https://pubmed.ncbi.nlm.nih.gov/15721829/.

14. Q. Yu, C. X. Yin, Y. Hui, J. Yu, F. F. He, J. Wei, and Y. Y. Wu, "Comparison of the Effect of Fluoxetine Combined with Hormone Replacement Therapy (HRT) and Single HRT in Treating Menopausal Depression," *Zhonghua Fu Chan Ke Za Zhi* 39, no. 7 (July 2004), 461–464, https://pubmed.ncbi.nlm.nih.gov/15347469/.

15. M. L. Morgan, I. A. Cook, A. J. Rapkin, and A. F. Leuchter, "Estrogen Augmentation of Antidepressants in Perimenopausal Depression: A Pilot Study," *Journal of Clinical Psychiatry,* 66, no. 6 (June 2005), 774–780, https://pubmed.ncbi.nlm.nih.gov/15960574/.

16. B. Mangweth-Matzek, H. W. Hoek, C. I. Rupp, G. Kemmler, H. G. Pope, and J. Kinzl, "The Menopausal Transition—A Possible Window of Vulnerability for Eating Pathology," *International Journal of Eating Disorders* 46, no. 6 (September 2013), 609–616, https://pubmed.ncbi.nlm.nih.gov/23847142/.

17. B. Mangweth-Matzek, C. I. Rupp, S. Vedova, V. Dunst, P. Hennecke, M. Daniaux, and H. G. Pope, "Disorders of Eating and Body Image During the Menopausal Transition: Associations with Menopausal Stage and with Menopausal Symptomatology," *Eating and Weight Disorders* 26, no. 8 (December 2021), 2763–2769, https://pubmed.ncbi.nlm.nih.gov/33595812/.

18. K. A. Thompson and A. M. Bardone-Cone, "Evaluating Attitudes About Aging and Body Comparison as Moderators of the Relationship Between Menopausal Status and Disordered Eating and Body Image Concerns Among Middle-aged Women," *Maturitas* 124 (June 2019), 25–31, https://pubmed.ncbi.nlm.nih.gov/31097174/.

19. M. D. Marcus, J. T. Bromberger, H. L. Wei, C. Brown, and H. M. Kravitz, "Prevalence and Selected Correlates of Eating Disorder Symptoms Among a Multiethnic Community Sample of Midlife Women," *Annals of Behavioral*

Medicine 33, no. 3 (June 2007), 269–277, https://pubmed.ncbi.nlm.nih.gov /17600454/.

20. K. L. Samuels, M. M. Maine, and M. Tantillo, "Disordered Eating, Eating Disorders, and Body Image in Midlife and Older Women," *Current Psychiatry Reports* 21, no. 8 (July 1, 2019), 70, https://pubmed.ncbi.nlm.nih.gov /31264039/.

21. J. G. Robinson, N. Ijioma, and W. Harris, "Omega-3 Fatty Acids and Cognitive Function in Women," *Women's Health* 6, no. 1 (January 2010), 119–134, https://www.ncbi.nlm.nih.gov/pmc/articles/PMC2826215/.

22. M. Chae and K. Park, "Association Between Dietary Omega-3 Fatty Acid Intake and Depression in Postmenopausal Women," *Nutrition Research and Practice* 15, no. 4 (August 2021), 468–478, https://www.ncbi.nlm.nih.gov /pmc/articles/PMC8313386/.

23. National Institutes of Health, Office of Dietary Supplements, "Choline," https://ods.od.nih.gov/factsheets/Choline-HealthProfessional/.

24. A. Yagi, R. Nouchi, L. Butler, and R. Kawashima, "Lutein Has a Positive Impact on Brain Health in Healthy Older Adults: A Systematic Review of Randomized Controlled Trials and Cohort Studies," *Nutrients* 13 (2021), 1746. https://mdpi-res.com/d_attachment/nutrients/nutrients-13–01746 /article_deploy/nutrients-13–01746.pdf.

25. E. M. Paolucci, D. Loukov, D. W. E. Bowdish, and J. J. Heisz, "Exercise Reduces Depression and Inflammation but Intensity Matters," *Biological Psychology* 133 (March 2018), 79–84, https://pubmed.ncbi.nlm.nih.gov/29408464/.

26. S. Gujral, H. Aizenstein, C. F. Reynolds, III, M. A. Butters, and K. I. Erickson, "Exercise Effects on Depression: Possible Neural Mechanisms" *General Hospital Psychiatry* 49 (November 2017), 2–10, https://www.ncbi.nlm.nih .gov/pmc/articles/PMC6437683/.

27. B. M. Hoffman, M. A. Babyak, W. E. Craighead, A. Sherwood, P. M. Doraiswamy, M. J. Coons, and J. A. Blumenthal, "Exercise and Pharmacotherapy in Patients With Major Depression: One-Year Follow-Up of the SMILE Study," *Psychosomatic Medicine* 73, no. 2 (February–March 2011), 127–133, https://www.ncbi.nlm.nih.gov/pmc/articles/PMC3671874/.

28. M. Dąbrowska-Galas and J. Dąbrowska, "Physical Activity Level and Self-Esteem in Middle-Aged Women," *International Journal of Environmental Research and Public Health* 18, no. 14 (July 2021), https://www.ncbi.nlm .nih.gov/pmc/articles/PMC8305857/.

29. L. Mandolesi, A. Polverino, S. Montuori, F. Foti, G. Ferraioli, P. Sorrentino, and G. Sorrentino, "Effects of Physical Exercise on Cognitive Functioning and Wellbeing: Biological and Psychological Benefits," *Frontiers in Psychology* 9 (2018), 509, https://www.ncbi.nlm.nih.gov/pmc/articles /PMC5934999/.

30. D. Anderson, C. Seib, and L. Rasmussen, "Can Physical Activity Prevent Physical and Cognitive Decline in Postmenopausal Women? A Systematic Review of the Literature," *Maturitas* 79, no. 1 (September 2014), 14–33, https://pubmed.ncbi.nlm.nih.gov/25008420/.

31. F. B. Schuch, S .S. Pinto, N. C. Bagatine, P. Zaffari, C. L. Alberton, E. L. Cadore, R. F. Silva, and L. F. M. Kruel, "Water-based Exercise and Quality of Life in Women: The Role of Depressive Symptoms," *Women & Health* 54, no. 2 (2014), 161–175, https://pubmed.ncbi.nlm.nih.gov/24329155/.

32. P. Abedi, P. Nikkhah, and S. Najar, "Effect of Pedometer-based Walking on Depression, Anxiety, and Insomnia Among Postmenopausal Women," *Climacteric* 18, no. 6 (2015), 841–845, https://pubmed.ncbi.nlm.nih.gov/26100101/.

33. A. Aibar-Almazán, F. Hita-Contreras, D. Cruz-Díaz, M. de la Torre-Cruz, J. D. Jiménez-García, and A. Martínez-Amat, "Effects of Pilates Training on Sleep Quality, Anxiety, Depression and Fatigue in Postmenopausal Women: A Randomized Controlled Trial," *Maturitas* 124 (June 2019), 62–67, https://pubmed.ncbi.nlm.nih.gov/31097181/.

34. M. P. Jorge, D. F. Santaella, I. M. O. Pontes, V. K. M. Shiramizu, E. B. Nascimento, A. Cabral, T. M. A. M. Lemos, R. H. Silva, and A. M. Ribeiro, "Hatha Yoga Practice Decreases Menopause Symptoms and Improves Quality of Life: A Randomized Controlled Trial," *Complementary Therapies in Medicine* 26 (June 2016), 128–135, https://pubmed.ncbi.nlm.nih.gov/27261993/.

35. C. Wong, B. H. K. Yip, T. Gao, K. Y. U. Lam, D. M. S. Woo, A. L. K. Yip, C. Y. Chin, W. P. Y. Tang, M. M. T. Choy, K. W. K. Tsang, S. C. Ho, H. S. W. Ma, and S. Y. S. Wong, "Mindfulness-Based Stress Reduction (MBSR) or Psychoeducation for the Reduction of Menopausal Symptoms: A Randomized, Controlled Clinical Trial," *Scientific Reports* 8 (2018), https://www.ncbi.nlm.nih.gov/pmc/articles/PMC5919973/.

36. C. Schwert, S. Aschenbrenner, M. Weisbrod, and A. Schröder, "Cognitive Impairments in Unipolar Depression: The Impact of Rumination," *Psychopathology* 50, no. 5 (2017), 347–354. https://pubmed.ncbi.nlm.nih.gov/28850956/.

37. D. Y. Koçak and Y. Varişoğlu, "The Effect of Music Therapy on Menopausal Symptoms and Depression: A Randomized-controlled Study," *Menopause,* 29, no. 5 (May 2022), 545–552, https://journals.lww.com/menopausejournal/Abstract/9000/The_effect_of_music_therapy_on_menopausal_symptoms.96827.aspx.

38. E. Morita, S. Fukuda, J. Nagano, N. Hamajima, H. Yamamoto, Y. Iwai, T. Nakashima, H. Ohira, and T. Shirakawa, "Psychological Effects of Forest Environments on Healthy Adults: Shinrin-yoku (Forest-air Bathing, Walking) as a Possible Method of Stress Reduction," *Public Health* 121, no. 1 (January 2007), 54–63, https://pubmed.ncbi.nlm.nih.gov/17055544/.

39. M. Konishi, B. Berberian, V. de Gardelle, and J. Sackur, "Multitasking Costs on Metacognition in a Triple-task Paradigm," *Psychonomic Bulletin & Review* 28, no. 6 (December 2021), 2075–2084, https://pubmed.ncbi.nlm.nih.gov/34173189/.

40. D. Bach, G. Groesbeck, P. Stapleton, R. Sims, K. Blickheuser, and D. Church, "Clinical EFT (Emotional Freedom Techniques) Improves Multiple Physiological Markers of Health," *Journal of Evidence-Based Integrative Medicine,* 24 (2019), https://www.ncbi.nlm.nih.gov/pmc/articles/PMC6381429/.

41. L. Mosconi, V. Berti, J. Dyke, E. Schelbaum, S. Jett, L. Loughlin, G. Jang, A. Rahman, H. Hristov, S. Pahlajani, R. Andrews, D. Matthews, O. Etingin, C. Ganzer, M. de Leon, R. Isaacson, and R. D. Brinton, "Menopause Impacts Human Brain Structure, Connectivity, Energy Metabolism, and Amyloid-beta Deposition," *Scientific Reports* 11 (2021), https://www.nature.com/articles/s41598-021-90084-y.

42. G. A. Greendale, M. H. Huang, R. G. Wight, T. Seeman, C. Luetters, N. E. Avis, J. Johnston, and A. S. Karlamangla, "Effects of the Menopause Transition and Hormone Use on Cognitive Performance in Midlife Women," *Neurology* 72, no. 21 (May 26, 2009), 1850–1857, https://www.ncbi.nlm.nih.gov/pmc/articles/PMC2690984/.

Chapter 9: The Seemingly Never-Ending Menopause Type

1. M. DiBonaventura, X. Luo, M. Moffatt, A. G. Bushmakin, M. Kumar, and J. Bobula, "The Association Between Vulvovaginal Atrophy Symptoms and Quality of Life Among Postmenopausal Women in the United States and Western Europe," *Journal of Women's Health* 24, no. 9 (September 2015), 713–722, https://pubmed.ncbi.nlm.nih.gov/26199981/.

2. E. Moyneur, K. Dea, L. R. Derogati, F. Vekeman, A. Y. Dury, and F. Labrie, "Prevalence of Depression and Anxiety in Women Newly Diagnosed with Vulvovaginal Atrophy and Dyspareunia," *Menopause* 27, no. 2 (February 2020), 134–142, https://pubmed.ncbi.nlm.nih.gov/31688416/.

3. C. E. Kline, A. B. Colvin, K. P. Gabriel, C. A. Karvonen-Gutierrez, J. A. Cauley, M. H. Hall, K. A. Matthews, K. M. Ruppert, G. S. Neal-Perry, E. S. Strotmeyer, and B. Sternfeld, "Associations Between Longitudinal Trajectories of Insomnia Symptoms and Sleep Duration with Objective Physical Function in Postmenopausal Women: The Study of Women's Health Across the Nation," *Sleep* 44, no. 8 (August 2021), https://www.ncbi.nlm.nih.gov/pmc/articles/PMC8361301/.

4. M. A. Grandner, S. Nowakowski, J. D. Kloss, and M. L. Perlis, "Insomnia Symptoms Predict Physical and Mental Impairments Among Postmeno-

pausal Women," *Sleep Medicine* 16, no. 3 (March 2015), 317–318, https://www.ncbi.nlm.nih.gov/pmc/articles/PMC4375439/.

5. N. Mili, S. A. Paschou, A. Armeni, N. Georgopoulos, D. G Goulis, and I. Lambrinoudaki, "Genitourinary Syndrome of Menopause: A Systematic Review on Prevalence and Treatment," *Menopause* 28, no. 6 (March 15, 2021), 706–716, https://pubmed.ncbi.nlm.nih.gov/33739315/.

6. I. Pérez-Herrezuelo, A. Aibar-Almazán, A. Martínez-Amat, R. Fábrega-Cuadros, E. Díaz-Mohedo, R. Wangensteen, and F. Hita-Contreras, "Female Sexual Function and Its Association with the Severity of Menopause-Related Symptoms," *International Journal of Environmental Research and Public Health* 17, no. 19 (October 2020), 7235, https://www.ncbi.nlm.nih.gov/pmc/articles/PMC7579461/.

7. N. E. Avis, S. L. Crawford, G. Greendale, J. T. Bromberger, S. A. Everson-Rose, E. B. Gold, R. Hess, H. Joffe, H. M. Kravitz, P. G. Tepper, R. C. Thurston, "Duration of Menopausal Vasomotor Symptoms Over the Menopause Transition," *JAMA Internal Medicine,* 175, no. 4 (April 1, 2015), 531–539, https://www.ncbi.nlm.nih.gov/pmc/articles/PMC4433164/.

8. N. F. Woods, E. S. Mitchell, D. B. Percival, and K. Smith-DiJulio, "Is the Menopausal Transition Stressful? Observations of Perceived Stress from the Seattle Midlife Women's Health Study," *Menopause* 16, no. 1 (January–February 2009), https://www.ncbi.nlm.nih.gov/pmc/articles/PMC3842691/.

9. G. Kołodyńska, M. Zalewski, and K. Rożek-Piechura, "Urinary Incontinence in Postmenopausal Women—Causes, Symptoms, Treatment," *Przegląd Menopauzalny* 18, no. 1 (April 2019), 46–50, https://www.ncbi.nlm.nih.gov/pmc/articles/PMC6528037/.

10. E. Shih, H. Hirsch, and H. L. Thacker, "Medical Management of Urinary Incontinence in Women," *Cleveland Clinic Journal of Medicine* 84, no. 2 (February 2017), 151–158, https://www.ccjm.org/content/84/2/151.long.

11. The North American Menopause Society, "Urinary Incontinence," https://www.menopause.org/for-women/sexual-health-menopause-online/causes-of-sexual-problems/urinary-incontinence.

12. S. J. Parish and S. R. Hahn, "Hypoactive Sexual Desire Disorder: A Review of Epidemiology, Biopsychology, Diagnosis, and Treatment," *Sexual Medicine Reviews* 4, no. 2 (April 2016), 103–120, https://pubmed.ncbi.nlm.nih.gov/27872021/.

13. A. Greenstein, L. Abramov, H. Matzkin, and J. Chen, "Sexual Dysfunction in Women Partners of Men with Erectile Dysfunction," *International Journal of Impotence Research* 18 (2006), 44–46, https://www.nature.com/articles/3901367.

14. The North American Menopause Society, "Vaginal Dryness," https://www.menopause.org/docs/default-source/for-women/mn-vaginal-dryness.pdf.

15. Mayo Clinic, "Kegel Exercises: A How-to Guide for Women," https://www.mayoclinic.org/healthy-lifestyle/womens-health/in-depth/kegel-exercises/art-20045283.

16. The North American Menopause Society, "The North American Menopause Society Statement on Continuing Use of Systemic Hormone Therapy After Age 65," http://www.menopause.org/docs/default-source/2015/2015-nams-hormone-therapy-after-age-65.pdf.

17. C. L. Drake, D. A. Kalmbach, J. T. Arnedt, P. Cheng, C. V. Tonnu, A. Cuamatzi-Castelan, and C. Fellman-Couture, "Treating Chronic Insomnia in Postmenopausal Women: A Randomized Clinical Trial Comparing Cognitive-behavioral Therapy for Insomnia, Sleep Restriction Therapy, and Sleep Hygiene Education," *Sleep* 42, no. 2 (February 2019), https://academic.oup.com/sleep/article/42/2/zsy217/5179856.

18. S. Sahni, A. Lobo-Romero, and T. Smith, "Contemporary Non-hormonal Therapies for the Management of Vasomotor Symptoms Associated with Menopause: A Literature Review," *touchREVIEWS in Endocrinology* 17, no. 2, 133–137, https://www.touchendocrinology.com/reproductive-endocrinology/journal-articles/contemporary-non-hormonal-therapies-for-the-management-of-vasomotor-symptoms-associated-with-menopause-a-literature-review/.

19. M. C. Pingarrón Santofimia, S. P. González Rodríguez, M. Lilue, and S. Palacios, "Experience with Ospemifene in Patients with Vulvar and Vaginal Atrophy: Case Studies with Bone Marker Profiles," *Drugs in Context* 9 (2020), https://www.ncbi.nlm.nih.gov/pmc/articles/PMC7337603/.

20. National Institutes of Health, Office of Dietary Supplements, "Vitamin B6," https://ods.od.nih.gov/factsheets/VitaminB6-HealthProfessional/.

21. N. Pereira, M. F. Naufel, E. B. Ribeiro, S. Tufik, and H. Hachul, "Influence of Dietary Sources of Melatonin on Sleep Quality: A Review," *Journal of Food Science* 85, no. 1 (January 2020), 5–13, https://ift.onlinelibrary.wiley.com/doi/full/10.1111/1750–3841.14952.

22. National Institutes of Health, Office of Dietary Supplements, "Black Cohosh," https://ods.od.nih.gov/factsheets/BlackCohosh-HealthProfessional/.

23. F. Halis, P. Yildirim, R. Kocaaslan, K. Cecen, and A. Gokce, "Pilates for Better Sex: Changes in Sexual Functioning in Healthy Turkish Women After Pilates Exercise," *Journal of Sex & Marital Therapy* 42, no. 4 (May 18, 2016), 302–308, https://pubmed.ncbi.nlm.nih.gov/25826474/.

24. L. Brown, C. Bryant, V. Brown, B. Bei, and F. Judd, "Investigating how Menopausal Factors and Self-compassion Shape Well-being: An Exploratory Path Analysis," *Maturitas* 81, no. 2 (June 2015), 293–299, https://pubmed.ncbi.nlm.nih.gov/25818770/.

25. A. A. Motzer and V. Hertig, "Stress, Stress Response, and Health," *The Nursing Clinics of North America* 39, no. 1 (March 2004), 1–17, https://pubmed.ncbi.nlm.nih.gov/15062724/.

26. American Physiological Society, "Anticipating A Laugh Reduces Our Stress Hormones, Study Shows," (April 10, 2008), https://www.sciencedaily.com/releases/2008/04/080407114617.htm.

27. J. Berg, "The Stress of Caregiving," *The North American Menopause Society: The Female Patient* 36 (July 2011), 33–36, http://www.menopause.org/docs/default-document-library/careberg.pdf?sfvrsn=2.

Chapter 10: The Silent Menopause Type

1. Cleveland Clinic, "Postmenopause," https://my.clevelandclinic.org/health/diseases/21837-postmenopause.

2. H. Currie and C. Williams, "Menopause, Cholesterol and Cardiovascular Disease," *US Cardiology* 5, no. 1 (2008), 12–14, https://www.uscjournal.com/articles/menopause-cholesterol-and-cardiovascular-disease-0.

3. S. Swarup, A. Goyal, Y. Grigorova, and R. Zeltser, "Metabolic Syndrome," *StatPearls,* https://www.ncbi.nlm.nih.gov/books/NBK459248/.

4. Mayo Clinic, "Metabolic Syndrome," https://www.mayoclinic.org/diseases-conditions/metabolic-syndrome/diagnosis-treatment/drc-20351921.

5. Centers for Disease Control and Prevention, "Diabetes Tests," https://www.cdc.gov/diabetes/basics/getting-tested.html.

6. Centers for Disease Control and Prevention, "Prediabetes—Your Chance to Prevent Type 2 Diabetes," https://www.cdc.gov/diabetes/basics/prediabetes.html.

7. M. Varacallo, T. J. Seaman, J. S. Jandu, and P. Pizzutillo, "Osteopenia," *StatPearls,* https://www.ncbi.nlm.nih.gov/books/NBK499878/.

8. B. A. Edwards, D. M. O'Driscoll, A. Ali, A. S. Jordan, J. Trinder, and A. Malhotra, "Aging and Sleep: Physiology and Pathophysiology," *Seminars in Respiratory and Critical Care Medicine* 31, no. 5 (October 2010), 618–633, https://www.ncbi.nlm.nih.gov/pmc/articles/PMC3500384/.

9. B. Miner and M. H. Kryger, "Sleep in the Aging Population," *Sleep Medicine Clinics* 15, no. 2 (June 2020), 311–318, https://pubmed.ncbi.nlm.nih.gov/32386704/.

10. S. Zolfaghari, C. Yao, C. Thompson, N. Gosselin, A. Desautels, T. T. Dang-Vu, R. B. Postuma, and J. Carrier, "Effects of Menopause on Sleep Quality and Sleep Disorders: Canadian Longitudinal Study on Aging," *Menopause* 27, no. 3 (March 2020), 295–304, https://pubmed.ncbi.nlm.nih.gov/31851117/.

11. MedlinePlus, "Obstructive Sleep Apnea," https://medlineplus.gov/genetics/condition/obstructive-sleep-apnea/.

12. M. V. Seeman, "Why Are Women Prone to Restless Legs Syndrome?" *International Journal of Environmental Research and Public Health* 17, no. 1 (January 2020), 368, https://www.ncbi.nlm.nih.gov/pmc/articles/PMC6981604/.

13. Cleveland Clinic, "Restless Legs Syndrome," https://my.clevelandclinic.org/health/diseases/9497-restless-legs-syndrome.

14. S. Romero-Peralta, I. Cano-Pumarega, C. Garcia-Malo, L. A. Ramos, and D. García-Borreguero, "Treating Restless Legs Syndrome in the Context of Sleep Disordered Breathing Comorbidity," *European Respiratory Review* 28 (2019), https://err.ersjournals.com/content/28/153/190061.

15. Cleveland Clinic Health Essentials, "Statins Giving You Achy Muscles? Ask Your Doctor About These 4 Potential Fixes," https://health.clevelandclinic.org/statins-giving-you-achy-muscles-ask-your-doctor-about-these-4-potential-fixes/.

16. H. Qu, M. Guo, H. Chai, W. T. Wang, Z-y. Gao, and D. Z. Shi, "Effects of Coenzyme Q10 on Statin-Induced Myopathy: An Updated Meta-Analysis of Randomized Controlled Trials," *Journal of the American Heart Association* 7, no. 19 (September 25, 2018), https://www.ahajournals.org/doi/10.1161/JAHA.118.009835.

17. P. Ockermann, L. Headley, R. Lizio, and J. Hansmann, "A Review of the Properties of Anthocyanins and Their Influence on Factors Affecting Cardiometabolic and Cognitive Health," *Nutrients* 13, no. 8 (August 2021), 2831, https://www.ncbi.nlm.nih.gov/pmc/articles/PMC8399873/.

18. N. G. Hord, Y. Tang, and N. S. Bryan, "Food Sources of Nitrates and Nitrites: The Physiologic Context for Potential Health Benefits," *The American Journal of Clinical Nutrition* 90, no. 1 (July 2009), 1–10, https://academic.oup.com/ajcn/article/90/1/1/4596750.

19. Mayo Clinic, "Nutrition and Healthy Eating: 3 Diet Changes Women Over 50 Should Make Right Now," https://www.mayoclinic.org/healthy-lifestyle/nutrition-and-healthy-eating/in-depth/3-diet-changes-women-over-50-should-make-right-now/art-20457589.

20. National Institutes of Health, Office of Dietary Supplements, "Calcium," https://ods.od.nih.gov/factsheets/Calcium-HealthProfessional/.

21. National Institutes of Health, Office of Dietary Supplements, "Vitamin D," https://ods.od.nih.gov/factsheets/VitaminD-HealthProfessional/.

22. National Institutes of Health, Office of Dietary Supplements, "Vitamin K," https://ods.od.nih.gov/factsheets/vitaminK-HealthProfessional/.

23. National Institutes of Health, Office of Dietary Supplements, "Vitamin C," https://ods.od.nih.gov/factsheets/VitaminC-HealthProfessional/.

24. J. B. Nelson, "Mindful Eating: The Art of Presence While You Eat," *Diabetes Spectrum* 30, no. 3 (August 2017), 171–174, https://www.ncbi.nlm.nih.gov /pmc/articles/PMC5556586/.

25. S. Musich, S. S. Wang, S. Kraemer, K. Hawkins, and E. Wicker, "Purpose in Life and Positive Health Outcomes Among Older Adults," *Population Health Management* 21, no. 2 (April 1, 2018), 139–147, https://www.ncbi .nlm.nih.gov/pmc/articles/PMC5906725/.

26. Greater Good in Action, "Body Scan Meditation," https://ggia.berkeley.edu /practice/body_scan_meditation.

27. Mayo Clinic Health System, "5, 4, 3, 2, 1: Countdown to Make Anxi- ety Blast Off," (June 6, 2020), https://www.mayoclinichealthsystem.org /hometown-health/speaking-of-health/5–4–3–2–1-countdown-to-make -anxiety-blast-off.

28. N. Morrow-Howell, J. Hinterlong, P. A. Rozario, and F. Tang, "Effects of Volunteering on the Well-being of Older Adults," *The Journals of Gerontol- ogy. Series B, Psychological Sciences and Social Sciences* 58, no. 3 (May 2003), S137–145, https://pubmed.ncbi.nlm.nih.gov/12730314/.

29. M. Huo, L. M. S. Miller, K. Kim, and S. Liu, "Volunteering, Self- Perceptions of Aging, and Mental Health in Later Life," *Gerontologist* 61, no. 7 (September 13, 2021), 1131–1140, https://pubmed.ncbi.nlm.nih.gov /33103726/.

Chapter 11: Prioritizing Relief and Your Safety

1. R. Leproult and E. Van Cauter, "Role of Sleep and Sleep Loss in Hormonal Release and Metabolism," *Endocrine Development* 17 (2010), 11–21, https: //www.ncbi.nlm.nih.gov/pmc/articles/PMC3065172/.

2. Women's Health Network, "Talking to Your Doctor About Hormone Therapy," https://www.womenshealthnetwork.com/hrt/hormone-therapy -talking-to-your-doctor/.

Chapter 12: Personalizing Your Treatment Plan

1. N. Khunger and K. Mehrotra, "Menopausal Acne—Challenges And Solu- tions," *International Journal of Women's Health* 11 (2019), 555–567, https: //www.ncbi.nlm.nih.gov/pmc/articles/PMC6825478/.

2. E. Aylett, N. Small, and P. Bower, "Exercise in the Treatment of Clinical Anxiety in General Practice—A Systematic Review and Meta-analysis," *BMC Health Services Research* 18 (2018), 559, https://www.ncbi.nlm.nih.gov /pmc/articles/PMC6048763/.

3. N. M. Simon, S. G. Hofmann, D. Rosenfield, S. S. Hoeppner, E. A. Hoge, E. Bui, and S. B. S. Khalsa, "Efficacy of Yoga vs Cognitive Behavioral Therapy vs Stress Education for the Treatment of Generalized Anxiety Disorder: A Randomized Clinical Trial," *JAMA Psychiatry* 78, no. 1 (January 1, 2021), 13–20, https://pubmed.ncbi.nlm.nih.gov/32805013/.

4. A. Aibar-Almazán, F. Hita-Contreras, D. Cruz-Díaz, M. de la Torre-Cruz, J. D. Jiménez-García, and A. Martínez-Amat, "Effects of Pilates Training on Sleep Quality, Anxiety, Depression, and Fatigue in Postmenopausal Women: A Randomized Controlled Trial," *Maturitas* 124 (June 2019), 62–67, https://pubmed.ncbi.nlm.nih.gov/31097181/.

5. M. Gong, H. Dong, Y. Tang, W. Huang, and F. Lu, "Effects of Aromatherapy on Anxiety: A Meta-analysis of Randomized Controlled Trials," *Journal of Affective Disorders* 274 (September 1, 2020), 1028–1040, https://www.sciencedirect.com/science/article/abs/pii/S016503271933160X.

6. B. Mahdood, B. Imani, and S. Khazaei, "Effects of Inhalation Aromatherapy With Rosa damascena (Damask Rose) on the State Anxiety and Sleep Quality of Operating Room Personnel During the COVID-19 Pandemic: A Randomized Controlled Trial," *Journal of PeriAnesthesia Nursing* (October 29, 2021), https://www.ncbi.nlm.nih.gov/pmc/articles/PMC8554138/.

7. F. Barati, A. Nasiri, N. Akbari, and G. Sharifzadeh, "The Effect of Aromatherapy on Anxiety in Patients," *Nephro-Urology Monthly* 8, no. 5 (September 2016), https://www.ncbi.nlm.nih.gov/pmc/articles/PMC5111093/.

8. V. L. Katz, L. Rozas, R. Ryder, and R. C. Cefalo, "Effect of Daily Immersion on the Edema of Pregnancy," *American Journal of Perinatalogy* 9, no. 4 (July 1992), 225–227, https://pubmed.ncbi.nlm.nih.gov/1627208/.

9. C. Gurvich, C. Zhu, and S. Arunogiri, "'Brain Fog' During Menopause is Real—It Can Disrupt Women's Work and Spark Dementia Fears," *The Conversation* (December 13, 2021), https://theconversation.com/brain-fog-during-menopause-is-real-it-can-disrupt-womens-work-and-spark-dementia-fears-173150.

10. F. L. Balci, C. Uras, and S. Feldman, "Clinical Factors Affecting the Therapeutic Efficacy of Evening Primrose Oil on Mastalgia," *Annals of Surgical Oncology* 27, no. 12 (November 2020), 4844–4852, https://pubmed.ncbi.nlm.nih.gov/32748152/.

11. P. Dahiya, R. Kamal, M. Kumar, M. Niti, R. Gupta, and K. Chaudhary, "Burning Mouth Syndrome and Menopause," *International Journal of Preventive Medicine* 4, no. 1 (January 2013), 15–20, https://www.ncbi.nlm.nih.gov/pmc/articles/PMC3570906/.

12. A. Teruel and S. Patel, "Burning Mouth Syndrome: A Review of Etiology, Diagnosis, and Management," *General Dentistry* (March/April 2019), 25–29,

https://www.agd.org/docs/default-source/self-instruction-(gendent)/gen
dent_ma19_patel.pdf?sfvrsn=266273b1_0.

13. National Institute of Dental and Craniofacial Research, "Burning Mouth
Syndrome," https://www.nidcr.nih.gov/health-info/burning-mouth.

14. J. Khan, M. Anwer, N. Noboru, D. Thomas, and M. Kalladka, "Topical
Application in Burning Mouth Syndrome," *Journal of Dental Sciences* 14,
no. 4 (December 2019), 352–357, https://www.sciencedirect.com/science
/article/pii/S1991790219301692.

15. Sexual Medicine Society of North America (SMSNA), "What Is Sensate
Focus and How Does It Work?," https://www.smsna.org/patients/did-you
-know/what-is-sensate-focus-and-how-does-it-work.

16. B. N. Seal and C. M. Meston, "The Impact of Body Awareness on Women's
Sexual Health: A Comprehensive Review," *Sexual Medicine Reviews* 8, no. 2
(April 2020), 242–255, https://pubmed.ncbi.nlm.nih.gov/29678474/.

17. J. L. Shifren, "Patient Education: Sexual Problems in Women (Beyond the
Basics)," UpToDate, https://www.uptodate.com/contents/sexual-problems
-in-women-beyond-the-basics.

18. The North American Menopause Society, "MenoNote: Vaginal Dryness,"
https://www.menopause.org/docs/default-source/for-women/mn-vaginal
-dryness.pdf.

19. D. Herbenick and J. D. Fortenberry, "Exercise-induced Orgasm and Pleasure Among Women," *Sexual and Relationship Therapy* 26, no. 4 (2011),
378–388, https://www.tandfonline.com/doi/abs/10.1080/14681994.2011
.647902.

20. E. M. Gortner, S. S. Rude, and J. W. Pennebaker, "Benefits of Expressive
Writing in Lowering Rumination and Depressive Symptoms," *Behavior
Therapy* 37, no. 3 (September 2006), 292–303, https://pubmed.ncbi.nlm
.nih.gov/16942980/.

21. L. Tao, R. Jiang, K. Zhang, Z. Qian, P. Chen, Y. Lv, and Y. Yao, "Light Therapy
in Non-seasonal Depression: An Update Meta-Analysis," *Psychiatry Research*
291 (September 2020), 113247, https://pubmed.ncbi.nlm.nih.gov/32622169/.

22. L. F. Cunha, L. C. Pellanda, and C. T. Reppold, "Positive Psychology and
Gratitude Interventions: A Randomized Clinical Trial," *Frontiers in Psychology* 10 (March 21, 2019), 584, https://pubmed.ncbi.nlm.nih.gov/30949102/.

23. J. L. Gordon, M. Halleran, S. Beshai, T. A. Eisenlohr-Moul, J. Frederick, and
T. S. Campbell, "Endocrine and Psychosocial Moderators of Mindfulness-
based Stress Reduction for the Prevention of Perimenopausal Depressive
Symptoms: A Randomized Controlled Trial," *Psychoneuroendocrinology* 130
(August 2021), 105277, https://pubmed.ncbi.nlm.nih.gov/34058560/.

24. J. P. C. Chang, K. P. Su, V. Mondelli, and C. M. Pariante, "Omega-3 Poly-
unsaturated Fatty Acids in Youths with Attention Deficit Hyperactivity

Disorder: A Systematic Review and Meta-Analysis of Clinical Trials and Biological Studies," *Neuropsychopharmacology* 43, no. 3 (February 2018), 534–545, https://www.ncbi.nlm.nih.gov/pmc/articles/PMC5669464/.

25. M. Terauchi, T. Odai, A. Hirose, K. Kato, M. Akiyoshi, M. Masuda, R. Tsunoda, H. Fushiki, and N. Miyasaka, "Dizziness in Peri-and Post-menopausal Women Is Associated with Anxiety: A Cross-sectional Study," *BioPsychoSocial Medicine* 12 (2018), 21. https://www.ncbi.nlm.nih.gov/pmc/articles/PMC6291970/.

26. Medical News Today, "Does menopause cause dizziness?," https://www.medicalnewstoday.com/articles/319860.

27. Mayo Clinic, "Orthostatic Hypotension (Postural Hypotension)," https://www.mayoclinic.org/diseases-conditions/orthostatic-hypotension/diagnosis-treatment/drc-20352553.

28. Cleveland Clinic, "Low Blood Pressure (Orthostatic Hypotension)," https://my.clevelandclinic.org/health/diseases/9385-low-blood-pressure-orthostatic-hypotension.

29. Cleveland Clinic, "Vestibular Rehabilitation," https://my.clevelandclinic.org/health/treatments/15298-vestibular-rehabilitation.

30. T. Peck, L. Olsakovsky, and S. Aggarwal, "Dry Eye Syndrome in Meno-pause and Perimenopausal Age Group," *Journal of Mid-Live Health* 8, no. 2 (April–June 2017), 51–54, https://www.ncbi.nlm.nih.gov/pmc/articles/PMC5496280/.

31. Mayo Clinic, "Dry Eyes," https://www.mayoclinic.org/diseases-conditions/dry-eyes/symptoms-causes/syc-20371863.

32. K. Boyd, "What Is Dry Eye? Symptoms, Causes, and Treatment," American Academy of Ophthalmology (September 15, 2021), https://www.aao.org/eye-health/diseases/what-is-dry-eye#treatment.

33. American Academy of Dermatology Association, "Caring For Your Skin in Menopause," https://www.aad.org/public/everyday-care/skin-care-secrets/anti-aging/skin-care-during-menopause.

34. Cleveland Clinic, "Here's How Menopause Affects Your Skin and Hair," https://health.clevelandclinic.org/heres-how-menopause-affects-your-skin-and-hair/.

35. A. El Hajj, N. Wardy, S. Haidar, D. Bourgi, M. El Haddad, D. El Cham-mas, N. El Osta, L. R. Khabbaz, and T. Papazian, "Menopausal Symptoms, Physical Activity Level and Quality of Life of Women Living in the Med-iterranean Region," *PLoS ONE* 15, no. 3, https://journals.plos.org/plosone/article?id=10.1371/journal.pone.0230515.

36. C. L. Ward-Ritacco, A. L. Adrian, P. J. O'Connor, J. A. Binkowski, L. Q. Rogers, M. A., Johnson, and E. M. Evans, "Feelings of Energy Are Associated with Physical Activity and Sleep Quality, but not Adiposity,

in Middle-aged Postmenopausal Women," *Menopause* 22, no. 3 (March 2015), 304–311, https://journals.lww.com/menopausejournal/Abstract/2015/03000/Feelings_of_energy_are_associated_with_physical.11.aspx.

37. Gaiam, "1-Minute Breathing Exercise for Energy and Productivity," https://www.gaiam.com/blogs/discover/1-minute-breathing-exercise-for-energy-and-productivity.

38. S. M. Lenger, M. S. Bradley, D. A. Thomas, M. H. Bertolet, J. L. Lowder, and S. Sutcliffe, "D-mannose vs Other Agents for Recurrent Urinary Tract Infection Prevention in Adult Women: A Systematic Review and Meta-analysis," *American Journal of Obstetrics and Gynecology* 223, no. 2 (August 2020), 265.e1–265.e.13, https://www.ncbi.nlm.nih.gov/pmc/articles/PMC7395894/.

39. S. Chaikittisilpa, N. Rattanasirisin, R. Panchaprateep, N. Orprayoon, P. Phutrakul, A. Suwan, and U. Jaisamrarn, "Prevalence of Female Pattern Hair Loss in Postmenopausal Women: A Cross-sectional Study," *Menopause* 29, 4 (April 2022), 415–420, https://journals.lww.com/menopausejournal/Abstract/2022/04000/Prevalence_of_female_pattern_hair_loss_in.7.aspx.

40. Z. S. Goluch-Koniuszy, "Nutrition of Women with Hair Loss Problem During the Period of Menopause," *Menopause Review* 15, no. 1 (March 2016), 56–61, https://www.ncbi.nlm.nih.gov/pmc/articles/PMC4828511/.

41. Cleveland Clinic, "Women and Heart Rate," https://my.clevelandclinic.org/health/diseases/17644-women—abnormal-heart-beats.

42. L. L. Sievert, and C. M. Obermeyer, "Symptom Clusters at Midlife: A Four-Country Comparison of Checklist and Qualitative Responses," *Menopause* 19, no. 2 (February 2012), 133–144, https://www.ncbi.nlm.nih.gov/pmc/articles/PMC3267011/.

43. The North American Menopause Society, "Menopause FAQS: Hot Flashes," https://www.menopause.org/for-women/menopause-faqs-hot-flashes.

44. R. Bansal and N. Aggarwal, "Menopausal Hot Flashes: A Concise Review," *Journal of Mid-Life Health* 10, no. 1 (January–March 2019), 6–13, https://www.ncbi.nlm.nih.gov/pmc/articles/PMC6459071/.

45. T. Li, Y. Zhang, Q. Cheng, M. Hou, X. Zheng, Q. Zheng, and L. Li, "Quantitative Study on the Efficacy of Acupuncture in the Treatment of Menopausal Hot Flashes and its Comparison with Nonhormonal Drugs," *Menopause* 28, no. 5 (March 15, 2021), 564–572, https://pubmed.ncbi.nlm.nih.gov/33739313/.

46. F. C. Baker, M. de Zambotti, I. M. Colrain, and B. Bei, "Sleep Problems During the Menopausal Transition: Prevalence, Impact, and Management Challenges," *Nature and Science of Sleep* 10 (2018), 73–95, https://www.ncbi.nlm.nih.gov/pmc/articles/PMC5810528/.

47. S. Sharma and M. Kavuru, "Sleep and Metabolism: An Overview," *International Journal of Endocrinology* (2010), https://www.ncbi.nlm.nih.gov/pmc/articles/PMC2929498/.

48. M. Magliano, "Menopausal Arthralgia: Fact or Fiction," *Maturitas* 67, no. 1 (September 2010), 29–33, https://pubmed.ncbi.nlm.nih.gov/20537472/.

49. K. L. Clark, W. Sebastianelli, K. R. Flechsenhar, D. F. Aukermann, F. Meza, R. L. Millard, J. R. Deitch, P. S. Sherbondy, and A. Albert, "24-Week Study on the Use of Collagen Hydrolysate as a Dietary Supplement in Athletes with Activity-Related Joint Pain," *Current Medical Research and Opinion* 24, no. 5 (May 2008), 1485–1496, https://pubmed.ncbi.nlm.nih.gov/18416885/.

50. S. R. Davis, C. Castelo-Branco, P. Chedraui, M. A. Lumsden, R. E. Nappi, D. Shah, P. Villaseca, "Understanding Weight Gain at Menopause," *Climacteric* 15, no. 5 (September 2012), 419–429, https://www.tandfonline.com/doi/full/10.3109/13697137.2012.707385.

51. E. Kapoor, M. L. Collazo-Clavell, and S. S. Faubion, "Weight Gain in Women at Midlife: A Concise Review of the Pathophysiology and Strategies for Management," *Mayo Clinic Proceedings* 92, no. 10 (October 2017), 1552–1558, https://pubmed.ncbi.nlm.nih.gov/28982486/.

52. Mayo Clinic, "Chart of High-Fiber Foods," https://www.mayoclinic.org/healthy-lifestyle/nutrition-and-healthy-eating/in-depth/high-fiber-foods/art-20050948.

53. N. C. Howarth, E. Saltzman, and S. B. Roberts, "Dietary Fiber and Weight Regulation," *Nutrition Reviews* 59, no. 5 (May 2001), 129–139, https://pubmed.ncbi.nlm.nih.gov/11396693/.

54. The North American Menopause Society, "Decreased Desire," https://www.menopause.org/for-women/sexual-health-menopause-online/sexual-problems-at-midlife/decreased-desire.

55. The North American Menopause Society, "Effective Treatments for Sexual Problems," https://www.menopause.org/for-women/sexual-health-menopause-online/effective-treatments-for-sexual-problems.

56. F. Sanaati, S. Najafi, Z. Kashaninia, and M. Sadeghi, "Effect of Ginger and Chamomile on Nausea and Vomiting Caused by Chemotherapy in Iranian Women with Breast Cancer," *Asian Pacific Journal of Cancer Prevention* 17, no. 8 (2016), 4125–4129, https://pubmed.ncbi.nlm.nih.gov/27644672/.

57. N. M. Steele, J. French, J. Gatherer-Boyles, S. Newman, and S. Leclaire, "Effect of Acupressure by Sea-Bands on Nausea and Vomiting of Pregnancy," *Journal of Obstetric, Gynecologic, and Neonatal Nursing* 30, no. 1 (January–February 2001), 61–70, https://pubmed.ncbi.nlm.nih.gov/11277163/.

58. F. Sharifzadeh, M. Kashanian, J. Koohpayehzadeh, F. Rezaian, N. Sheikhansari, and N. Eshraghi, "A Comparison Between the Effects of Ginger, Pyridox-

ine (Vitamin B6), and Placebo for the Treatment of the First Trimester Nausea and Vomiting of Pregnancy (NVP)," *Journal of Maternal-Fetal and Neonatal Medicine* 31, no. 19 (October 2018), 2509–2514, https://pubmed .ncbi.nlm.nih.gov/28629250/.

59. National Institutes of Health, Office of Dietary Supplements, "Vitamin B6," https://ods.od.nih.gov/factsheets/VitaminB6-Consumer/.

60. H. K. Kim, S. Y. Kang, Y. J. Chung, J. H. Kim, and M. R. Kim, "The Recent Review of the Genitourinary Syndrome of Menopause," *Journal of Menopausal Medicine* 21, no. 2 (August 2015), 65–71, https://www.ncbi .nlm.nih.gov/pmc/articles/PMC4561742/.

61. R. Naseri, V. Farnia, K. Yazdchi, M. Alikhani, B. Basanj, and S. Salemi, "Comparison of Vitex Agnus-castus Extracts with Placebo in Reducing Menopausal Symptoms: A Randomized Double-Blind Study," *Korean Journal of Family Medicine* 40, no. 6 (November 2019), 362–367, https://www .ncbi.nlm.nih.gov/pmc/articles/PMC6887765/.

62. F. Kazemi, A. Z. Masoumi, A. Shayan, and K. Oshvandi, "The Effect of Evening Primrose Oil Capsule on Hot Flashes and Night Sweats in Postmenopausal Women: A Single-Blind Randomized Controlled Trial," *Journal of Menopausal Medicine* 27, no. 1 (April 2021), 8–14, https://www.ncbi .nlm.nih.gov/pmc/articles/PMC8102809/.

63. F. Farzaneh, S. Fatehi, M. R. Sohrabi, and K. Alizadeh, "The Effect of Oral Evening Primrose Oil on Menopausal Hot Flashes: A Randomized Clinical Trial," *Archives of Gynecology and Obstetrics* 288, no. 5 (November 2013), 1075–1079, https://pubmed.ncbi.nlm.nih.gov/23625331/.

64. P. A. Komesaroff, C. V. Black, V. Cable, and K. Sudhir, "Effects of Wild Yam Extract on Menopausal Symptoms, Lipids and Sex Hormones in Healthy Menopausal Women," *Climacteric* 4, no. 2 (June 2001), 144–150, https://pubmed.ncbi.nlm.nih.gov/11428178/.

Chapter 13: Self-Care Going Forward

1. National Institutes of Health, Office of Dietary Supplements, "Probiotics," https://ods.od.nih.gov/factsheets/Probiotics-HealthProfessional/.

2. National Institutes of Health, Office of Dietary Supplements, "Dietary Supplements: What You Need to Know," https://ods.od.nih.gov/factsheets /WYNTK-Consumer/.

3. J. Corley, S. R. Cox, A. M. Taylor, M. V. Hernandez, S. M. Maniega, L. Ballerini, S. Wiseman, R. Meijboom, E. V. Backhouse, M. E. Bastin, J. M. Wardlaw, and I. J. Deary, "Dietary Patterns, Cognitive Function, and Structural Neuroimaging Measures of Brain Aging," *Experimental Gerontol-*

ogy 142 (December 2020), https://www.sciencedirect.com/science/article/abs/pii/S0531556520304654.

4. T. R. P. De Brito, D. P. Nunes, L. P. Corona, T. da Silva Alexandre, and Y. A. de Oliveira Duarte, "Low Supply of Social Support as Risk Factor for Mortality in the Older Adults," *Archives of Gerontology and Geriatrics* 73 (November 2017), 77–81, https://pubmed.ncbi.nlm.nih.gov/28783514/.

5. G. L. Smith, L. Banting, R. Eime, G. O'Sullivan, J. G. Z. van Uffelen, "The Association Between Social Support and Physical Activity in Older Adults: A Systematic Review," *International Journal of Behavioral Nutrition and Physical Activity* 14, no. 1 (April 27, 2017), 56, https://www.ncbi.nlm.nih.gov/pmc/articles/PMC5408452/.

6. B. M. Hoffman, M. A. Babyak, W. E. Craighead, A. Sherwood, P. M. Doraiswamy, M. J. Coons, and J. A. Blumenthal, "Exercise and Pharmacotherapy in Patients With Major Depression: One-Year Follow-Up of the SMILE Study," *Psychosomatic Medicine* 73, no. 2 (February–March 2011), 127–133, https://www.ncbi.nlm.nih.gov/pmc/articles/PMC3671874/.

7. R. A. Asbjørnsen, J. Wentzel, M. L. Smedsrød, J. Hjelmesæth, M. M. Clark, L. S. Nes, and J. E. W. C. Van Gemert-Pijnen, "Identifying Persuasive Design Principles and Behavior Change Techniques Supporting End User Values and Needs in eHealth Interventions for Long-Term Weight Loss Maintenance: Qualitative Study," *Journal of Medical Internet Research* 22, no. 11 (November 2020), e22598, https://www.ncbi.nlm.nih.gov/pmc/articles/PMC7735908/.

8. Medical News Today, "What to Know About Menopause and High Blood Pressure," https://www.medicalnewstoday.com/articles/menopause-and-high-blood-pressure-link-and-treatment.

9. H. Currie and C. Williams, "Menopause, Cholesterol and Cardiovascular Disease," *US Cardiology* 5, no. 1 (2008), 12–14, https://www.uscjournal.com/articles/menopause-cholesterol-and-cardiovascular-disease-0.

10. American Heart Association, "Heart-Health Screenings," https://www.heart.org/en/health-topics/consumer-healthcare/what-is-cardiovascular-disease/heart-health-screenings.

11. H. Currie and C. Williams, "Menopause, Cholesterol and Cardiovascular Disease," *US Cardiology* 5, no. 1 (2008), 12–14, https://www.uscjournal.com/articles/menopause-cholesterol-and-cardiovascular-disease-0.

12. National Heart, Lung, and Blood Institute, "Blood Cholesterol: Diagnosis," https://www.nhlbi.nih.gov/health/blood-cholesterol/diagnosis.

13. National Institute of Diabetes and Digestive and Kidney Diseases, "What is Diabetes?," https://www.niddk.nih.gov/health-information/diabetes/overview/what-is-diabetes.

14. American Diabetes Association, "Diabetes Overview: The Path to Understanding Diabetes Starts Here," https://www.diabetes.org/diabetes.

15. U.S. Preventive Services Task Force, "Prediabetes and Type 2 Diabetes: Screening," (August 24, 2021), https://www.uspreventiveservicestaskforce .org/uspstf/recommendation/screening-for-prediabetes-and-type-2 -diabetes.

16. H. Currie and C. Williams, "Menopause, Cholesterol and Cardiovascular Disease," *US Cardiology* 5, no. 1 (2008), 12–14, https://www.uscjournal .com/articles/menopause-cholesterol-and-cardiovascular-disease-0.

17. Centers for Disease Control and Prevention, "Diabetes Tests," https://www .cdc.gov/diabetes/basics/getting-tested.html.

18. National Institute of Diabetes and Digestive and Kidney Diseases, "The A1C Test & Diabetes," https://www.niddk.nih.gov/health-information /diagnostic-tests/a1c-test.

19. National Institute of Diabetes and Digestive and Kidney Diseases, "Diabetes Tests & Diagnosis," https://www.niddk.nih.gov/health-information /diabetes/overview/tests-diagnosis#who.

20. S. R. El Khoudary, B. Aggarwal, T. M. Beckie, H. N. Hodis, A. E. Johnson, R. D. Langer, M. C. Limacher, J. E. Manson, M. L. Stefanick, M. A. Allison, "Menopause Transition and Cardiovascular Disease Risk: Implications for Timing of Early Prevention: A Scientific Statement From the American Heart Association," *Circulation* 142, no. 25 (November 30, 2020), e506-e532, https: //www.ahajournals.org/doi/10.1161/CIR.0000000000000912.

21. A. Gesing, "The Thyroid Gland and the Process of Aging," *Thyroid Research* 8 (June 22, 2015), A8, https://www.ncbi.nlm.nih.gov/pmc/articles /PMC4480281/.

22. Y. Kim, Y. Chang, I. Y. Cho, R. Kwon, G. Y. Lim, J. H. Jee, S. Ryu, and M. Kang, "The Prevalence of Thyroid Dysfunction in Korean Women Undergoing Routine Health Screening: A Cross-Sectional Study," *Thyroid* (May 16, 2022), https://pubmed.ncbi.nlm.nih.gov/35293242/.

23. American Cancer Society, "American Cancer Society Guidelines for the Early Detection of Cancer," https://www.cancer.org/healthy/find -cancer-early/american-cancer-society-guidelines-for-the-early-detection -of-cancer.html.

24. Centers for Disease Control and Prevention, "Breast Cancer Screening Guidelines for Women," https://www.cdc.gov/cancer/breast/pdf/breast -cancer-screening-guidelines-508.pdf.

25. Centers for Disease Control and Prevention, "Breast Cancer: What Is a Mammogram?," https://www.cdc.gov/cancer/breast/basic_info/mammograms .htm.

26. Centers for Disease Control and Prevention, "Breast Cancer Statistics," https://www.cdc.gov/cancer/breast/statistics/index.htm.

27. American Cancer Society, "Key Statistics for Cervical Cancer," https://www.cancer.org/cancer/cervical-cancer/about/key-statistics.html.

28. American Cancer Society, "The Pap (Papanicolaou) Test," https://www.cancer.org/cancer/cervical-cancer/detection-diagnosis-staging/screening-tests/pap-test.html.

29. American Cancer Society, "The HPV Test," https://www.cancer.org/cancer/cervical-cancer/detection-diagnosis-staging/screening-tests/hpv-test.html.

30. American College of Obstetricians and Gynecologists, "Updated Cervical Cancer Screening Guidelines," (April 2021), https://www.acog.org/clinical/clinical-guidance/practice-advisory/articles/2021/04/updated-cervical-cancer-screening-guidelines.

31. American Cancer Society, "Key Statistics for Colorectal Cancer," https://www.cancer.org/cancer/colon-rectal-cancer/about/key-statistics.html.

32. U.S. Preventive Services Task Force, "Colorectal Cancer: Screening," (May 18, 2021), https://www.uspreventiveservicestaskforce.org/uspstf/recommendation/colorectal-cancer-screening.

33. Centers for Disease Control and Prevention, "Colorectal Cancer Screening Tests," https://www.cdc.gov/cancer/colorectal/basic_info/screening/tests.htm.

34. U.S. Preventive Services Task Force, "Colorectal Cancer: Screening," May 18, 2021, https://www.uspreventiveservicestaskforce.org/uspstf/recommendation/colorectal-cancer-screening.

35. Mayo Clinic, "Colon Cancer," https://www.mayoclinic.org/diseases-conditions/colon-cancer/symptoms-causes/syc-20353669.

36. Endocrine Society, "Menopause and Bone Loss," (January 23, 2022), https://www.endocrine.org/patient-engagement/endocrine-library/menopause-and-bone-loss.

37. U.S. Preventive Services Task Force, "Osteoporosis to Prevent Fractures: Screening," (June 26, 2018), https://www.uspreventiveservicestaskforce.org/uspstf/recommendation/osteoporosis-screening#bootstrap-panel—6.

38. Ibid.

39. Bone Health and Osteoporosis Foundation, "What is Osteoporosis and What Causes It?," https://www.bonehealthandosteoporosis.org/patients/what-is-osteoporosis/.

40. Bone Health and Osteoporosis Foundation, "Evaluation of Bone Health/Bone Density Testing," https://www.bonehealthandosteoporosis.org/patients/diagnosis-information/bone-density-examtesting/.

41. M. D. Barber and C. Maher, "Epidemiology and Outcome Assessment of Pelvic Organ Prolapse," *International Urogynecology Journal* 24, no. 11 (November 2013), 1783–1790, https://pubmed.ncbi.nlm.nih.gov/2414 2054/.

Index